AF616138

Blood Loss and Shock

Blood Loss and Shock

Edited by

Niels H Secher
Department of Anaesthesia, Rigshospitalet, University of Copenhagen,
Copenhagen, Denmark

James A Pawelczyk
Cardiology Division, Department of Internal Medicine, University of Texas,
Southwestern Medical Center and Director, Autonomic and Exercise Physiology Laboratories,
Institute for Exercise and Environmental Medicine, Presbyterian Hospital of Dallas, Dallas, Texas, USA

and

John Ludbrook
Cardiovascular Research Laboratory, University of Melbourne Department of Surgery,
Royal Melbourne Hospital, Parkville, Australia

Edward Arnold
A member of the Hodder Headline Group
LONDON BOSTON MELBOURNE AUCKLAND

First published in Great Britain 1994

Distributed in the Americas by Little, Brown and Company,
34 Beacon Street, Boston, MA 02108

British Library Cataloguing in Publication Data

Secher, Neils
Blood Loss and Shock
I. Title
617.2

ISBN 0-340-56021-5

Typeset in 10/11pt Linotron Baskerville by
Rowland Phototypesetting Ltd, Bury St Edmunds, Suffolk.
Printed and bound in Great Britain for Edward Arnold,
a division of Hodder Headline PLC, Mill Road,
Dunton Green, Sevenoaks, Kent TN13 2YA by
Butler and Tanner Ltd, Frome and London

Foreword

Today we recognize the extraordinary complexity of the events at the vascular neuroeffector junctions that are the final arbitrators of the degree of constriction and relaxation of the systemic resistance and capacitance vessels. These events include the release of neurotransmitters, cotransmitters and modulators into the synaptic cleft; since the classic demonstration by von Euler in 1946 that noradrenaline is the sympathetic neurotransmitter, later studies have shown that adenosine triphosphate and neuropeptide Y may be coreleased with noradrenaline. Also numerous receptors have been demonstrated on the sympathetic varicosities that when activated can either increase or decrease the output of the neurotransmitters. In addition, numerous vasoactive substances can be released from the endothelial cells and some of these, in addition to causing relaxation or contraction of the vascular smooth muscle, can alter the output of neurotransmitters.[1]

This book *Blood Loss and Shock* makes it appropriate to mention the key original contributor to our knowledge of the sympathetic control of blood vessels in human limbs. I refer to Henry Barcroft, who came to The Queen's University of Belfast as Professor of Physiology 4 years before the outbreak of World War II in 1939. The antivivisection movement was active in the city at that time, so Barcroft decided to study the circulation in human limbs, using a water-filled plethysmograph to maintain a constant temperature, as devised by Lewis and Grant in 1925.[2]

Using this method, Barcroft and his colleagues first demonstrated that the blood vessels of human skeletal muscle are supplied by sympathetic vasoconstrictor fibres. This was done by demonstrating the increase in forearm blood flow that followed blocking of the deep arm nerves with local anaesthetic; following the same procedure there was no increase in the forearm that had been surgically sympathectomized while blood flow in the other forearm increased. The increase still occurred after intense constriction of the skin vessels by electrophoresis of adrenaline, indicating that the increase in flow occurred in the muscles.

These studies were followed, during the war years, by the accidental discovery of sympathetic vasodilator fibres to human muscle blood vessels. During an experiment on the circulatory effects of haemorrhage in a normal subject, the subject fainted; despite the abrupt decrease in arterial blood pressure, the forearm blood flow increased. Further studies in normal subjects who were bled until they fainted confirmed the vasodilatation. Since the blood flow to the hand, which is predominantly flow to the skin, decreased, it was concluded that the dilatation was occurring in the forearm muscles. By contrast in subjects with sympathectomized limbs the flow decreased; also during the faint the blood flow in the normal forearm was greater than in the opposite nerve-blocked forearm, indicating that there was active neurogenic vasodilatation as well as release of vasoconstrictor tone. Today the mechanism of this vasodilatation, which is also seen with emotional stress, is still undetermined. In addition to the possibility of activation of cholinergic nerves, the recent discovery that nitric oxide acts as a transmitter in non-adrenergic, non-cholinergic vasodilator nerves offers another possibility to account for the vasodilatation.[3]

Additional studies in which cardiac output and right atrial pressure were shown to be appreciably unchanged during the faint, excluded the previously held opinion that cardiac syncope, due to the cardiac vagal inhibition, was the cause of the faint and established a decrease in systemic vascular resistance as the primary mechanism. Later studies by Sharpey-Schaffer and his colleagues and by Greenfield, Barcroft's successor at The Queen's University Medical School, confirmed that emotional fainting also was due predominantly to vasodilatation in the skeletal muscles.

These classic studies also demonstrated the initial compensatory increase in systemic vascular resist-

ance during the early minutes of venesection, the sympathoexcitatory phase, interrupted by the rapid decrease that caused the faint.

These early studies demonstrate the continued importance of human studies in the understanding of the circulatory events in blood loss and shock. In this regard, the development, in 1969, of the microneurographic technique for intraneural recording of sympathetic nerve activity to human limbs has added an important new dimension to our understanding of the role of the sympathetic nervous system in circulatory regulation in humans, both in health and disease.[4] With this technique, it has been shown that just prior to syncope there is an abrupt inhibition of sympathetic outflow to muscle vessels. This shows that withdrawal of sympathetic vasoconstrictor activity contributes to the muscle vasodilation.[4]

While various theories have been enunciated to explain the fainting mechanism(s), this remains a key challenge for the future. Gaining this understanding will be important for the management of patients with hypovolemic shock.

John T Shepherd

References

1. Shepherd JL and Hainsworth R: Future challenges: from introspection to prospection. In Hainsworth R and Mark AL (eds): *Cardiovascular Reflex Control in Health and Disease.* WB Saunders Co., 1993; 491–510.
2. Barcroft H and Swan HJC: *Sympathetic Control of Human Blood Vessels.* Edward Arnold: London, 1953; 165.
3. Dinerman JL, Lowenstein CH and Snyder SH: Molecular mechanisms of nitric oxide regulation. Potential relevance to cardiovascular disease. *Circulation Research*, 1993; **73**: 217–22.
4. Wallin BG: Assessment of sympathetic mechanisms from recordings of postganglionic efferent nerve activity. In Hainsworth R and Mark EL (eds): *Cardiovascular Reflex Control in Health and Disease.* WB Saunders Co., 1993; 65–93.

Preface

Haemorrhage is not itself a disease, but it is a manifestation – and often a life-threatening one – of many injuries and diseases. As a result, most medical practitioners have had the experience of treating bleeding patients. Yet despite the knowledge of the effects of haemorrhage that has accumulated over the centuries, and though careful monitoring of heart rate and blood pressure in patients who are bleeding has been the rule since the classic work of Cushing, there are vitally important aspects of the haemodynamic and other consequences of acute blood loss that are not mentioned in textbooks of surgery, anaesthesia, intensive care, or even physiology.

During World War II Henry Barcroft and his colleagues made fundamental observations of the haemodynamic events that accompanied acute blood loss in human volunteers. In particular, they recognized that a first, compensatory or vasoconstrictor, stage in which blood pressure is well maintained is succeeded by a decompensatory stage in which heart rate, peripheral resistance and blood pressure fall abruptly and drastically. These observations have been confirmed and expanded upon a great many times since then, in humans and in conscious laboratory animals, yet these stages, and in particular the latter, scarcely seem to have entered the consciousness of clinicians. One of our prime goals in putting together this book has been to revive the findings of Barcroft and his colleagues and to emphasize the importance of a stage of hypovolaemic shock in which there is relative bradycardia, and hypotension due to peripheral vasodilatation.

However, we believe that this book has a good deal more to offer than this. Our contributors are clinical scientists from a variety of disciplines and cardiovascular physiologists. They have reviewed the observations that have been made in humans and animals on the haemodynamic, humoral and other changes associated with acute blood loss or acute reduction in central blood volume. They have provided authoritative accounts of the physiological mechanisms that underlie these changes, both central and peripheral. They have discussed the important interactions that occur in clinical practice between acute hypovolaemia and such factors as hypoxaemia, anaesthesia and splanchnic ischaemia. And, finally, they have evaluated the methods used in clinical practice for treating hypovolaemic shock and for monitoring the efficacy of those treatments.

We hope that the information contained in this book will be of interest to, and will influence, clinicians who are called upon to diagnose and treat acute hypovolaemia, especially that which results from blood loss. We also hope that it will provide a useful review of the subject for physiologists and for those engaged in research into shock.

We know how busy the authors are and thank them for taking the time which has been required to prepare a text for this book. Also, we acknowledge the initiative and support from Edward Arnold Publishers, in particular Diana Waha and Carol Baker, without which the present text would not have appeared.

Niels H Secher
James A Pawelczyk
John Ludbrook

Contents

List of contributors

Warwick P Anderson, PhD, Senior Principal Research Fellow of the National Health and Medical Research Council of Australia; Deputy Director of the Baker Medical Research Institute; and Associate Professor in Physiology at Monash University, Melbourne, Australia

Richard L Converse Jr, MD, Fellow, Cardiology Division, Department of Internal Medicine, University of Texas, Southwestern Medical Center, Dallas, Texas, USA

Murray D Esler, MB, BS, BMedSc(Melb), PhD(ANU), FRACP, NH & MRC Senior Principal Research Fellow, Baker Medical Research Institute, Melbourne, Australia

Daniel B Friedman, MD, Assistant Professor, Cardiology Division, Department of Internal Medicine, University of Texas, Southwestern Medical Center, Dallas, Texas, USA

Stig Haunsø, PhD, MD, Professor, Department of Medicine B, Rigshospitalet, University Hospital, Copenhagen, Denmark

John Jacobsen, MD, Department of Anaesthesia, Herlev Hospital, University Hospital, Copenhagen, Denmark

Tage N Jacobsen, MD, Fellow, Cardiology Division, Department of Internal Medicine, University of Texas, Southwestern Medical Center, Dallas, Texas, USA

John M Johnson, PhD, Professor, Department of Physiology, University of Texas Health Science Center, San Antonio, Texas, USA

Ferdinand Jónsson Medical student, University of Reykjavik, Reykjavik, Iceland

Charles M T Jost, MD, Fellow, Cardiology Division, Department of Internal Medicine, University of Texas, Southwestern Medical Center, Dallas, Texas, USA

Emrys Kirkman, BSc(Hons), PhD, MRC Scientific (Non-Clinical) Staff Member, MRC Trauma Group and North Western Injury Research Centre; and Honorary Lecturer, Department of Physiological Sciences, University of Manchester, Manchester, UK

Mads Klokker, MD, Department of Infectious Diseases, Rigshospitalet, Copenhagen; and Danish Armed Forces Health Services, Jaegersborg Kaserne, Gentofte, Denmark

Niels A Lassen, PhD, MD, Chief, Department of Clinical Physiology and Nuclear Medicine, Bispebjerg Hospital, Copenhagen, Denmark

Roderick A Little, BSc(Hons), PhD, MRCPath, Head of MRC Trauma Group; and Director, North Western Injury Research Centre, Manchester, UK

John Ludbrook, DSc, MD(Otago), ChM, BMedSc(NZ), FRCS, FRACS, NH & MRC Senior Principal Research Fellow, Cardiovascular Research Laboratory, University of Melbourne Department of Surgery, Parkville, Australia

Per Madsen, Medical student, Department of Anaesthesia, Rigshospitalet, University of Copenhagen, Copenhagen, Denmark

Steen Matzen, MD, Fellow, Department of Plastic Surgery, Rigshospitalet, Copenhagen, Denmark

Ole Michael Nielsen, DrMedSc, MD, Senior Registrar, Department of Vascular Surgery RK, Rigshospitalet, University Hospital, Copenhagen, Denmark

Olaf B Paulson, PhD, MD, Professor, Head of Department, Department of Neurology, Copenhagen University Hospital, Copenhagen, Denmark

James A Pawelczyk, PhD, Assistant Professor, Cardiology Division, Department of Internal Medicine, University of Texas, Southwestern Medical Center; and Director, Autonomic and Exercise Physiology Laboratories, Institute for Exercise and Environmental Medicine, Presbyterian Hospital, Dallas, Texas, USA

Bente K Pedersen, PhD, MD, Department of Infectious Diseases, Rigshospitalet, University of Copenhagen, Copenhagen, Denmark

Goazina Perko, MD, Registrar, Department of Anaesthesia, Hillerød Hospital, Hillerød, Denmark

Loring B Rowell, PhD, MD, Professor, School of Medicine, Department of Physiology and Biophysics, University of Washington, Seattle, Washington, USA

James C Schadt, PhD, Research Investigator, Dalton Cardiovascular Research Center and Department of Veterinary Biomedical Sciences, University of Missouri, Columbia, Missouri, USA

Jes F Schmidt, PhD, MD, Head of Department, Department of Anaesthesia, Copenhagen University Hospital, Glostrup, Denmark

Niels H Secher, PhD, MD, Associate Professor, Department of Anaesthesia, Rigshospitalet, University of Copenhagen, Copenhagen, Denmark

Gabor Szénási, CD, Senior Research Fellow, Department of Pharmacology, EGIS Pharmaceuticals, Budapest, Hungary; Visiting Scientist at the Baker Medical Research Institute, Melbourne, Australia, 1991–92; and Former Fellow of the Hungarian Academy of Sciences, Semmelweiss University School of Medicine, Budapest, Hungary

Else Tønnesen, PhD, MD, Department of Anaesthesia – Intensive Care, Odense University Hospital, Odense, Denmark

Ronald G Victor, MD, Associate Professor of Medicine, Cardiology Division, Department of Internal Medicine, University of Texas, Southwestern Medical Center, Dallas, Texas, USA

B Gunnar Wallin, MD, Professor of Clinical Neurophysiology, Sahlgren Hospital, University of Goteborg, Goteborg, Sweden

Part 1
Experimental observations

1

Changing concepts of hypovolaemic shock

John Jacobsen and Niels H Secher

In 1743 a French physician used the word 'choc' to describe sudden collapse in patients following serious traumatic episodes.[1] Major surgery at that time, and for the next 100 years, involved the amputation of extremities, and this was especially true for battlefield injuries. The English physician John Hunter[2] described in 1794 a patient who was treated with a medical method popular for many years: blood-letting. During this procedure the patient fainted and the color of the venous blood changed from dark to a fine scarlet. In several patients no changes were noted in pulse rate. In 1867 Edwin Morris[3] first used the word shock systematically in a monograph entitled '*Shock or A Practical Treatise on Shock After Surgical Operations and Injuries: With Especial Reference to Shock Caused by Railway Accidents*'. Morris found evidence for a description of shock dating as far back as the beginning of the eighteenth century in a '*Treatise on Gun-shot Wounds*' by the surgeon Guthrie.

According to Morris, the symptoms of shock included:

> 'a deathlike paleness, followed by sickness and vomiting, and afterwards succeeded by shakes and abundant perspiration, and the whole frame becomes shaken by an universal tremor. The pulse is small, feeble and slow. The patient is perfectly senseless and the respiration scarcely perceptible.'

If the condition is prolonged the pulse becomes

> 'more and more feeble, irregular and intermitting, the extremities becomes cold.'

The connection between loss of blood and the incidence of shock in relation to severe trauma and surgery was unclear. The most important cause of the patient's condition was considered to be a 'shock' of the central nervous system with accompanying organic symptoms.

In the years to come there was quiet regarding this condition. Even the great wars in the beginning of this century did not evoke any new thinking relevant to shock, though an investigation committee (Medical Research Committee) on wound and surgical shock was formed after World War I. There were some animal experiments designed to parallel the situations observed in patients during the war, but the results were obscured by misinterpretation. McMichael[4] stated in 1944:

> 'From the historical point of view, therefore, we may note and learn that good clinical evidence of the last war was forced into the background in favor of speculation based on experimental work.'

It should be mentioned that a condition with falling blood pressure and pulse rate followed by collapse had been previously described in soldiers with 'irritable hearts' by Cotton and Lewis[5] in 1918–20, and in healthy subjects by Starr and Collins[6] in 1930. This condition was termed 'vasovagal syncope' by Lewis in 1932 and could be observed in healthy individuals under special conditions such as emotional stress.[7] This description likely paralleled the clinical descriptions of shock given by Morris[3] in 1867.

It was not until during World War II that renewed interest led to a classification of clinical signs related to organ responses during haemorrhage. Clinical observations from the great number of injured soldiers and civilians inspired many experimental investigations. It was noted in clinical situations by McMichael[4] that pulse rate was not always inversely related to the fall in blood pressure. Sometimes a fall in pulse rate was noted together with a fall in blood pressure. This led to the suggestion that pulse rate was far less reliable than blood pressure in serving as a guide for estimating either the severity of a given case of shock or the results of treatment. Grant and Reeve[8] reported clinical observations on air-raid victims in 1941. Based on their observations they divided shock into three stages. Stages I and II related to blood pressure while stage III, subdivided into A, B and C, was related to a combination of blood pressure and heart rate. In stage III blood pressure fell to below 100 mmHg, while in stage IIIA heart rate was below 70 beats/min, in IIIB between 70 and 100 beats/min, and in IIIC greater than 100 beats/min. Patients in stage IIIA were all pale with nausea, eventually vomiting and sweating. One of the concluding remarks of the study was that the term shock was used too broadly by physicians given that the condition was still poorly understood.

Since 1945 there has been an abundant amount of both clinical and experimental investigations covering different aspects of shock, and descriptions of the condition are given in most textbooks. However, only in the last decade has a connection between the so-called 'vasovagal syncope' and the clinical condition of shock been established.

Textbook descriptions of shock

The term shock is often used loosely to describe conditions characterized by failing circulation due to hypovolaemia, sepsis, trauma, anaphylactic reactions or failed pumping (cardiogenic shock).

As described by Guyton,[9] haemorrhagic shock can be divided into a non-progressive (compensated) and a progressive phase, ending in irreversible shock. The compensated shock is characterized by an intense sympathetic stimulation of the circulation triggered by the baroreceptors. This gives rise to constriction of arterioles, increased peripheral resistance and tachycardia (to a maximum value of 200 beats/min). Both heart and brain circulation are maintained via reductions in flow to non-vital organs such as the splanchnic area and skin. There is a stress-induced production of several hormones including angiotensin and vasopressin (antidiuretic hormone) along with a compensatory reabsorbtion of interstitial – and intestinal – fluid to restore the blood volume.

If central blood volume (CBV) is not restored the shock will continue into the progressive phase, with myocardial depression due to reductions in coronary blood flow and influences from toxic by-products of ischaemic tissue and endotoxins from the intestinal flora which penetrate the ischaemic intestinal wall. If the vasomotor centre ceases to function there will be clotting of blood in small vessels and an increased capillary permeability; the shock will then progress into the irreversible phase. The exact mechanism of this phase is still unknown, but beyond a certain point the tissue damage is so great that even the restoration of cardiac output by transfusion will have only a temporary effect. The sympathetic reactions are observed immediately, while other compensatory mechanisms have a latency from 10 min to several hours. In the progressive phase bradycardia may be related to hypoxia and cerebral ischaemia.[9]

Ganong describes tachycardia as a characteristic of simple hypovolaemic shock, and a fall in heart rate as an element of the refractory (irreversible) shock.[10]

In physiology textbooks there is general agreement concerning this pattern of reaction; as mentioned by Scher,[11] Keele *et al.*[12] and Weiss,[13] the baroreceptor reflex is the background for the reduction of the inhibitory influence on the vasomotor centre during bleeding. Yet, Holcroft and Trunkey[14] and Shires[15] mention that heart rate is an unreliable measure of the degree of blood loss in the bleeding patient.

Abboud[16] divided reactions during shock into three stages: stage I – *Compensated shock*, characterized by hypotension, low cardiac output or vasodilatation, but with effective compensatory mechanisms capable of restoring the circulation; stage II – *Decompensated shock*, when compensatory mechanisms are failing and reduced perfusion of vital organs is evident; and stage III – *Irreversible shock*, excessive vasoconstriction causing cellular damage to vital organs. Bacterial toxins will also contribute to the deterioration of the patient's condition.

In other forms of shock such as anaphylatic reactions there is a release of histamine and other vasoactive mediators from the mast cells after contact with the antigen–allergen complex. This leads to an increase in capillary permeability and peripheral vasodilatation with a redistribution of the circulating blood volume resulting in central hypovolaemia and shock, a situation similar to the one described for shock induced by bleeding.[17]

Taken together, there seems to be nearly universal agreement in textbooks of physiology, medicine, surgery and anaesthesiology, that central hypovolaemia gives rise to a characteristic elevation of heart rate (tachycardia) and that bradycardia is mentioned only when shock is irreversible. However, this conclusion is reached only when excluding the simultaneous decrease in heart rate and blood pressure which takes place with a reduction of CBV by approximately 30 per cent.[18] When the cardiovascular responses to procedures performed for reduction of CBV have been reviewed, the hypotensive bradycardic phase has not been included.[19,20] When attempts have been made to define a role for bradycardia during hypovolaemic shock, tachycardia is considered to be the normal response while bradycardia is confined to severe haemorrhage.[21,22] However, when confining bradycardia to severe haemorrhage, one finds a discrepancy between the experimental findings and the well-established clinical experience that patients in severe shock have tachycardia.

A concomitant decrease in heart rate and blood pressure is mentioned in textbooks under headings such as 'vasovagal syncope' or 'fainting', thus reflecting how the early experience was summarized without considering that hypovolaemic shock may be the most clinically relevant cause for the reaction.[10] As a result, bradycardia during haemorrhage has not been recognized by the clinician and bleeding patients with bradycardia are in danger of being examined for heart disease, myxoedema or head trauma before haemorrhage is diagnosed and accepted as causal. Most importantly, the diagnosis of haemorrhage may be critically delayed and the irreversible stage of hypovolaemic shock reached before appropriate measures are taken to stop the bleeding and institute fluid therapy.

During experimental investigations on humans where the circulatory response to an increased gravity – lower body negative pressure (LBNP), head-up tilt (anti-Trendelenburg's position) – has been examined, physiological reactions to a reduced CBV have been reevaluated.[18]

Stages of shock

Haemorrhage

Studies involving haemorrhage in the rat, cat, dog, rabbit and pig have shown that the small initial

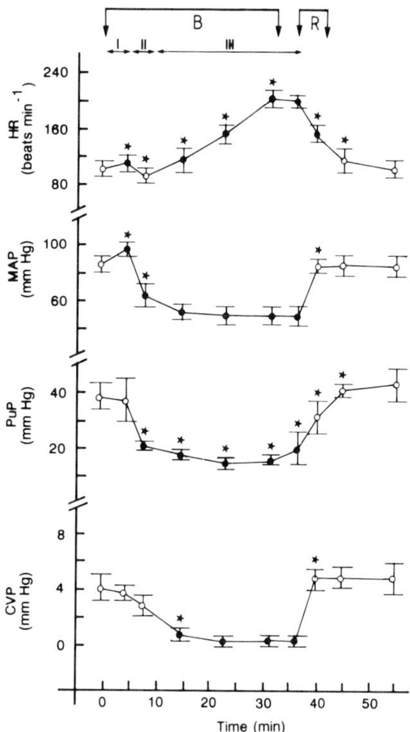

Fig. 1.1. Heart rate (HR), mean arterial pressure (MAP), pulse pressure (PuP) and central venous pressure (CVP) in six pigs at rest, during bleeding (B) to a MAP of 50 mmHg and after retransfusion (R) of the shed blood. I, II, and III refer to stages of haemorrhage. Values are expressed as means ± SE. ●, Different from rest ($P < 0.05$); ★, different from preceding value ($P < 0.05$). From Jacobsen et al.,[23] with permission.

increase in heart rate most often is followed by a reduction in heart rate and then by tachycardia as hypotension becomes more severe or prolonged with transition to the irreversible stage of shock (Fig. 1.1).[23,24] An exception exists for rats of the Swedish germ-free strain, which always show tachycardia.

In humans several methods have been employed to induce a transient decrease in CBV of sufficient magnitude to elicit presyncopal symptoms (nausea, light-headedness, heat, paleness, sweating) with associated bradycardia and hypotension. The most commonly applied models include LBNP, head-up tilt, positive pressure breathing, venous congestion of the legs with or without venesection, spinal or epidural anaesthesia and the lordotic posture. Heart rate seldom exceeds 100 beats/min during the initial response to these manoeuvres and blood pressure may be elevated. During presyncope a decrease in heart rate and blood pressure is observed.

The typical finding is that heart rate decreases toward resting values at the time when the experiment has to be terminated. However, if termination of the intervention is delayed, extreme bradycardia, e.g. 1–2 beats/min, may occur.[18]

A low heart rate has also been demonstrated in volunteers after bleeding of approximately 1 litre, in patients with a blood loss of approximately 2 litres, and also during anaesthesia. The finding that the patients appear to have a larger blood loss than the volunteers at the time when a low heart rate appears reflects that fluid therapy, albeit inadequate, delays the response in the patients. Patients in hypovolaemic shock may also present with tachycardia following the bradycardic stage, and it is usually associated with a lower blood pressure. Table 1.1 presents a comparison of 34 consecutive bleeding, hypotensive patients with either a low (<100 beats/min) or a high (>100 beats/min) heart rate. Those patients presenting with tachycardia had a blood loss approximately 60 per cent larger than those with a low heart rate. They also had lower blood pressure. All patients who had a low heart rate when haemorrhage was recognized recovered. In the tachycardic group, 6 of the 21 patients died, either during operation (three patients) or during postoperative intensive care treatment due to multiple organ failure (three patients).[25] These findings support the hypothesis that tachycardia during hypovolaemic shock represents a more severe degree of shock than bradycardia. Coupled with the experience gained from studies in animals, tachycardia during haemorrhage in humans may represent a situation where a transition to the irreversible stage of shock has to be anticipated.

In terms of the stages of shock, it may be relevant to include the first circulatory changes seen after withdrawal of approximately 10–15 per cent of blood, namely moderate tachycardia and peripheral vasoconstriction. This *stage I* could be considered 'preshock' as the patient or subject has a near normal blood pressure and no symptoms. *Stage II*, with a blood loss of 20–30 per cent, represents a simultaneous decrease in heart rate and blood pressure, and in *stage III* manifest hypotension is associated with tachycardia.

Evidence that the three stages follow one other during progressive depletion of CBV is supported by the finding that the succession may be reversed. The hypotensive and bradycardic phase (stage II) reverts to normotension with a moderately elevated heart rate (stage I) before the resting heart rate is reached during expansion of the circulating blood volume.[26] This response could be classified as a Bainbridge reflex with tachycardia following central volume loading.[26] Thus, volume expansion of patients after haemorrhage should continue until heart rate decreases after this initial increase. However, in stage III of hypovolaemic shock the increased heart rate most often remains during resuscitation. During volume loading of patients in stage III of hypovolaemic shock, only one of those patients presented in Table 1.1 had a slowing of heart rate followed by a new increase in heart rate before the resting value was reestablished (Fig. 1.2).

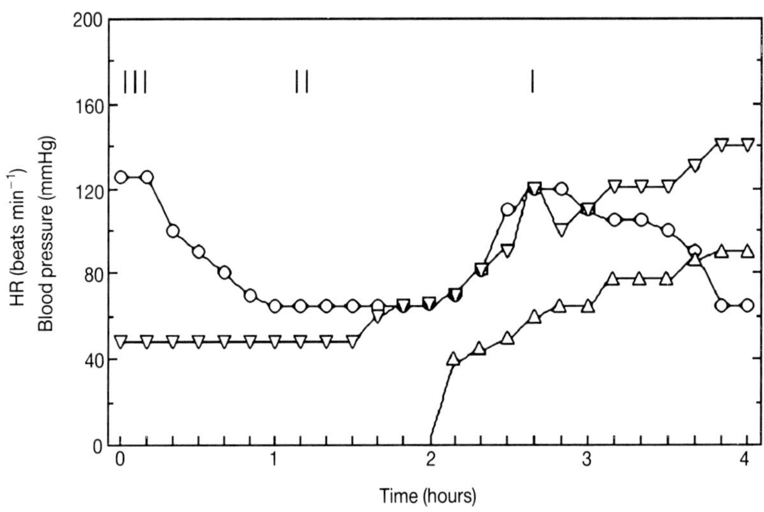

Fig. 1.2. Heart rate (HR, ○), and arterial blood pressure (systolic, ▽; diastolic, △) during resuscitation from hypovolaemic shock (stage III). During volume loading a decrease in HR (stage II) is seen followed by an increase (stage I, preshock) as blood pressure starts to increase and before the resting HR is reestablished. From Jacobsen and Secher,[25] with permission.

Table 1.1 Clinical characteristics for 34 consecutive patients in circulatory shock due to haemorrhage with either a low (<100 beats/min; n = 13) or a high (>100 beats/min; n = 21) heart rate when the diagnosis was established.

	Heart rate (beats/min)	
	79	129
Age (years)	55	53
Blood pressure (mmHg)	60	48
Blood loss (litres)	2.3	3.6
Volume replacement (litres)		
Blood products	2.0	3.4
Crystaloids	2.7	2.5
Survived	13/13	15/21

Values are expressed as medians with ranges.

Injury

Where injury is the cause of haemorrhage it has not been possible to use heart rate as an indicator of the condition of the patient.[4,8,27] With knowledge of the normal variations in heart rate during haemorrhage, a lack of correlation between the condition of the patient and heart rate may be self-evident, e.g. a heart rate of 70 beats/min may be seen after a blood loss of 1.5 litres but also after the loss has been replaced. Thus, heart rate registration is only useful when coupled with clinical observations and blood pressure monitoring. Additionally, in diseased states a high sympathetic tone elicited from the injured area overrides the normal decrease in heart rate described above and an increase in heart rate is manifest from the first blood loss (Fig. 1.3). It should also be noted that no decrease in heart rate takes place following haemorrhage in diabetics with impaired vagal function.

Regional anaesthesia

A decrease in heart rate and blood pressure during epidural and spinal anaesthesia has been attributed to blockade of the sympathetic nerves to the heart and thus to unbalanced vagal activity.[28] However, if unbalanced vagal activity is established by acute β-blockade, resting blood pressure is not affected and heart rate decreases only by approximately 10–15 beats/min.[29] During epidural and spinal anaesthesia bradycardia is not seen without a concomitant decrease in blood pressure. Furthermore, during regional anaesthesia heart rate can reach extremely low values and may be associated with complete (third degree) heart block, and volume

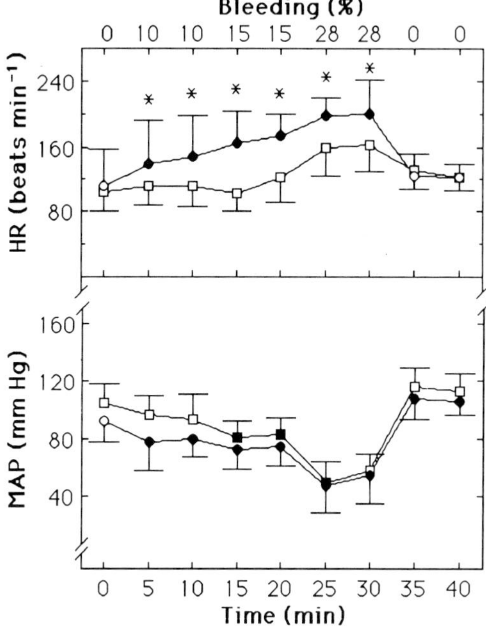

Fig. 1.3. Heart rate (HR) and mean arterial pressure (MAP) in 10 pigs at rest, during bleeding and after retransfusion of the shed blood. Values are expressed as means ± SD. □, Before ileus; □, after ileus; ■/●, different from rest ($P < 0.05$); *, difference before and after ileus ($P < 0.05$). From Jacobsen et al.,[42] with permission.

expansion alone increases both heart rate and blood pressure, even during high epidural and spinal anaesthesia. During epidural anaesthesia, leg blood volume increases while the blood volume in other regions including the thorax decreases. If anaesthesia extends more proximally the blockade induces an increase in the blood volume of the splanchnic area as well, suggesting that vasodilatation in this large vascular bed may induce central hypovolaemia to the extent that provokes the decrease in heart rate and blood pressure.

Taken together these findings suggest that an increase in vagal activity rather than a blockade of sympathetic activity is responsible for the cardiovascular depression during epidural and spinal anaesthesia. This has been demonstrated by measuring the hormone pancreatic polypeptide, which can be used as a marker of vagal parasympathetic activity in plasma (Fig. 1.4).[43]

Similar reactions

A cardioinhibitory–vasodepressor reaction that is characteristic of stage II of central hypovolaemia

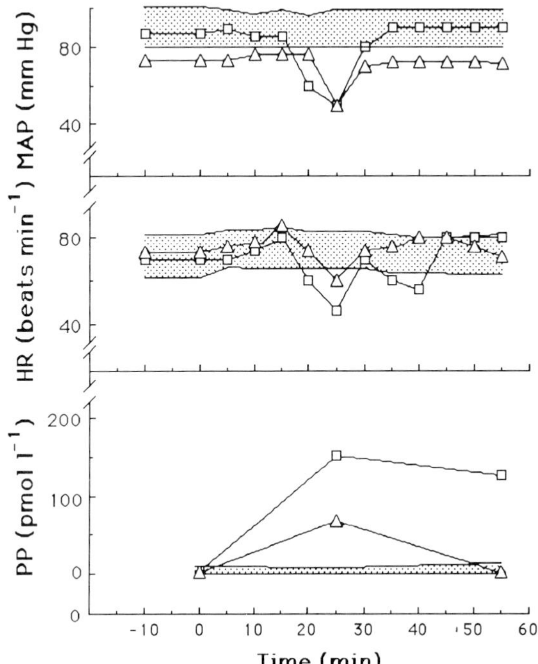

Fig. 1.4. Mean arterial pressure (MAP), heart rate (HR) and plasma concentration of the hormone pancreatic polypeptide (PP) in eight healthy volunteers given lumbar epidural anaesthesia with a level of analgesia at Th_{8-10}. In two of the volunteers (□ and △) a concomitant fall in HR and MAP was observed 25 min after injection of the local anaesthetic. The increase in PP indicates parasympathetic (vagal) activation. The dotted area indicates the range of six cardiovascular stable volunteers. From Jacobsen et al.,[43] with permission.

also may be observed during other circumstances such as emotional stress (vasovagal syncope), anaphylactic reactions, release of an arterial tourniquet and stimulation of the nasopharynx.[5,6,7,30–35] Of these reflexes the emotional elicitation of the vasovagal syncope may be the most relevant in association with the cardioinhibitory–vasodepressor reflex response to a reduced CBV since vasovagal fainting often follows blood sampling. However, the cardioinhibitory–vasodepressor reaction occurs with a probability that increases with the amount of blood withdrawn, and conversely with a given blood loss, fasting subjects and those with the smallest blood volume are affected most often.[36] Although the reactions taking place during CBV depletion may be similar to those elicited during a 'vasovagal syncope', the trigger mechanisms appear to be different. It should be emphasized that the important common denominator in the cardiovascular reactions to central hypovolaemia and the other reactions is peripheral vasodilatation (see below) and not the associated bradycardia which, as mentioned, need not be severe. In accordance with the classical description of the vasovagal syncope, atropine administration or cutting or cooling the vagi produce an increase in heart rate but do not affect blood pressure in stage II of shock.[5–7] To the contrary, the use of cardiac pacing in treatment of patients with recurrent syncope has been proposed to prevent extreme bradycardia, but this would not prevent the associated vasodilatation.

Severe hypoxaemia may also result in a decrease in heart rate, blood pressure and total peripheral resistance that resembles stage II of haemorrhage.[37] However, the cardioinhibitory–vasodepressor reaction during central hypovolaemia is preceded by an increase in ventilation and patients in stage II of shock are not hypoxaemic, although they may be cyanotic which can be explained by venoconstriction.[30]

Conclusion

There is no obvious reason for a decrease in heart rate during moderately severe haemorrhage, and this may explain why the finding has not been included in textbook descriptions of hypovolaemic shock.[18] A teleological explanation for the decrease in heart rate during central hypovolaemia could be that it prevents the ventricles from emptying with the markedly reduced preload. It could also be speculated that a decrease in blood pressure during haemorrhage would act to reduce the amount of blood lost. Perhaps the reflex-inducing hypotension and bradycardia during haemorrhage have a protective effect in the circulatory system, their aim as the degree of haemorrhage increases to preserve organ perfusion, possibly through a β_2-adrenergic mechanism, at the expense of arterial blood pressure.[38,39] Sjöstrand[40,41] argued that rats with severed cardiac nerves, and thus without the ability to elicit the reflex involving hypotension and bradycardia, reached the irreversible stage of shock before control animals.

The above mentioned observations can be integrated into a model explaining the cardiovascular changes that occur during haemorrhage (Fig. 1.1). The reactions seen during stage I of shock correspond to the effect of stimulation of myelinated cardiopulmonary afferents rather than to an arterial baroreceptor reflex. With the first decrease in blood pressure and/or pulse pressure the arterial baroreceptors also contribute to the increase in heart rate. Further haemorrhage leads to the hypotensive bradycardic (second) stage of shock, due to stimulation of unmyelinated left ventricular afferents activated by mechanical distortion. It follows that a Bainbridge-type reflex, elicited during central volume loading of patients in stage II of hypovolaemic shock, can be explained by unloading of unmyelinated cardiac afferents. Furthermore, the decrease in heart rate with continuous volume loading corresponds to unloading of the arterial baroreceptors and myelinated cardiac afferents. In stage III of shock tachycardia is established by a classical baroreceptor reflex together with activity in myelinated cardiopulmonary afferents associated with fatigue of unmyelinated cardiac afferents. With a critically reduced cerebral blood flow (CBF), brain ischaemia determines the elevated pulse rate. Accordingly, the heart rate excursions seen during haemorrhage are not generally reversable during resuscitation from stage III of shock.

References

1. le Dran HF: *A Treatise, or Reflections Drawn from Practice on Gunshot Wounds*, translated. London, Clarke, 1743.
2. Palmer JF: *The Works of John Hunter, F.R.S. with Notes*. London, Longman, Rees, Orme, Brown, Green, and Longman, 1837.
3. Morris E: Symptoms of shock. In Morris E (ed.): *A Practical Treatise on Shock After Operations and Injuries*. London, Hardwicke, 1867, 31–41.
4. McMichael J: Clinical aspects of shock. *Journal of the American Medical Association*, 1944; **124,** 275–81.
5. Cotton TF and Lewis T: Observations upon fainting attacks due to inhibitory cardiac impulses. *Heart*, 1918–20; **vii,** 23–6.
6. Starr I and Collins LH: Physiological studies of faintness and syncope. *Journal of Clinical Investigation*, 1931; **9,** 561–76.
7. Lewis T: Vasovagal syncope and the carotid sinus mechanism. *British Medical Journal*, 1932; **i,** 873–6.
8. Grant RT, Reeve EB: Clinical observations on air-raid casualties. *British Medical Journal*, 1941; **ii,** 293–7, 329–32.
9. Guyton AC: Shock. In Guyton AC (ed.): *Textbook of Medical Physiology*. Philadelphia, PA, WB Saunders Co., 1986, 327–32.
10. Ganong WF: Cardiovascular homeostasis in health and disease. In Ganong WF (ed.): *Review of Medical Physiology*. East Norwalk, CT, Appleton & Lange, 1991, 589–97.
11. Scher AM: Control of arterial blood pressure. In Ruch TC and Patton HD (eds): *Physiology and Biophysics*. Philadelphia, PA, WB Saunders Co., 1974, 146–69.
12. Keele CA, Neil E and Joels N: *Samson Wright's Applied Physiology*. Oxford, Oxford University Press, 1982, 151.
13. Weiss C: Loss of blood. In Schmidt RF and Thews G (eds): *Human Physiology*. New York, NY, Springer, 1983, 444–6.
14. Holcroft JW and Trunkey DD: Shock. In Douphy JE and Way LW (eds): *Current Surgical Diagnosis and Treatment*. Los Altos, Lange, 1979, 196–8.
15. Shires GT: Classification and clinical signs. In Shires GT (ed.): *Shock and Related Problems*. Edinburgh, Churchill Livingstone, 1984, 4–11.
16. Abboud FM: Shock. In Wyngarden JB and Smith LH (eds): *Cecil Textbook of Medicine*. Philadelphia, PA, WB Saunders Co., 1985, 211–25.
17. Guyton AC: Shock. In Guyton AC (ed.): *Textbook of Medical Physiology*. Philadelphia, PA, WB Saunders Co., 1986, 332–3.
18. Secher NH and Bie P: Bradycardia during reversible haemorrhagic shock – a forgotten observation? *Clinical Physiology*, 1985; **5,** 316–23.
19. Mark AL and Mancia G: Cardiopulmonary baroreflexes in humans. In Shepherd JH and Abboud FM (eds): *Handbook of Physiology. Section 2: The Cardiovascular System, Volume 3*. Bethesda, MD, American Physiological Society, 1983, 795–813.
20. Rowell LB: In *Human Circulation Regulation During Physical Stress*. New York, NY, Oxford University Press, 1986, 136–73.
21. Bishop VS, Malliani A and Thorén P: Cardiac mechanoreceptors. In Shepherd JH and Abboud FM (eds): *Handbook of Physiology. Section 2: The Cardiovascular System, Volume 3*. Bethesda, MD, American Physiological Society, 1983, 497–555.
22. van Leeuwen AF, Evans RG, Ludbrook J: Haemodynamic responses to acute blood loss: new roles for heart, brain and endogenous opioids. *Anaesthesia and Intensive Care*, 1989; **17,** 312–19.
23. Jacobsen J, Søfelt S, Sheikh S, Warberg J and Secher NH: Cardiovascular and endocrine responses to haemorrhage in the pig. *Acta Physiologica Scandinavica*, 1990; **133,** 167–73.
24. Secher NH, Jacobsen J, Friedman DB and Matzen S: Bradycardia during reversible hypovolaemic shock: associated neural reflex mechanisms and clinical implications. *Clinical and Experimental Pharmacology and Physiology*, 1992; **19**, 733–43.
25. Jacobsen J and Secher NH: Heart rate during haemorrhagic shock. *Clinical Physiology*, 1992; **12,** 659–66.

26. Bainbridge FA: The influence of venous filling upon the rate of the heart. *Journal of Physiology*, 1915; **50,** 65–84.
27. Beecher HK: *Resuscitation and Anesthesia for Wounded Men, the Management of Traumatic Shock*. Springfield, IL, CC Thomas, 1949.
28. Murphy TM: Spinal, epidural, and caudal anesthesia. In Miller RD (ed.): *Anesthesia*. New York, NY, Churchill Livingstone, 1986, 1061–111.
29. Mitchell JH, Reeves DR, Rogers HB, Secher NH and Victor RG: Autonomic blockade and cardiovascular responses to static exercise in partially curarized man. *Journal of Physiology*, 1989; **413,** 433–45.
30. Wallin BG and Sundlöf G: Sympathetic outflow to muscles during vasovagal syncope. *Journal of the Autonomic Nervous System*, 1982; **6,** 287–91.
31. Sander-Jensen K, Garne S and Schwartz TW: Pancreatic polypeptide release during emotionally induced vasovagal syncope. *Lancet*, 1985; **ii,** 1132.
32. Ziegler MG, Echon C, Wilner KD, Specho P, Lake CR and McCutchen JA: Sympathetic nervous withdrawal in the vasodepressor (vasovagal) reaction. *Journal of the Autonomic Nervous System*, 1986; **17,** 273–8.
33. Jacobsen J and Secher NH: Slowing of the heart during anaphylactic shock. A report of five cases. *Acta Anaesthesiologica Scandinavica*, 1988; **32,** 401–3.
34. Jacobsen J, Rørsgaard S and Secher NH: Bradycardia during hypotension following release of a tourniquet in orthopedic surgery. *Acta Anaesthesiologica Scandinavica*, 1988; **30,** 511–14.
35. James JEA and de Burgh Daly M: Nasal reflexes. *Proceedings of the Royal Society of Medicine*, 1969; **62,** 1287–93.
36. Poles FC and Boycott M: Syncope in blood donors. *Lancet*, 1942; **ii,** 531–5.
37. Anderson DP, Allen WJ, Barcroft H, Edholm OG and Manning GW: Circulatory changes during fainting and coma caused by oxygen lack. *Journal of Physiology*, 1946; **104,** 426–34.
38. Gustafsson D and Lundvall J: β_2-Adrenergic vascular control in hemorrhage and its influence on cardiac performance. *American Journal of Physiology*, 1984; **246,** H351–9.
39. Chen HI, Stinnett HO, Peterson DF and Bishop VS: Enhancement of vagal restraint on systemic blood pressure during hemorrhage. *American Journal of Physiology*, 1978; **234,** H192–8.
40. Sjöstrand T: Circulatory control via vagal afferents V. Impairment of the circulatory adjustment to hemorrhage by vagal deafferentation and prolonged hypotension. *Acta Physiologica Scandinavica*, 1973; **87,** 228–39.
41. Sjöstrand T: Circulatory control via vagal afferents VI. The bleeding bradycardia in the rat, its elicitation and relation to the release of vasopressin. *Acta Physiologica Scandinavica*, 1973; **89,** 39–50.
42. Jacobsen J, Hansen OB, Sztuk F, Warberg J, Knigge U and Secher NH: Enhanced heart rate response to haemorrhage by ileus in the pig. *Acta Physiologica Scandinavica*; in press.
43. Jacobsen J, Søfelt S, Brocks V, Fernandes A, Warberg J and Secher NH. Reduced left ventricular diameters at onset of bradycardia during epidural anaesthesia. *Acta Anaesthesiologica Scandinavica*, 1992; **36**: 831–6.

2

Experimental observations – animals

James C Schadt

This chapter will review the neurohumoral and haemodynamic adjustments associated with acute blood loss in conscious animals other than humans. Human hypovolaemic shock, the emphasis of this volume, is a pathological situation that develops after a significant period of hypovolaemia. Why is a discussion of the immediate adjustments to blood loss in animals relevant to human hypovolaemic shock? First, studies in a variety of animals including humans have demonstrated more similarities than differences in terms of the response to blood loss.[1] In addition, some of the experimental studies discussed could not have been carried out in humans. Finally, the immediate adjustments that the organism makes during blood loss set the stage for all subsequent adjustments. Indeed, these initial changes may determine whether the organism even has the opportunity to put long-term homeostatic mechanisms into effect.

When an animal loses blood sensory receptors detect changes in blood pressure and/or volume. This sensory information is sent to the central nervous system and produces changes in efferent systems. These efferent changes are designed to maintain arterial blood pressure through changes in cardiovascular parameters such as vascular resistance and heart rate.

Two groups of sensory receptors, arterial baroreceptors and cardiopulmonary baroreceptors, are important in this response. Arterial baroreceptors are concentrated around the bifurcation of the carotid artery and in the aortic arch. Cardiopulmonary receptors are found in all four chambers of the heart as well as in blood vessels in and around the heart and lungs. Rather than pressure, the stimulus that activates both groups of receptors is stretch. Increased stretch due to increases in blood pressure and/or volume causes increased discharge of these receptors. Decreases in blood pressure and/or volume decrease their discharge. In general increased afferent input from these receptors results in changes designed to lower arterial blood pressure. These changes include vasodilatation, decreased heart rate and decreased contractile function of the heart. Decreased input from these receptors produces changes designed to increase pressure, such as vasoconstriction, increased heart rate and increased contractile function of the heart.

The available efferent mechanisms in terms of cardiovascular control include the sympathetic and parasympathetic branches of the autonomic nervous system as well as humoral mechanisms such as vasopressin and the renin–angiotensin system. Peripheral sympathetic nerves innervate the heart and blood vessels. They release noradrenaline as their neurotransmitter. Increased activity in these nerves increases release of noradrenaline and results in increased heart rate and force of contraction, and constriction of blood vessels. There are also some sympathetic nerves that produce vasodilatation, but they do not seem to be involved in the response to blood loss and will not be discussed here.

The adrenal medulla is part of the sympathetic nervous system but is specialized to function as an endocrine organ. It releases mostly adrenaline, but also releases some noradrenaline. The ratio of released adrenaline to noradrenaline varies among species. Adrenaline and noradrenaline have similar effects on blood vessels and the heart. Therefore, we might expect activation of the adrenal medulla and peripheral sympathetic nerves to have similar cardiovascular effects.

The parasympathetic nervous system innervates

the heart but not blood vessels. The cardiac innervation is via the vagus nerves. Parasympathetic effects on the heart include decreased rate and force of contraction.

Blood loss is also likely to bring about release of vasopressin from the pituitary and renin from the kidney. Renin is an enzyme that catalyses the conversion of angiotensinogen to angiotensin I. Angiotensin I (AI) is converted to AII by angiotensin converting enzyme (ACE). AII and vasopressin are potent vasoconstrictors. They also affect cardiovascular reflexes and interact with the sympathetic nervous system at several levels. In addition, vasopressin and AII promote fluid retention by the kidney and, thus, have profound long-term effects on fluid balance and blood volume.

Studies carried out near the end of World War II in conscious human volunteers were the first to demonstrate the biphasic nature of the response to acute haemorrhage. Groups on both sides of the Atlantic[2,3] showed that while the response to haemorrhage initially involves vasoconstriction and maintenance of arterial blood pressure, this is followed by a precipitous fall in blood pressure due to a decrease in total peripheral resistance. In other words, a paradoxical vasodilatation occurs at a time when increased vasoconstriction is essential for blood pressure maintenance.

The biphasic nature of the haemodynamic response to acute blood loss has more recently been documented in other conscious animals.[4–7] The response in animals, as in humans, involves an initial period of arterial blood pressure maintenance followed by a precipitous decrease. This decrease is due primarily to a fall in vascular resistance (Fig. 2.1). Thus, in animals as well as humans, the initial priority during haemorrhage is maintenance of perfusion pressure. After a critical blood loss this priority appears to be replaced by efforts to maintain perfusion or blood flow. An additional benefit of this approach, at least in the case of traumatic blood loss, is that decreased arterial blood pressure probably results in decreased blood loss.

This review will attempt to contrast the haemo-

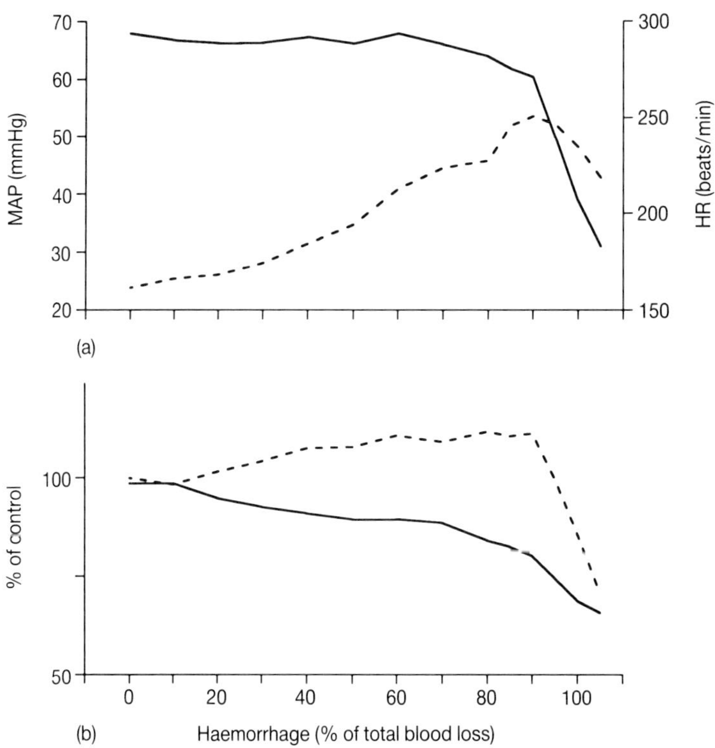

Fig. 2.1. The haemodynamic effects of blood loss in the conscious rabbit. (a) MAP, mean arterial pressure (—) and HR, heart rate (– – –); (b) CO, cardiac output (—); TPR, total peripheral resistance (– – –); total blood loss, blood loss required to reduce MAP to <40 mmHg.

dynamic and neurohumoral adjustments to non-hypotensive (arterial pressure maintained) and hypotensive (arterial pressure not maintained) haemorrhage. It will discuss the roles of the various efferent and afferent systems in each. Finally, there will be a brief discussion of some potential mediators of the response to blood loss and other factors that may influence the response in animals as well as humans. The data shown in the Figures are taken from experiments carried out in the author's laboratory. While New Zealand white rabbits were used in these experiments, the haemodynamic and neurohumoral responses shown here are qualitatively similar in a variety of animals, including humans.[1] This review will concentrate on studies in conscious animals since anaesthesia alters the haemodynamic and neurohumoral response to haemorrhage.

Non-hypotensive blood loss

The majority of studies carried out prior to 1967 emphasized the important role of vasoconstriction in the haemodynamic response to haemorrhage.[8] Although most of these studies relied on information gathered from experiments on anaesthetized animals, many studies since then in conscious animals support this emphasis during non-hypotensive haemorrhage. In unanaesthetized dogs,[7,9,10] rabbits,[4,11–15] rats[16–19] and non-human primates[20] vasoconstriction is the major mechanism by which arterial pressure is maintained during moderate haemorrhage. However, there appears to be some regional and species variability in the pattern of change. There has been general agreement that, early in blood loss, muscle and skin vasculature constrict.[4,11] The reported responses of the gastrointestinal vasculature have ranged from no change[4] or a slight increase[11] to a substantial increase in vascular resistance.[9] Similarly, renal vascular resistance has been reported to decrease[4,9] or to increase.[11,13,20–22] The cerebral vasculature apparently dilates,[13,20] while coronary vascular resistance has been reported to increase,[9,23] decrease[13] or stay the same.[20] Technical difficulties associated with measurement of blood flow in conscious animals as well as species and protocol differences probably account for these apparent discrepancies. Despite these differences, there is general agreement that early in haemorrhage the fall in cardiac output is closely matched by an increase in systemic vascular resistance (Fig. 2.1). The result is that mean arterial pressure is well maintained.

In most experiments this period of arterial blood pressure maintenance lasts until haemorrhage exceeds 20–30 per cent of blood volume. The most prominent feature of this phase is activation of the sympathetic nervous system, with the resultant vasoconstriction and increase in heart rate. Renal sympathetic nerve activity (RSNA) increases during non-hypotensive haemorrhage in conscious dogs[6] and rabbits[24–26] (Fig. 2.2). Measurements of plasma noradrenaline, the transmitter released by peripheral sympathetic nerves, serve as an indirect indicator of sympathetic outflow. Plasma levels of

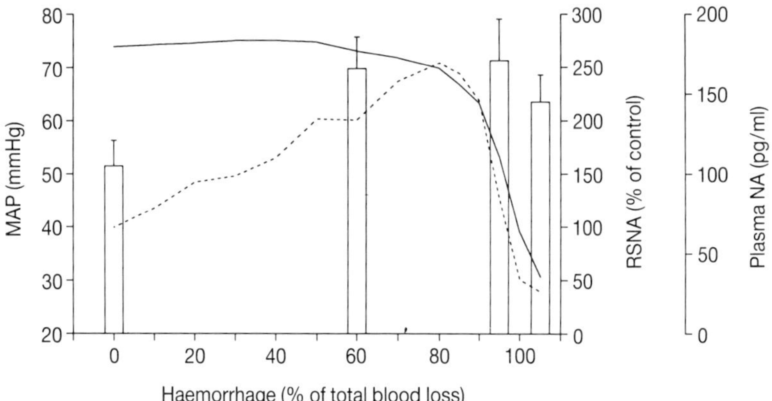

Fig. 2.2. The effects of blood loss on sympathetic nervous system outflow. The mean arterial pressure (MAP, —) effects are shown for reference. RSNA, renal sympathetic nerve activity (– – –); NA, noradrenaline (□); total blood loss, blood loss required to reduce MAP to <40 mmHg. *Source*: Hasser and Schadt[26] and Schadt and Gaddis.[27]

noradrenaline increase during non-hypotensive blood loss (Fig. 2.2) in conscious rabbits[27,28] but not in conscious rats.[16,18,19] Finally, pharmacological blockade of sympathetic vasoconstriction during blood loss limits the rise in vascular resistance as well as the animal's ability to control arterial blood pressure.[9]

The increase in heart rate that occurs during this phase is due to withdrawal of existing cardiac vagal activity and increases in cardiac sympathetic activity.[10,29,30] There appears to be some species variability in the heart rate response as rats show almost no increase in heart rate during non-hypotensive haemorrhage.[16,18,19] It might be expected that sympathetically mediated increases in heart rate and myocardial contractility help maintain cardiac output during moderate haemorrhage. This is apparently not true in unanaesthetized animals. Total blockade of cardiac autonomic efferent systems during blood loss in conscious rabbits does not affect the rate of fall of cardiac output.[15] In addition, non-hypotensive haemorrhage in conscious dogs increases heart rate but has little effect on left ventricular contractility, and the pattern of arterial blood pressure changes is unaffected by β-adrenergic blockade.[10]

The principal sympathetic contribution during non-hypotensive blood loss originates in cardiac and vascular sympathetic nerves and not from the adrenal medulla. Since adrenaline is only released by the adrenal medulla, its plasma level is a good indicator of increased adrenal medullary activity. During non-hypotensive blood loss there is little if any change in plasma adrenaline in conscious dogs,[31] rabbits[27,28] or rats.[18] In addition, removal of the adrenal gland, adrenal medullectomy or adrenal denervation has no effect on the haemodynamic adjustments during non-hypotensive haemorrhage in conscious rabbits.[27,32]

Although renin release increases during non-hypotensive haemorrhage (Fig. 2.3) in conscious dogs,[35,36] rabbits,[33,37–39] rats[18] and sheep,[40] the contribution of the renin–angiotensin system to the haemodynamic response to acute blood loss is still uncertain. In studies employing ACE inhibition during haemorrhage the results are somewhat contradictory. In one study AII appeared to be necessary for a normal increase in vascular resistance during blood loss.[33] In addition, hypotension occurred after a smaller blood loss in the presence of the ACE inhibitor. However, other studies failed to demonstrate an effect of ACE inhibition on the response to acute blood loss.[12,41]

Vasopressin is another humoral agent that might be important in the cardiovascular adjustments to haemorrhage. However, non-hypotensive haemorrhage does not increase plasma levels of vasopressin (Fig. 2.3) in conscious rabbits,[34,37,39,42] rats,[18] monkeys,[43] dogs[35,36] or sheep.[40] The potential role of vasopressin during blood loss has also been tested by performing haemorrhage with and without prior blockade of vascular vasopressin re-

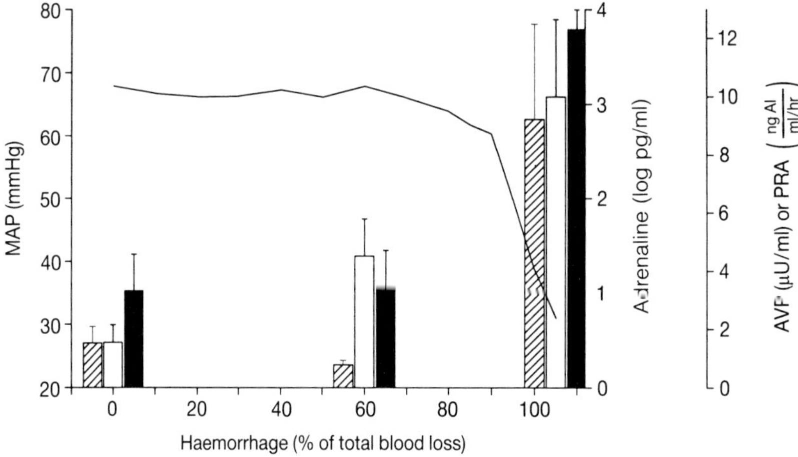

Fig. 2.3. The effects of blood loss on humoral mechanisms involved with cardiovascular control. The mean arterial pressure (MAP, —) effects are shown for reference. AVP, vasopressin (▨); PRA, plasma renin activity (□); Adrenaline (■); AI, angiotensin I; total blood bloss, blood loss required to reduce MAP to <40 mmHg. *Source*: Schadt and Gaddis[33] and Schadt and Hasser.[34]

ceptors. Blockade of these receptors has no effect in conscious rabbits[12,34] during non-hypotensive haemorrhage. However, there is a premature fall in arterial pressure during haemorrhage in conscious dogs after similar blockade.[44] In addition, a smaller decrease in arterial pressure appears to be necessary in dogs to cause an increase in plasma vasopressin.[35,45]

In summary, the primary efferent mechanism involved with the haemodynamic changes associated with non-hypotensive haemorrhage is activation of the sympathetic nerves to blood vessels. Circulating levels of the humoral agents, vasopressin and adrenaline, appear to be relatively unimportant to blood pressure maintenance during this phase of the response to blood loss. Renin release and the subsequent generation of AII may have some role during this phase, perhaps as a facilitator of sympathetic vasoconstrictor mechanisms.[33] Similarly, all three agents may have facilitatory interactions with one another and with the sympathetic nervous system. In conscious rabbits release of renin and vasopressin increases earlier during haemorrhage in the presence of autonomic blockade.[38] In addition, in the absence of functional sympathetic efferents, AII and vasopressin help to maintain peripheral resistance.[12]

Arterial baroreceptors appear to be the most important group of receptors involved during non-hypotensive blood loss. Acute denervation of these receptors causes an increase in heart rate and systemic vascular resistance, and regional vascular resistance in skin, skeletal muscle, visceral organs and the kidneys.[46] In intact dogs and rabbits arterial blood pressure is well maintained even after blood loss greater than 20 per cent of total blood volume.[4,7,15,47] After surgical denervation of arterial baroreceptors the response to blood loss is a fall in blood pressure that is directly related to the volume of blood removed. In addition, hypotension develops after a smaller blood loss.[7,48] The normal increases in heart rate, vascular resistance and release of noradrenaline during haemorrhage are abolished or reversed.[7,15,48] One exception is the increase in renin release, which is unaffected by removal of arterial baroreceptors.[7,37,45]

The other group of receptors of potential importance in the response to haemorrhage are the cardiopulmonary receptors. Compared to arterial baroreceptors these receptors appear to be of little importance to the haemodynamic and neurohumoral response to non-hypotensive haemorrhage. Acute blockade of cardiac afferents (and efferents) with intrapericardial procaine[15,25,37,47,49] or chronic surgical interruption by cardiac denervation[7,36] or vagotomy[6] has little effect on the pattern of haemodynamic and neurohumoral changes during non-hypotensive blood loss. Thus, afferent input from the heart appears to be relatively unimportant in the haemodynamic response of conscious animals to moderate blood loss.

Arterial baroreceptors appear to play the major role in coordinating the haemodynamic and neurohumoral response to non-hypotensive haemorrhage in conscious animals. Cardiopulmonary receptors, particularly cardiac receptors, appear to contribute little to the haemodynamic and neurohumoral adjustments associated with non-hypotensive blood loss.

Hypotensive blood loss

Laboratory studies in conscious animals have shown that arterial blood pressure is well maintained during haemorrhage until blood loss reaches a critical level. Once blood loss reaches this level there is a rapid decrease in arterial pressure (Fig. 2.1). This phenomenon has been shown in conscious dogs[6,7] and rabbits.[4,5,24,25,42,49,50] The response appears to be slightly different in conscious rats,[16,19,51] where arterial pressure falls from the beginning of haemorrhage. Although heart rate decreases coincident with arterial pressure, the pressure decrease is independent of the change in heart rate. Blockade of muscarinic cholinergic receptors with atropine abolishes the bradycardia but not the hypotension.[2,52] In addition, cardiac output decreases throughout haemorrhage and the change during the sudden onset of hypotension is relatively small.[2,4,5,7,53,54]

The sudden decrease in arterial pressure during blood loss in unanaesthetized rabbits, dogs and humans is due to a decrease in systemic vascular resistance.[2–5,7,53,54] Vascular beds that are under sympathetic control all appear to dilate, and the decrease in vascular resistance appears to be global.[4,12]

As with the haemodynamic response during non-hypotensive haemorrhage, the chief determinant of the changes during hypotensive haemorrhage appears to be a change in efferent sympathetic activity. RSNA decreases during the hypotensive phase of haemorrhage in conscious dogs,[6] rabbits[24–26] and anaesthetized rats (Fig. 2.2).[51–55] This is at a time when maintained or increasing sympathetic activity is vital to pressure maintenance. The decrease is to near[6] or below control levels.[24–26,51] Plasma noradrenaline, an indirect indicator of sympathetic activity, does not increase further at the onset of hypotension (Fig. 2.2).[28] The lack of a decrease in plasma noradrenaline is probably due to the time lag between changes in release and the reflection of these changes in plasma levels and to a simultaneous increase in output by the adrenal medulla (see below).

Unlike peripheral sympathetic nerves, activity of the adrenal medulla increases at the transition to hypotension. Plasma adrenaline, an indicator of adrenal medullary activity, increases dramatically at the onset of hypotension (Fig. 2.3) in conscious dogs,[31] rabbits[27,28,32] and rats.[16,19] In addition, during hypotensive haemorrhage in anaesthetized rats, while RSNA is decreasing, adrenal sympathetic nerve activity is increasing.[55] Since the adrenal medulla releases both adrenaline and noradrenaline (the ratio varies in different species), release of some noradrenaline by the adrenal gland may account for the inability to show a decrease in plasma noradrenaline when arterial pressure falls, even though sympathetic nerve activity is decreasing. Consistent with this, adrenalectomized or adrenal denervated rabbits show a significant decrease in plasma noradrenaline at the transition to hypotension. If the adrenal glands are intact there is no significant change (Fig 2.2).[27]

The value to the organism of adrenal activation late in haemorrhage is not readily apparent. Increased release of adrenaline does not appear to be vital to maintenance of circulatory function during haemorrhage.[55] The changes in myocardial contractility and mean arterial pressure that occur during haemorrhage are not affected by β-adrenergic receptor blockade in conscious dogs.[10] In addition, blockade of cardiac β-adrenergic and muscarinic receptors does not affect the fall in cardiac output or mean arterial pressure during haemorrhage in conscious rabbits.[15] Finally, the haemodynamic response to haemorrhage is not altered by adrenal denervation or adrenalectomy in conscious rabbits.[27]

Release of renin continues to increase after hypotensive haemorrhage in conscious rabbits,[33,37–39,42] rats,[18] dogs[44] and sheep.[40] Prior autonomic blockade exaggerates this increase.[38] Although it does not appear to play a pivotal role during non-hypotensive haemorrhage, increased renin release after hypotensive haemorrhage is important to spontaneous recovery of arterial blood pressure. In conscious rabbits blockade of the production of AII delays and reduces spontaneous recovery of arterial pressure and vascular tone.[12,33] In addition, saralasin, an AII antagonist, limits blood pressure recovery after hypotensive blood loss in conscious monkeys and dogs.[56,57]

In conscious rabbits,[34,37–39,42] rats,[18] monkeys[43] and sheep[40] plasma vasopressin levels increase only after hypotensive blood loss. Thus, vasopressin apparently does not have a prominent role in maintaining blood pressure during an acute reduction in CBV. In dogs vasopressin may play a more important role (see above). Like AII, vasopressin may be more important during recovery from acute haemorrhagic hypotension. Blockade of vascular vasopressin receptors decreases the rate and degree of spontaneous recovery from acute haemorrhagic hypotension in conscious rabbits[34] and conscious rats.[58] In addition, vasopressin may limit the fall in arterial pressure after haemorrhage in conscious rabbits. With prior blockade of vascular vasopressin receptors arterial blood pressure and vascular resistance fall to lower levels after hypotensive haemorrhage.[12,34] Thus, a vasoconstrictive action of vasopressin is apparent only after arterial blood pressure decreases.

While a decrease in vascular resistance clearly accounts for the decrease in arterial pressure after hypotensive haemorrhage, the cause of the decrease is less clear. It is not due to decreased release of renin, vasopressin or adrenal catecholamines since these all increase as blood pressure falls. The inhibition of activity in peripheral sympathetic nerves could account for the decrease, but a causal relation has not been proven. However, the dramatic decrease in sympathetic nerve activity clearly must contribute to the fall in pressure and resistance during hypotensive blood loss. Increased release of vasopressin and renin probably contribute to the recovery of blood pressure after haemorrhage.

Although arterial baroreceptors are the dominant afferent signal during non-hypotensive haemorrhage, their role after hypotensive haemorrhage is clearly diminished. The simultaneous decrease in arterial pressure, heart rate and vascular resistance is hardly indicative of normal baroreflex function. In some species cardiac receptors that project centrally in the vagus nerve appear to be important. These receptors, when activated produce bradycardia and vasodilatation in resistance and capacitance vessels.[59] The vasodilatation is due to sympathoinhibition. While these receptors are normally thought to be more active during increases in blood pressure or volume, paradoxical increases in activity during decreases in blood pressure or volume might also be important. It has been suggested that these receptors might be stimulated during blood loss by the combination of increased sympathetic stimulation and decreased ventricular volume. If so, they might play a protective role by limiting cardiac contractile function and heart rate during times of poor diastolic filling.[59,60] An important role for these receptors during haemorrhage in conscious rabbits has recently been reported. Reversible blockade of the cardiac nerves with intrapericardial procaine abolishes the decrease in pressure and sympathetic nerve activity during haemorrhage.[25] This procedure also blocks the decrease in vascular resistance associated with the hypotension produced by gradual vena caval occlusion.[49] In rats the decrease in activity in peripheral sympathetic nerves[61,62] as well as the increase in activity in the adrenal nerve[55] during acute haemorrhagic hypotension are abolished by vagotomy. The situation in dogs is slightly different. In this species the sympathoinhibition associated with hypotensive haemorrhage is not blocked by cardiac and/or arterial baroreceptor denervation and is actually augmented by the combination of arterial baroreceptor denervation and vagotomy.[6] Thus, a signal from the heart may initiate the hypotensive phase of haemorrhage in rabbits, cats and rats. The afferent signal in dogs is unknown.

Although there is general agreement that plasma levels of vasopressin and renin are elevated after hypotensive haemorrhage, the source of the stimulus for this release is not so clear. In conscious dogs and rabbits renin release does not appear to require arterial or cardiac baroreceptors.[37,45] Normal increases in plasma levels of renin during haemorrhage occur in the absence of either group or both groups of receptors. Afferent input from cardiac baroreceptors is generally thought to be important for vasopressin release during haemorrhage.[37,45,63] However, there have also been reports which deemphasize the role of these receptors[64–66] and emphasize the role of arterial baroreceptors.[43,64]

Potential central mediators of the response to blood loss

Endogenous opioid peptides

Many neurotransmitters are involved with control of the cardiovascular response to haemorrhage. However, one group of compounds, endogenous opioid peptides, has received the most attention. Much of the evidence for a role for these peptides in the response to blood loss is based on observations of the cardiovascular effects of opioid antagonists after hypotensive haemorrhage or prior to blood loss.[1,67–69]

During hypotension associated with haemorrhage the opioid antagonist, naloxone, increases arterial blood pressure in conscious rabbits,[24,70,71] baboons,[72,73] and rats.[74–76] In some cases the increase in arterial pressure is accomplished through reversal of the effects of hypotensive blood loss. That is, it increases vascular resistance[4] and sympathetic nerve activity.[24,26,28,71] In addition, prophylactic administration of naloxone before haemorrhage blocks the decrease in sympathetic nerve activity, vascular resistance and arterial pressure.[5,25]

There are both peripheral and central mechanisms involving opioids that could account for some of the changes associated with blood loss. However, experimental evidence favours a central role for naloxone.[49,50,77–79] It follows that central nervous system mechanisms involving opioid peptides may mediate the response to hypotensive haemorrhage.

Serotonin

Serotonin may also be involved with the response to acute blood loss. Pharmacological depletion of serotonin in the central nervous system prior to haemorrhage attenuates the subsequent decreases in arterial pressure and heart rate as well as sympathetic nerve activity.[80] In addition, the serotonin antagonist, methysergide, increases arterial blood pressure during haemorrhagic hypotension.[80,81] There is also some evidence for a central nervous system interaction between opioid peptides and serotonin. Systemic administration of one opioid peptide, β-endorphin, produces a decrease in arterial blood pressure that can be abolished by opioid or serotonin antagonists.[82] In addition, depletion of serotonin abolishes the response while blockade of serotonin reuptake with fluoxetine potentiates the hypotension.

Other factors influencing the response to blood loss

Anaesthesia

General anaesthesia depresses central nervous system function and results ultimately in loss of consciousness. This depression also affects reflex mechanisms, such as arterial baroreflexes, which are important for blood pressure maintenance.[83–85] As a result, the ability of animals to maintain arterial blood pressure even after a small blood loss is severely compromised under general anaesthesia. The response to blood loss in pentobarbital or halothane anaesthetized dogs is virtually identical to that after baroreceptor denervation.[86] Pentobarbital also blunts the increase in sympathetic activity[9,87–89] but increases release of renin[87] during haemorrhage. Propofol, ketamine and alfentanil anaesthesia also reduce the vasoconstrictive response to decreases in CBV.[90] Furthermore, changes produced by anaesthetics are not only quantitative. In the conscious dog the vasodilatation seen in the kidney during haemorrhage is changed to a vasoconstriction if blood loss occurs during pentobarbital anaesthesia.[9] Thus, anaesthetics can have profound effects on the haemodynamic and neurohumoral response to acute haemorrhage.

Gender

There is not much information available on the influence of gender on the response to blood loss. However, it is known that receptors for gonadal steroids exist in the heart and blood vessels and also in central nervous system areas associated with cardiovascular control.[91] The effect of gender on vasopressin release is one area which has been addressed. Baseline as well as stimulated vasopressin release is influenced by gender. Baseline vasopressin release is greater in males than in females,[92] and vasopressin release during haemorrhage is generally greater in females.[93] However, this difference during blood loss is also influenced by the stage of oestrus cycle.[93] In sheep release of vasopressin during hypotension due to nitroprusside injection is augmented by ovariectomy while renin release in response to the same stimulus is decreased.[94] These differences appear to be due, at least in part, to differences in central mechanisms controlling vasopressin release.[95,96] There are apparently no gender differences in the blood pressure or heart rate response to blood loss in rats. However, vasopressin does appear to be more important to blood pressure recovery in females after hypotensive haemorrhage.[93]

Stress

While the response to haemorrhage in humans and other animals is well documented,[1] the effects of simultaneous stress on this response are not as well understood. With the exception of the situation in the laboratory, blood loss usually occurs in the presence of stressful sensory stimulation. Therefore, it is important to know what the effects of simultaneous stress are on the response to blood loss. Stress is known to increase sympathetic nerve activity and release of renin, vasopressin and adrenaline.[97–99] It seems likely that the response to a subsequent haemorrhage would be altered by these changes. Some studies have demonstrated an interaction between stressful stimuli and blood loss. For example, surgical stress augments the haemorrhage-induced release of vasopressin and renin,[100] and painful stimuli augment release of noradrenaline during haemorrhage.[101] In addition, preliminary reports indicate that stressful sensory stimulation can quantitatively and qualitatively alter the haemodynamic response to blood loss.[102,103] Stress also increases the blood loss necessary to produce hypotension.[102,103] That is, the animal's ability to maintain arterial pressure appears to be enhanced by stress.

Summary

The response to acute blood loss in conscious animals is biphasic and involves both sympathoexcitation and sympathoinhibition. The initial response involves an increase in sympathetic activity, heart rate and vascular resistance. As a result, arterial blood pressure is well maintained. If blood loss continues beyond 20–30 per cent of the animal's total blood volume, arterial pressure decreases dramatically due to a global decrease in vascular resistance. The decrease in resistance is due, at least in part, to a centrally mediated sympathoinhibition. The vasopressin and renin–angiotensin systems, while apparently not crucial to this initial response to blood loss, do come into play during hypotension and contribute significantly to spontaneous recovery of arterial blood pressure. The afferent signal that results in sympathoinhibition and ultimately hypotension appears to originate in the heart in most species studied. Central neurotransmitters that may be important in this response include endogenous opioid peptides and serotonin. Anaesthesia dramatically alters the response to blood loss and decreases the amount of blood loss necessary to produce hypotension. Gender or concomitant stressful sensory stimuli may affect the response to blood loss.

Acknowledgements

The work from this laboratory would not have been possible without my collaboration with Dr Ronald Gaddis and Dr Eileen Hasser. Support for this work has been provided by the National Heart, Lung and Blood Institute under Grant HL-31218 and by the National Science Foundation under Grant BNS-8719372. I am grateful to the American Physiological Society for allowing me to use data previously published in the *American Journal of Physiology*. I acknowledge the contribution of Professor John Ludbrook to this manuscript through our continuing discussions of this phenomenon. Finally, I thank Dr Eileen Hasser and Dr Curt Vogel for critically reviewing this manuscript.

References

1. Schadt JC and Ludbrook J: Hemodynamic and neurohumoral responses to acute hypovolemia in conscious mammals. *American Journal of Physiology*, 1991; **260,** H305–18.
2. Barcroft H, McMichael J, Edholm OG and Sharpey-Schafer EP: Posthaemorrhagic fainting. Study by cardiac output and forearm flow. *Lancet*, 1944; **i,** 489–91.
3. Warren JV, Brannon ES, Stead EA and Merrill AJ: The effect of venesection and the pooling of blood in the extremities on the atrial pressure and cardiac output in normal subjects with observations on acute circulatory collapse in three instances. *Journal of Clinical Investigation*, 1945; **24,** 337–44.
4. Schadt JC, McKown MD, McKown DP and Franklin D: Hemodynamic effects of hemorrhage and subsequent naloxone treatment in conscious rabbits. *American Journal of Physiology*, 1984; **247,** R497–508.
5. Ludbrook J and Rutter PC: Effect of naloxone on haemodynamic responses to acute blood loss in unanaesthetized rabbits. *Journal of Physiology (London)*, 1988; **400,** 1–14.
6. Morita H, Vatner SF: Effects of hemorrhage on renal nerve activity in conscious dogs. *Circulation Research*, 1985; **57,** 788–93.
7. Shen Y-T, Knight DR, Thomas JX and Vatner SF: Relative roles of cardiac receptors and arterial baroreceptors during hemorrhage in conscious dogs. *Circulation Research*, 1990; **66,** 397–405.
8. Chien S: Role of the sympathetic nervous system in hemorrhage. *Physiological Reviews*, 1967; **47,** 214–88.
9. Vatner SF: Effects of hemorrhage on regional blood flow distribution in dogs and primates. *Journal of Clinical Investigation*, 1974; **54,** 225–35.
10. Hintze TH and Vatner SF: Cardiac dynamics during hemorrhage: relative unimportance of adrenergic inotropic responses. *Circulation Research*, 1982; **50,** 705–13.
11. Chalmers JP, Korner PI and White SW: Effects of haemorrhage on the distribution of blood flow in the rabbit. *Journal of Physiology (London)*, 1967; **192,** 561–74.
12. Korner PI, Oliver JR, Zhu JL, Gipps J and Hanneman F: Autonomic, hormonal, and local circulatory effects of hemorrhage in conscious rabbits. *American Journal of Physiology*, 1990; **258,** H229–39.
13. Neutze JM, Wyler F and Rudolph AM: Changes in distribution of cardiac output after hemorrhage in rabbits. *American Journal of Physiology*, 1968; **215,** 857–64.
14. Chalmers JP, Korner PI and White SW: The effects of haemorrhage in the unanaesthetized rabbit. *Journal of Physiology (London)*, 1967; **189,** 367–91.
15. Ludbrook J and Graham WF: The role of cardiac receptor and arterial baroreceptor reflexes in control of the circulation during acute change of blood volume in the conscious rabbit. *Circulation Research*, 1984; **54,** 424–35.
16. Haggendal J: On the patterns of blood pressure, heart rate, and blood levels of noradrenaline and adrenaline during haemorrhage in the rat. *Acta Physiologica Scandinavica*, 1986; **127,** 513–22.
17. Skarphedinsson JO and Thoren P: The effects of naloxone on behavioural depression due to hypotensive haemorrhage in unanesthetized spontaneously hypertensive rats. *Acta Physiologica Scandinavica*, 1987; **129,** 27–34.
18. Fejes-Toth G, Brinck-Johnsen T and Naray-Fejes-Toth A: Cardiovascular and hormonal response to hemorrhage in conscious rats. *American Journal of Physiology*, 1988; **254,** H947–53.
19. Darlington DN, Shinsako J and Dallman MF: Responses of ACTH, epinephrine, norepinephrine, and cardiovascular system to hemorrhage. *American Journal of Physiology*, 1986; **251,** H612–18.
20. Forsyth RP, Hoffbrand BI and Melmon KL: Redis-

tribution of cardiac output during hemorrhage in the unanesthetized monkey. *Circulation Research*, 1970; **27,** 311–20.

21. Sondeen JL, Gonzaludo GA, Loveday JA, Deshon GE, Clifford CB, Hunt MM, Rodkey WG and Wade CE: Renal responses to graded hemorrhage in conscious pig. *American Journal of Physiology*, 1990; **259,** R119–25.
22. Courneya CA and Korner PI: Neurohumoral mechanisms and the role of arterial baroreceptors in the reno-vascular response to haemorrhage in rabbits. *Journal of Physiology (London)*, 1991; **437,** 393–407.
23. Granata L, Huvos A, Pasque A and Gregg DE: Left coronary hemodynamics during hemorrhagic hypotension and shock. *American Journal of Physiology*, 1969; **216,** 1583–9.
24. Morita H, Nishida Y, Motochigawa H, Uemura N, Hosomi H and Vatner SF: Opiate receptor-mediated decrease in renal nerve activity during hypotensive hemorrhage in conscious rabbits. *Circulation Research*, 1988; **63,** 165–72.
25. Burke SL and Dorward PK: Influence of endogenous opiates and cardiac afferents on renal nerve activity during haemorrhage in conscious rabbits. *Journal of Physiology (London)*, 1988; **402,** 9–27.
26. Hasser EM and Schadt JC: Sympathoinhibition and its reversal by naloxone during hemorrhage. *American Journal of Physiology*, 1992; **262,** R444–51.
27. Schadt JC and Gaddis RR: Role of adrenal medulla in hemodynamic response to hemorrhage and naloxone. *American Journal of Physiology*, 1988; **254,** R559–65.
28. Schadt JC and Gaddis RR: Endogenous opiate peptides may limit norepinephrine release during hemorrhage. *Journal of Pharmacology and Experimental Therapeutics*, 1985; **232,** 656–60.
29. Schadt JC and York DH: Involvement of both adrenergic and cholinergic receptors in the cardiovascular effects of naloxone during hemorrhagic hypotension in the conscious rabbit. *Journal of the Autonomic Nervous System*, 1982; **6,** 237–51.
30. Sander-Jensen K, Mehlsen J, Stadeager C, Christensen NJ, Fahrenkrug J, Schwartz TW, Warberg J and Bie P: Increase in vagal activity during hypotensive lower-body negative pressure in humans. *American Journal of Physiology*, 1988; **255,** R149–56.
31. Engeland WC, Dempsher DP, Byrnes GJ, Presnell K and Gann DS: The adrenal medullary response to graded hemorrhage in awake dogs. *Endocrinology*, 1981; **109,** 1539–44.
32. Rutter PC, Potocnik SJ and Ludbrook J: Sympathoadrenal mechanisms in cardiovascular responses to naloxone after hemorrhage. *American Journal of Physiology*, 1987; **252,** H40–46.
33. Schadt JC, Gaddis RR: Renin–angiotensin system and opioids during acute hemorrhage in conscious rabbits. *American Journal of Physiology*, 1990; **258,** R543–51.
34. Schadt JC and Hasser EM: Interaction of vasopressin and opioids during rapid hemorrhage in the conscious rabbit. *American Journal of Physiology*, 1991; **260**, R373–81.
35. Wang BC, Flora-Ginter G, Leadley RJ and Goetz KL: Ventricular receptors stimulate vasopressin release during hemorrhage. *American Journal of Physiology*, 1988; **254,** R204–11.
36. Wang BC, Sundet WD, Hakumaki MOK and Goetz KL: Vasopressin and renin responses to hemorrhage in conscious, cardiac-denervated dogs. *American Journal of Physiology*, 1983; **245,** H399–405.
37. Quail AW, Woods RL and Korner PI: Cardiac and arterial baroreceptor influences in release of vasopressin and renin during hemorrhage. *American Journal of Physiology*, 1987; **252,** H1120–26.
38. Oliver JR, Korner PI, Woods RL and Zhu JL: Reflex release of vasopressin and renin in hemorrhage is enhanced by autonomic blockade. *American Journal of Physiology*, 1990; **258,** H221–8.
39. Matsukawa S, Keil LC and Reid IA: Role of renal nerves in regulation of vasopressin secretion and blood pressure in conscious rabbits. *American Journal of Physiology*, 1990; **258,** F821–30.
40. Hjelmqvist H, Ullman J, Gunnarsson U, Lundberg JM and Rundgren M: Haemodynamic and humoral responses to repeated hypotensive haemorrhage in conscious sheep. *Acta Physiologica Scandinavica*, 1991; **143,** 55–64.
41. Matsukawa S, Keil LC and Reid IA: Role of endogenous angiotensin II in the control of vasopressin secretion during hypovolemia and hypotension in conscious rabbits. *Endocrinology*, 1991; **128,** 204–10.
42. Ludbrook J, Potocnik SJ and Woods RL: Simulation of acute haemorrhage in unanesthetized rabbits. *Clinical and Experimental Pharmacology and Physiology*, 1988; **15,** 575–84.
43. Arnauld E, Czernichow P, Fumoux F and Vincent J-D: The effects of hypotension and hypovolaemia on the liberation of vasopressin during haemorrhage in the unanaesthetized monkey (*Macaca mulatta*). *Pflügers Archiv. European Journal of Physiology*, 1977; **371,** 193–200.
44. Schwartz J, Reid IA: Effect of vasopressin blockade on blood pressure regulation during hemorrhage in conscious dogs. *Endocrinology*, 1981; **109,** 1778–80.
45. Goetz KL, Wang BC, Sundet WD: Comparative effects of cardiac receptors and sinoaortic baroreceptors on elevations of plasma vasopressin and renin activity elicited by haemorrhage. *Journal of Physiology (Paris)*, 1984; **79,** 440–45.
46. Hales JRS, Ludbrook J: Baroreflex participation in redistribution of cardiac output at onset of exercise. *Journal of Applied Physiology*, 1988; **64,** 627–34.
47. Courneya CA, Korner PI, Oliver JR and Woods

RL: Afferent vascular resistance control during hemorrhage in normal and autonomically blocked rabbits. *American Journal of Physiology*, 1991; **261,** H380–91.
48. Schadt JC and Gaddis RR: Cardiovascular responses to hemorrhage and naloxone in conscious barodenervated rabbits. *American Journal of Physiology*, 1986; **251,** R909–15.
49. Evans RG, Ludbrook J and Potocnik SJ: Intracisternal naloxone and cardiac nerve blockade prevent vasodilatation during simulated haemorrhage in awake rabbits. *Journal of Physiology (London)*, 1989; **409**, 1–14.
50. Evans RG, Ludbrook J, van Leeuwen AF: Role of central opiate receptor subtypes in the circulatory responses of awake rabbits to graded caval occlusions. *Journal of Physiology (London)*, 1989; **419,** 15–31.
51. Skarphedinsson JO, Stage L and Thoren P: Cerebral function during hypotensive haemorrhage in spontaneously hypertensive rats and Wistar–Kyoto rats. *Acta Physiologica Scandinavica*, 1986; **128,** 445–52.
52. Murray RH and Shropshire S: Effect of atropine on circulatory responses to lower body negative pressure and vasodepressor syncope. *Aerospace Medicine*, 1970; **41,** 717–22.
53. Epstein SE, Stampfer M and Beiser GD: Role of the capacitance and resistance vessels in vasovagal syncope. *Circulation*, 1968; **37,** 524–33.
54. Murray RH, Thompson LJ, Bowers JA and Albright CD: Hemodynamic effects of graded hypovolemia and vasodepressor syncope induced by lower body negative pressure. *American Heart Journal*, 1968; **76,** 799–811.
55. Victor RG, Thoren P, Morgan DA and Mark AL: Differential control of adrenal and renal sympathetic nerve activity during hemorrhagic hypotension in rats. *Circulation Research*, 1989; **64,** 686–94.
56. Freeman RH, Davis JO, Johnson JA, Spielman WS and Zatzman ML: Arterial pressure regulation during hemorrhage: homeostatic role of angiotensin II. *Proceedings of the Society for Experimental Biology and Medicine*, 1975; **149,** 19–22.
57. Cornish KG, Barazanji MW and Iaffaldano R: Neural and hormonal control of blood pressure in conscious monkeys. *American Journal of Physiology*, 1990; **258,** H107–12.
58. Johnson JV, Bennett GW, Hatton R: Central and systemic effects of a vasopressin V_1 antagonist on MAP recovery after haemorrhage in rats. *Journal of Cardiovascular Pharmacology*, 1988; **12,** 405–12.
59. Oberg B and Thoren P: Circulatory responses to stimulation of left ventricular receptors in the cat. *Acta Physiologica Scandinavica*, 1973; **88,** 8–22.
60. Oberg B and Thoren P: Increased activity in left ventricular receptors during hemorrhage or occlusion of caval veins in the cat. – A possible cause of the vaso-vagal reaction. *Acta Physiologica Scandinavica*, 1972; **85,** 164–73.
61. Skoog P, Mansson J and Thoren P: Changes in renal sympathetic outflow during hypotensive haemorrhage in rats. *Acta Physiologica Scandinavica*, 1985; **125,** 655–60.
62. Morgan DA, Thoren P, Wilczynski EA, Victor RG and Mark AL: Serotonergic mechanisms mediate renal sympathoinhibition during severe hemorrhage in rats. *American Journal of Physiology*, 1988; **255,** H496–502.
63. Oliver JR, Courneya CA, Woods RL and Korner PI: Role of cardiac and sinoaortic baroreceptors in enhanced vasopressin (AVP) and plasma renin activity (PRA) responses during haemorrhage after total autonomic blockade (TAB). *Proceedings of the International Union of Physiological Sciences*, 1989; **17,** 63 (abstract).
64. Shen Y-T, Cowley AW Jr and Vatner SF: Relative roles of cardiac and arterial baroreceptors in vasopressin regulation during hemorrhage in conscious dogs. *Circulation Research*, 1991; **68,** 1422–36.
65. Shen Y-T, Knight DR, Thomas JX, Cowley AW and Vatner SF: Cardiac receptors are not the major regulators of vasopressin release during hemorrhage in conscious dogs. *Circulation*, 1988; **7 (suppl. II),** 522.
66. Thrasher TN, O'Donnell CP and Keil LC: Role of cardiac receptors in the stimulation of vasopressin secretion in response to hypovolemia. *Proceedings of the International Union of Physiological Sciences*, 1989; **17,** 490 (abstract).
67. Holaday JW, d'Amato RJ, Ruvio BA and Faden AI: Action of naloxone and TRH on the autonomic regulation of circulation. *Advances in Biochemical Psychopharmacology*, 1982; **33,** 353–61.
68. Holaday JW: Cardiovascular consequences of endogenous opiate antagonism. *Biochemical Pharmacology*, 1983; **32,** 573–85.
69. Holaday JW: Cardiovascular effects of endogenous opiate systems. *Annual Review of Pharmacology and Toxicology*, 1983; **23,** 541–94.
70. Schadt JC and York DH: The reversal of hemorrhagic hypotension by naloxone in conscious rabbits. *Canadian Journal of Physiology and Pharmacology*, 1981; **59,** 1208–13.
71. Rutter PC, Potocnik SJ and Ludbrook J: Factors influencing the effects of intravenous naloxone on arterial pressure and heart rate after haemorrhage in conscious rabbits. *Clinical and Experimental Pharmacology and Physiology*, 1986; **13,** 383–97.
72. Golanov EV, Cherkovich GM and Suchkov VV: Effect of naloxone in hypotension induced by acute blood loss in baboons (*Papio hamadryas*). *Bulletin of Experimental Biology and Medicine*, 1983; **96,** 1428–31.
73. McIntosh TK, Palter M, Grasberger R, Vezina R,

Yseton NS and Egdahl RH: Effect of an opiate antagonist (naloxone) and an agonist/antagonist (nalbuphine) in primate hemorrhagic shock: relationship to catecholamine release. *Circulatory Shock*, 1985; **17,** 313–25.

74. Feuerstein G, Chiueh CC and Kopin IJ: Effect of naloxone on the cardiovascular and sympathetic response to hypovolemic hypotension in the rat. *European Journal of Pharmacology*, 1981; **75,** 65–9.
75. Bennett T and Gardiner SM: The influence of naloxone on haemorrhagic hypotension in Brattleboro rats. *Journal of Physiology (London)*, 1982; **332,** 69–70P.
76. Faden AI and Holaday JW: Opiate antagonists: a role in the treatment of hypovolemic shock. *Science*, 1979; **205,** 317–18.
77. Holaday JW, O'Hara M and Faden AI: Hypophysectomy alters cardiorespiratory variables: central effects of pituitary endorphins in shock. *American Journal of Physiology*, 1981; **241,** H479–85.
78. Jang W, Schadt JC and Gaddis RR: Peripheral opioidergic mechanisms do not mediate naxolone's pressor effect in the conscious rabbit. *Circulatory Shock*, 1993; **39,** 121–7.
79. d'Amato R and Holaday JW: Multiple opioid receptors in endotoxic shock: evidence for δ involvement and μ–δ interactions *in vivo*. *Proceedings of the National Academy of Sciences (USA)*, 1984; **81,** 2898–901.
80. Elam R, Bergmann F and Feuerstein G: The use of antiserotonergic agents for the treatment of acute hemorrhagic shock of cats. *European Journal of Pharmacology*, 1985; **107,** 275–8.
81. Hasser EM, Schadt JC and Grove KJ: Serotonergic and opioid interactions during acute hemorrhagic hypotension in the conscious rabbit. *FASEB Journal*, 1989; **3,** A1014 (abstract).
82. Lemaire I, Tseng R and Lemaire S: Systemic administration of beta-endorphin: Potent hypotensive effect involving a serotonergic pathway. *Proceedings of the National Academy of Sciences (USA)*, 1978; **75,** 6240–42.
83. Vatner SF, Franklin D and Braunwald E: Effects of anesthesia and sleep on circulatory response to carotid sinus nerve stimulation. *American Journal of Physiology*, 1971; **220,** 1249–55.
84. Duke PC, Fownes D and Wade JG: Halothane depresses baroreflex control of heart rate in man. *Anesthesiology*, 1977; **46,** 184–7.
85. Vatner SF, Braunwald E: Cardiovascular control mechanisms in the conscious state. *New England Journal of Medicine*, 1975; **293,** 970–76.
86. Vatner SF: Effects of anesthesia on cardiovascular control mechanisms. *Environmental Health Perspectives*, 1978; **26,** 193–206.
87. Zimpfer M, Manders WT, Barger AC and Vatner SF: Pentobarbital alters compensatory neural and humoral mechanisms in response to hemorrhage. *American Journal of Physiology*, 1982; **243,** H713–21.
88. Adamicza A, Tarnoky K, Nagy A and Nagy S: The effect of anaesthesia on the haemodynamic and sympathoadrenal response of the dog in experimental haemorrhagic shock. *Acta Physiologica Hungarica*, 1985; **65,** 239–54.
89. Gaddis RR, Schadt JC, McKown MD and Franklin D: Pentobarbital anesthesia reduces plasma catecholamines in control and hemorrhaged rabbits. *Federation Proceedings*, 1983; **42,** 379.
90. van Leeuwen AF, Evans RG and Ludbrook J: Effects of halothane, ketamine, propofol and alfentanil anesthesia on circulatory control in rabbits. *Clinical and Experimental Pharmacology and Physiology*; in press.
91. Stumpf WE: Steroid hormones and the cardiovascular system: direct actions of estradiol, progesterone, testosterone, gluco- and mineral-corticoids, and soltriol [vitamin D] on central nervous regulatory and peripheral tissues. *Experientia*, 1990; **46,** 13–25.
92. Crofton JT, Share L and Brooks DP: Pressor responsiveness to and secretion of vasopressin during the estrous cycle. *American Journal of Physiology*, 1988; **255,** R1041–8.
93. Crofton JT and Share L: Sexual dimorphism in vasopressin and cardiovascular response to hemorrhage in the rat. *Circulation Research*, 1990; **66,** 1345–53.
94. Keller-Wood M and Wood CE: Effect of ovariectomy on vasopressin, ACTH, and renin activity responses to hypotension. *American Journal of Physiology*, 1991; **261,** R223–30.
95. Stone JD, Crofton JT and Share L: Sex differences in central adrenergic control of vasopressin release. *American Journal of Physiology*, 1989; **257,** R1040–45.
96. Stone JD, Crofton JT and Share L: Sex differences in central adrenoreceptor-mediated vasopressin response to hemorrhage. *American Journal of Physiology*, 1991; **260,** E780–86.
97. Meyerhoff JL, Oleshansky MA, Kalogeras KT, Mougey EH, Chrousos GP and Granger LG: Neuroendocrine responses to emotional stress: possible interactions between circulating factors and anterior pituitary hormone release. *Advances in Experimental Medicine and Biology*, 1990; **274,** 91–112.
98. Herd JA: Cardiovascular response to stress. *Physiological Reviews*, 1991; **71,** 305–30.
99. Kapusta DR, Jones SY and DiBona GF: Opioids in the systemic hemodynamic and renal responses to stress in conscious spontaneously hypertensive rats. *Hypertension*, 1989; **13,** 808–16.
100. McNeill JR and Pang CCY: Effect of pentobarbital anesthesia and surgery on the control of arterial pressure and mesenteric resistance in cats: role of

vasopressin and angiotensin. *Canadian Journal of Physiology and Pharmacology*, 1982; **60,** 363–8.

101. Bereiter DA, Benetti AP and Thrivikraman KV: Thermal nociception potentiates the release of ACTH and norepinephrine by blood loss. *American Journal of Physiology*, 1990; **259,** R1236–42.
102. Schadt J, Hasser E and Taylor J: Environmental stimuli modify the response to blood loss in conscious rabbits. *FASEB Journal*, 1991; **5,** A1405 (abstract).
103. Schadt JC, Hasser EM, Astorino ME and Taylor JS: Stress alters the renal vascular response to hemorrhage. *FASEB Journal*, 1992; **6,** A1527 (abstract).

3

Cardiovascular and hormonal responses to central hypovolaemia in humans

James A Pawelczyk, Steen Matzen, Daniel B Friedman and Niels H Secher

Introduction

The physiological manifestations of hypovolaemia clearly depend on the amount of blood loss and the clinical status of the patient. It is the intent of this chapter to focus on the former effect, by considering the various models of volume loss that mimic bleeding and the cardiovascular and hormonal adaptations that result from central hypovolaemia. By providing controlled circumstances the phases of shock previously outlined may be delineated and investigated more thoroughly. Such experiments help to define better the haemodynamic and the hormonal consequences of hypovolaemia.

The largest body of information on *human* cardiovascular regulation during hypovolaemic shock is derived not from recording of variables in patients during haemorrhage but from experimental models eliciting 'functional haemorrhage'. Procedures meant to reduce CBV include LBNP, head-up tilt (reverse Trendelenburg's position), pressure breathing and venous congestion of the legs. Also, loop flying or placing a subject in a centrifuge with the legs oriented in the centrifugal field ($+G_z$ position) produces a shift of blood from the thorax to the legs. These techniques share a common theoretical basis to pool or remove blood from the central circulation mechanically without altering compensatory blood pressure regulatory mechanisms.

Other types of procedures, such as inhalation anaesthesia, regional nerve block, or ganglionic receptor blockade, reduce CBV by increasing venous pooling secondary to sympatholysis. As these perturbations share the common effect of causing blood to pool away from the central circulation secondary to vasodilatation, results obtained using these models are relevant to the manifestations seen in bleeding patients. Such experiments illustrate the importance of sympathetically mediated vasoconstriction for blood pressure maintenance and echo the authors' consensus that effective management of CBV and vasodilatation is essential to successful recovery from hypovolaemic shock.

In this chapter these models of hypovolaemic shock will be reviewed. The goal is to provide the reader with a foundation upon which to investigate research that might not otherwise be considered relevant to the clinical condition of hypovolaemic shock. As a prelude to the chapters discussing specific aspects of cardiovascular regulation, general features of the haemodynamic and hormonal responses to 'functional haemorrhage' will be considered. Related information is available in recent reviews.[1,2]

Overview of models of haemorrhage

Rigorous experimental study of the cardiovascular responses to haemorrhage evolved from investigations conducted during World War II. Fig. 3.1 represents a generalization of data from these studies[3–6] assuming that the subjects had normal blood volumes (estimated at 5.2 litres) when venesection commenced. The results define a line indicating that virtually all patients with rapid haemorrhage will lose consciousness when approximately 30 per cent of their circulating blood volume (approximately 1500 ml) is lost.

This line of research is notable not just for determining quantitatively the extent of haemorrhage that can be tolerated, but for determining the mechanisms of the cardiovascular responses to progressive blood loss. Much of the credit for this effort can be given to Barcroft and his colleagues.[7] As Fig. 3.2 illustrates, venesection approaching 1 litre of blood produced a biphasic response in heart rate and peripheral resistance. Bleeding was characterized by moderate tachycardia and vasoconstriction, with a transition to another phase characterized by bradycardia and vasodilatation.

This investigation provided the first quantitative evidence that vasodilatation accompanied severe blood loss. Barcroft's own studies, and those of others,[8,9] demonstrated that it is vasodilatation that is most important in producing the profound hypotension associated with the second (and probably tertiary) phases of haemorrhage, as blockade of the bradycardic response with atropine fails to ameliorate the hypotension.

The use of bleeding to study haemorrhage has obvious clinical relevance. However, it is unlikely that experimental perturbations of this nature would meet with approval from a modern day ethical review panel. The study of patients with haemorrhagic shock offers a second avenue of study,[10] but must be constrained by the requirements for proper patient care. As a result, a variety of alternative procedures have been used to mimic the volume status of the haemorrhagic patient. These procedures offer the general advantages that: (1) they are graded and controlled, allowing precise

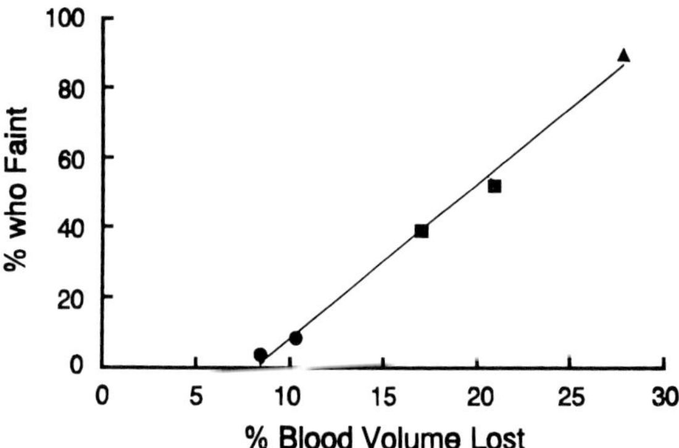

Fig. 3.1. Relation between incidence of fainting (prelude to progression to stage II of haemorrhagic shock) and per cent of blood volume lost by combinations of rapid venesection and venous congestion (leg tourniquets). *Source*: Poles and Boycott (●)[4], Barcroft and Edholm (▲)[5] and Barcroft and Edholm (■),[7] assuming a basal blood volume of 5.25 litres and that 700 ml of blood are trapped in the legs by the application of tourniquets to the thighs. Virtually all subjects succumb when rapid blood loss exceeds 30 per cent of total blood volume.

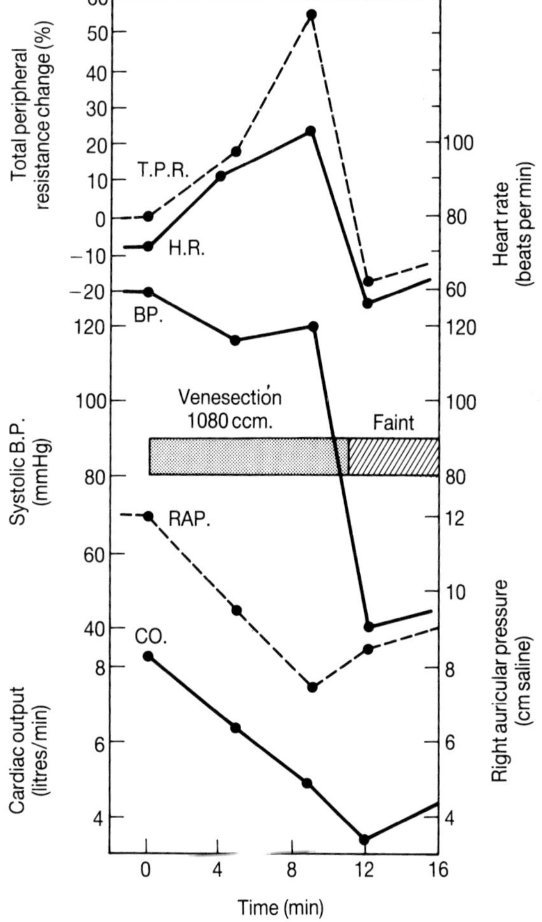

Fig. 3.2. Illustration of sympathetic activation and deactivation during the first two stages of hypovolaemic shock. Rapid venesection initially resulted in tachycardia and vasoconstriction, with relatively well-maintained blood pressure (BP). With further blood loss, heart rate (HR), blood pressure, and total peripheral resistance (TPR) suddenly fell, indicating that vasodilatation occurred. Note that an increase in right atrial pressure (RAP) preceded fainting, indicating that this measure is a poor indication of blood volume status during beyond the initial minutes of blood loss. CO, cardiac output. From Barcroft *et al.*,[7] with permission.

measurements to be made; and (2) the manifest responses are easily reversed when the procedure is terminated. A description of these procedures follows.

Lower body negative pressure

In this manoeuver subjects are enclosed in a rigid container from the level of the iliac crests' caudad. A seal is formed with a flexible rubber or cloth dam to prevent loss of vacuum and the pressure inside the chamber is gradually decreased by evacuation of air. Pressures in excess of −100 mmHg relative to ambient may be achieved, although exposure to pressures of −50 to −60 mmHg produces syncope in a large proportion of subjects. Haemorrhage is mimicked not just by peripheral pooling of blood, as haemoconcentration also occurs, indicating that the relative increase in vascular transmural pressure favours fluid extravasation equivalent to approximately 10 per cent of the vascular fluid compartment.[11,12] A potential drawback to the technique is the fact that repeated exposures to LBNP improves tolerance to the procedure.[13] Whether this response represents physiological adaptation or a learning effect remains to be determined.

Head-up tilting (reverse Trendelenburg's position)

Cardiovascular strain resulting from assuming the head-up or standing position was observed early by Lewis and associates in 1932.[14] Since that time, tilting has been used often as a simple method to study cardiovascular responses to loss of CBV. A subject is placed on a bed or table which is gradually tilted to a head-up position. In the head-up position subjects either support their own weight by standing or are suspended with a saddle or harness to minimize venous return from the legs via muscle pumping of dependent veins. Since the magnitude of the gravitational vector causing venous pooling varies directly with the sine of the angle of the tilt table, venous pooling with tilting in excess of 50° differs little from 90° tilting. However, true vertical is typically avoided because of the tendency for some subjects to experience vertigo. Reductions in CBV of 300–800 ml have been reported with tilting[15,16] and, when more prolonged, a further reduction of circulating blood volume results from extravasation of fluid to interstitial spaces, causing haemoconcentration of approximately 10 per cent.[17,18]

Some renewed interest in this procedure comes from its use, coupled with the simultaneous infusion of an inotropic agent (e.g. isoproterenol), to evaluate patients with syncope.[19] However, because syncope (resulting from progression to stage II of hypovolaemia) can be induced with this procedure even with normal patients, the specificity of this procedure for syncope must be questioned. It is more likely to be useful for identifying patients prone to orthostatic intolerance and guiding patient management with interventional therapy (e.g. sympathomimetic and cardiac sympatholytic agents, support hose, volume expansion, etc.). Thus, while the procedure has a place in clinical practice, its clinical utility can been challenged.

Pressure breathing

Although pressure breathing has rarely been employed as a model to understand central hypovolaemia, the procedure is effective at displacing blood from the chest and/or reducing venous return by increasing intrathoracic pressure. Cruz *et al.*[20] calculated that this procedure would cause cardiac output to cease if an airway pressure in excess of 30 cm H_2O were maintained for extended periods. The fact that this does not occur may be explained by the pronounced hyperventilation that often accompanies voluntary pressure breathing, which increases thoracic–abdominal pumping of venous return.[20] Thus, pressures in this range may reduce cardiac output by approximately 40 per cent.[21] Some humans, such as military pilots, are able to sustain pressures in excess of 80 cm H_2O for brief periods to displace blood from the thorax to maintain cerebral perfusion and consciousness during high performance manoeuvers in fighter aircraft.[22]

Venous congestion of the legs

In supine or semirecumbent subjects approximately 1.2–1.4 litres blood are located in the legs.[23,24] Thus, trapping blood in the legs by venous congestion with loose tourniquets or pneumatic cuffs inflated to pressures less than systolic arterial pressure traps approximately 700 ml blood in the legs.[25,26] A new steady-state is achieved when venous pressure exceeds congesting pressure. In the early half of this century this procedure figured quite prominently in the treatment of patients suffering with congestive heart failure as an effective 'bloodless' method to reduce ventricular preload.[25] This procedure has been used effectively to produce central hypovolaemia in humans[25–27] or to exacerbate the effects of venesection.[26,27] It is quite simple to perform and allows one to induce venous pooling in supine subjects to an extent similar to or exceeding that which occurs with standing.

Whole body centrifugation

If the primary force that causes venous pooling is the acceleration of one's body in the earth's gravitational field then greater pooling may be induced by increasing the magnitude of the gravitational field along the body's long axis in a head-to-foot direction. By convention this is referred to as acceleration along a vector oriented in the z axis with respect to body position, or the $+G_z$ condition.[22] This field is commonly increased by placing a subject on a moving arm centrifuge with the subject's head oriented towards the axis of rotation, so that angular acceleration of the moving arm substitutes for the acceleration of gravity.[22] The force is then expressed in multiples of earth gravity. In relaxed humans, loss of vision typically occurs at approximately $+4.0\ G_z$ and syncope ensues at $+4.5\ G_z$, the point at which arterial pressure driving cerebral perfusion approaches zero.[28]

Blockade of efferent compensatory mechanisms

Three pharmacological methods for blocking efferent sympathetic activity can be used to produce hypotension that mimics haemorrhage. The first is receptor blockade, which may be produced at one of two locations; sympathetic ganglia or the neuroeffector junction with vascular smooth muscle. At present the former is rarely used to study healthy conscious volunteers, although older investigations report profound orthostatic hypotension after administration of tetra-ethylammonium.[29] Neuroeffector receptor blockade may be produced by blockade of α_1-adrenergic receptors, which prevents neurally released noradrenaline from maintaining or inducing vascular smooth muscle contraction. Both oral and intravenous administration of adrenergic antagonists are effective methods for producing hypotension.[30]

The second method by which sympathetic activity may be blocked is through the use of regional anaesthesia, such as epidural or regional nerve blockade.[31] Epidural anaesthesia with sensory blockade at the level of T_4–T_8 effectively reduces muscle sympathetic nerve activity (MSNA) to the legs, with concomitant skin vasodilatation and loss of sudomotor responsiveness in the foot,[32] while anaesthesia with sensory blockade at the level of T_{10}–T_{11} is only partially effective.[32,33] The technique produces a relative shift of blood away from the chest, with resultant increases in splanchnic and leg blood volume.[34]

Finally, sympathetic activity may be reduced by pharmacological manipulation of supraspinal mechanisms initiating sympathetic activity. Perhaps the most relevant example is treatment with the α_2-adrenergic receptor agonist clonidine HCl, which decreases peripheral constrictor responses by central sympatholytic activity. The marked hypotension resulting from clonidine treatment is not caused by stimulation of inhibitory presynaptic α-adrenergic receptors since clonidine affects neither blood pressure responses in tetraplegic patients[35] nor the relation between sympathetic activity and spillover of noradrenaline from sympathetic nerve terminals.[36]

The efficacy of these procedures for producing states analogous to hypovolaemic shock illustrates the importance of adrenergic vasoconstriction for blood pressure and volume regulation. Conversely, patients with Shy–Drager syndrome (a progressive dysautonomia with Parkinsonian-like characteristics in its more severe stages) demonstrate profound orthostatic hypotension and virtually no change in their MSNA response to changes in posture, and improved cardiovascular and MSNA responses to postural stress after treatment with L-threo,-3,4-dihydroxyphenylserine (L-threo-DOPS), a synthetic precursor of noradrenaline.[37]

Compensatory cardiovascular responses to hypovolaemia

As indicated in the Preface of this book, the induction of central hypovolaemia in humans is characterized by a normotensive vasoconstrictor phase (stage I) and a hypotensive vasodilator phase (stage II). In stage I heart rate is generally stable, though elevated, and blood pressure is well maintained by concomitant vasoconstriction. This stage is sympathoexcitatory in nature. As central hypo-

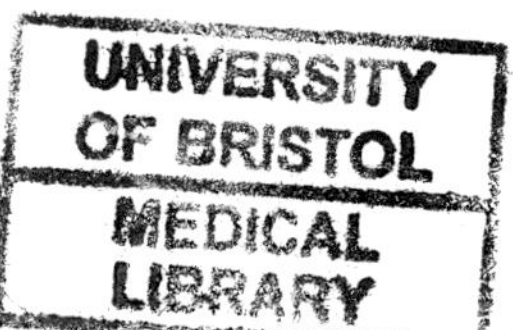

volaemia worsens, heart rate decreases and blood pressure falls as vascular resistance decreases. Thus, this stage is characterized by sympatho-inhibition. In the tertiary stage severe hypotension and tachycardia develop. The potential causes of these changes are the foci of later chapters.

Generally the cardiovascular responses to central hypovolaemia are similar among the procedures outlined. The reduction in CBV is accompanied by a reduction in cardiac filling, producing a fall in stroke volume and cardiac output. An exception to this generalization must be made with respect to central venous pressure (CVP). During positive pressure breathing, CVP, being influenced by the increase in thoracic pressure, increases while CBV falls. The decrease in CBV is revealed by the fact that plasma levels of atrial natriuretic peptide (ANP), which are directly related to atrial size, decrease during positive pressure breathing, head-up tilt and LBNP, despite the fact that CVP increases during positive pressure breathing but not the other two procedures.[38,39]

The often presumed direct relation between CVP and CBV exists only when the compliance of the central circulation, and the operating point on a given compliance curve, are constant. The point is illustrated by the fact that among individuals with higher compliance (for example, elite athletes), a reduction in left ventricular end-diastolic volume is associated with a smaller change in CVP than that among control subjects.[40] Another case is that of volume expanded patients, when the compliance curve tends to reach a volume plateau.[40] When these assumptions are violated CVP may not be an accurate index of cardiac filling volume or central volume status.

This hypothesis is confirmed by the observations that the changes in CVP and CBV (the sum of the pulmonary and cardiac blood volumes) during head-up tilt or LBNP are not proportional.[8,15] Figs 3.3 and 3.4 illustrate the point. The data in Fig. 3.3 were generated from 12 separate head-up tilt tests in which subjects had central venous catheters positioned in the superior vena cava near the right atrium, and arterial catheters advanced from the axillary artery to the aorta, which permitted the determination of CBV by dye dilution technique as the product of cardiac output and the catheter tip-to-tip transit time.[41] As the Figure illustrates, there was no relation between the quantitative change in CBV and the quantitative change in CVP.

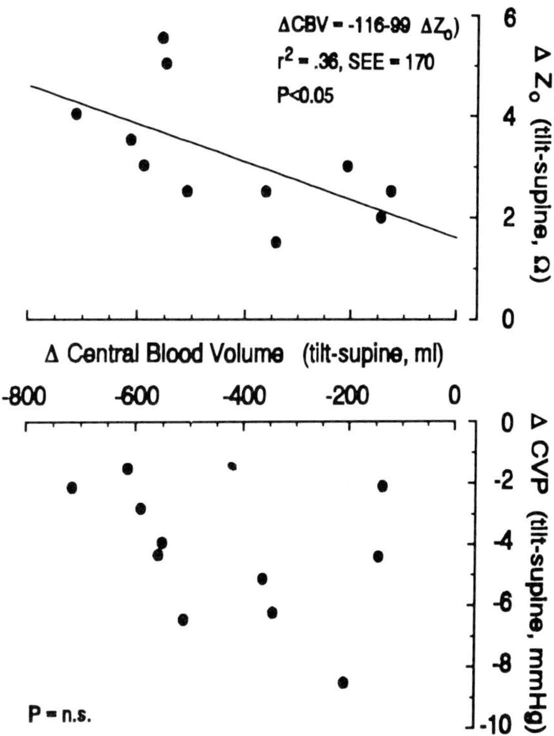

Fig. 3.3. Relation between thoracic impedance, central venous pressure (CVP) and central blood volume (CBV) during head-up tilt. CVP was measured from a catheter placed in the superior vena cava; CBV was determined using dye dilution technique. Thoracic impedance was measured using a 70 kHz excitation current passed through surface electrodes. Note that as CBV decreased thoracic impedance increased proportionally because blood (a more electrically conductive medium than tissue) was lost from the chest. No statistical relationship (n.s.) existed between changes in CBV and CVP.

Murray *et al.*[8] performed a similar experiment using LBNP as the model of haemorrhage. As illustrated in Fig. 3.4, although there appeared to be a proportionate relation between CBV and CVP with brief exposure to LBNP, during more prolonged LBNP, CVP tended to increase while CBV did not change.

This finding may have been provoked by the transition from stage I to stage II of haemorrhage, with the resultant vasodilatation occurring at the same time as venoconstriction.[42] Another possibility is that the increase in CVP reflects a reduction in the compliance of the central circulation, not necessarily a change in volume. Thus, the use of CVP to monitor long-term volume status, par-

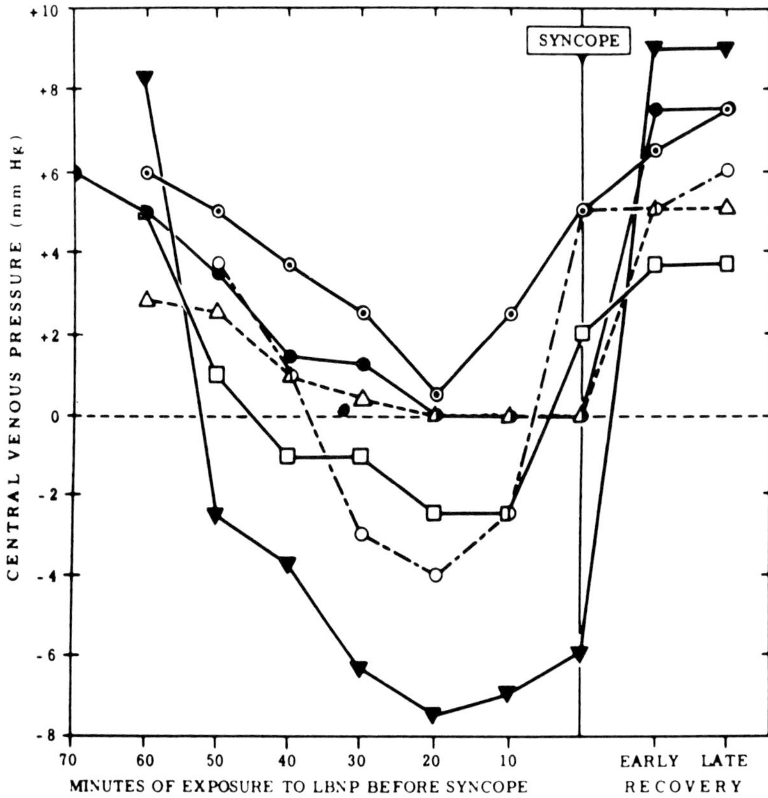

Fig. 3.4. Central venous pressure (CVP) changes prior to syncope (progression to stage II of haemorrhagic shock). Individual responses from six subjects. CVP failed to decrease immediately prior to syncope in all subjects, while it actually increased in four subjects. The conclusion may be drawn that CVP does not predict central blood volume status during this model of haemorrhagic shock. LBNP, lower body negative pressure. From Murray *et al.*,[8] with permission.

ticularly during stage II of shock, would result in erroneous conclusions.

The fact that for brief periods of time CVP and CBV appear to be related during LBNP, but not head-up tilt, deserves discussion. This difference may be resolved by the fact that during either of these stresses the heart moves caudally approximately 1–4 cm, depending on the individual subject. During LBNP this is of little concern with respect to pressure measurement as the hydrostatic gradient lies perpendicular to the direction in which the heart moves. However, during head-up tilt these vectors are aligned; thus, the point to which a fluid-filled catheter is referenced (typically the right atrium or the tricuspid valve) moves as well. Coupled with the fact that the theoretical 'hydrostatic indifferent point' (a location at which there is no hydrostatic influence on the measured pressure) may change with neurohumoral activation, unpredictable pressure changes result. This concept is reinforced by the observation that CVP *decreased* in one subject upon whom the measurement was performed during spaceflight, despite the apparent *increase* in CBV resulting from exposure to microgravity.[43]

The conclusion may be reached that CVP is a relative indicator of volume status only when: (1) the perturbation is brief; (2) the pressure measurement is unaffected by the perturbation; and (3) compliance of the cardiac and pulmonary circulations is fixed and unvaried. These limitations to pressure measurement preclude the use of CVP as an accurate measure of central volume status in any monitoring situation exceeding a few minutes.

Compensatory hormonal responses to hypovolaemia

Coincident to the cardiovascular responses outlined above, hormonal adjustments occur rapidly during hypovolaemia. Generally these responses are complimentary, and in both stages numerous reflex and humoral actions occur that affect blood pressure, intravascular volume, vascular resistance and cardiac pumping. The hormonal responses to hypovolaemia have been considered less frequently, and for this reason will be outlined in detail. Our summary of these effects is provided in Table 3.1.

Sympathoexcitatory phase

Stage I of blood loss may be referred to as sympathoexcitatory, as evidenced predominately by increases in plasma noradrenaline. Coupled with an increase in systemic vascular resistance and mild tachycardia, blood pressure is usually well preserved, and may increase, as is often observed during head-up tilt. The hormonal responses during this stage are summarized as follows.

Sympathetic and parasympathetic activity

During this stage there is an overall increase in vasoconstrictor activity (indicated by an increase in plasma noradrenaline), which plays an important role for the maintenance of mean arterial pressure. Failure to increase noradrenaline during this phase results in rapid development of orthostatic hypotension.[37] Generally, there is moderate or no change in plasma adrenaline secreted from the adrenal medulla. Pancreatic polypeptide is secreted from endocrine cells in the pancreas and is an indicator of overall vagal efferent activity to the gut.[44] It remains unchanged during this stage of hypovolaemia.[9,45]

Renin–angiotensin system

There is a consistent rise in plasma renin activity (PRA), either a result of factors affecting the juxtaglomerular apparatus directly or by the action of systemically circulating catecholamines. The contribution of this change to the haemodynamic compensation to acute blood loss seems limited. During head-up tilt blockade of 5-hydroxytriptamine (5-HT_1) receptors with methylsergide abolishes the rise in PRA without affecting the progression to stage II central hypovolaemia.[46] However, because

Table 3.1 Cardiovascular and hormonal changes during progressive hypovolaemic shock. Findings are related to the stage of shock as presented in the text. Hormones are grouped according to their primary locus of origin during shock. Vasoconstriction predominates during the earliest stages of shock while in the later stages hormonal regulation is directed toward preservation of organ perfusion at the expense of blood pressure regulation. In the tertiary stages of shock local control probably dominates the observed responses.

Variable	Stage of shock		
	I	II	III
Cardiovascular:			
CVP	– ↓	– ↓	– ↓
CBV	↓	↓	↓
Heart rate	– ↑	↓ ↓	↑
Blood pressure	–	↓ ↓	↓ ↓
Cardiac output	↓	↓ ↓	↓ ↓
Muscle vascular resistance	↑	↓ ↓	?
Splanchnic vascular resistance	↑	?	?
Hormonal:			
Sympathetic nerve terminals			
Noradrenaline	↑	– ↓	↑ ↑ ↑
Renal/adrenal			
Renin	– ↑	↑	?
Angiotensin II	–	↑	?
Aldosterone	↑	↑ ↑	↑ ↑
Cortisol	–	↑	?
Pituitary axis			
Pancreatic polypeptide	–	↑	↑
β-endorphin	–	↑	?
Vasopressin	–	↑	–
Endothelin-1	↑	↑ ↑	?
CGRP	–	↑	?
VIP	–	–	–
ACTH	–	↑	?
Heart			
ANP	↓	↓ ↓	?
Local			
NO	?	?	↑ ↑ (?)

CVP, central venous pressure; CBV, central blood volume; CGRP, calcitonin gene-related peptide; VIP, vasoactive intestinal peptide; ACTH. adrenocorticotropic hormone; ANP, atrial natriuretic peptide; NO, nitric oxide (endothelially-derived relaxing factor).

methylsergide also exerts some direct vasoconstrictor action a possible effect of reduced PRA may have been masked.

Vasopressin

During stage I of hypovolaemia plasma vasopressin does not rise. The response of this hormone seems to be relatively insensitive to changes in CBV, increasing only when loss of blood becomes severe.

Pituitary–adrenal axis

During initial central hypovolaemia there is a slight

increase in plasma β-endorphin, adrenocorticotrophic hormone (ACTH) and cortisol. These changes can be inhibited by treatment with diazepam without affecting the tolerance to hypovolaemia.[46]

Calcitonin gene-related and atrial natriuretic peptides

Calcitonin gene-related peptide (CGRP) also shows a gradual increase during hypovolaemia.[47,48] The importance of an increase in this vasodilator peptide during haemorrhage is unknown. ANP is a moderate vasodilator and diuretic regulated by atrial stretch that decreases during simulated haemorrhage, helping to maintain intravascular volume by sodium retention.[49] Accordingly, plasma ANP decreases during simulated haemorrhage (head-up tilt), indicating the magnitude of change of CBV.[50]

Endothelial factors

There is a gradual increase in the endothelium derived vasoconstricting peptide endothelin-1 during hypovolaemia.[51–53] This effect likely contributes to a reduction in venous capacitance, as this peptide demonstrates greater efficacy for veins than arteries.[54] As this response is not observed in subjects with paraventricular hypothalamic lesions associated with diabetes insipidus, it is likely that the rise of endothelin-1 normally observed is of central origin.[54] The fact that the rise in plasma vasopressin parallels the rise in endothelin-1 tends to support this hypothesis. As the net effect of this phase is vasoconstriction, nitric oxide (NO), the putative endothelially derived relaxing factor (EDRF) probably exerts only a small modulatory role, although reductions in constitutive production of this vasomodulator to produce relative constriction cannot be ruled out.

Sympathoinhibitory phase

With the continuous reduction of CBV associated with the progression to stage II of shock, 'paradoxical' bradycardia and vasodilation ensue. This response has been demonstrated to be associated with the activation of unmyelinated left ventricular afferents in experimental animals, leading to the suggestion that it results from an 'empty heart' reflex.[55] The term is somewhat of a misnomer; left ventricular volume decreases only 10–20 per cent, which may be sufficient to cause isometric contraction of the left ventricle during systole.[56] The endocrine responses appear to be closely related to the cardiovascular responses in this phase.

Sympathetic and parasympathetic activity

The decrease in vascular resistance is associated with a decrease in sympathetic vasoconstrictor activity to skeletal muscle, as evidenced by the findings that: (1) microneurographic recordings from the peroneal nerve are virtually absent of activity,[57,58]; and (2) plasma noradrenaline decreases or remains unchanged.[9,16,27,45] This sympathetic withdrawal may be the primary determinant of peripheral vasodilation as treatment with the synthetic precursor of noradrenaline, L-threo-DOPS, ameliorates the effect.[37] Central opiate receptors are implicated in this response also, as their blockade with naloxone improves blood pressure in exsanguinated rabbits.[59] With humans, however, naloxone fails to increase, and may decrease, tolerance to hypovolaemia induced by head-up tilt (Klokker, personal communication, 1993). Pancreatic polypeptide increases during the sympathoinhibitory phase of shock,[9,45,60] consistent with the observation that the bradycardia can be eliminated with atropine, indicating increased parasympathetic activity.[9] Elimination of the bradycardia, however, does not improve blood pressure, emphasizing that the vasodepressor component is neither vagally mediated nor a result of bradycardia.[8,9,14,26]

Renin–angiotensin system

A further moderate increase in PRA occurs at the onset of hypotension, which helps to maintain blood pressure in experimental animals. Using rabbits, Schadt and Gaddis[61] demonstrated that ACE inhibition delayed the recovery from hypotensive blood loss, and augmented the reduction in blood pressure.

Vasopressin

The development of hypotension is followed by a large increase in plasma concentrations of the systemic pressor agent vasopressin.[9,45] Cardiopulmonary or vagal afferent mechanisms have been shown to be an important part of this reflex arc, as cardiac denervation abolishes the vasopressin increase to hypotension in dogs.[62]

Pituitary–adrenal axis

Profound activation of this system occurs at the onset of hypotension. Animal investigations have shown that afferent vagal activity is crucial for the ACTH response to hypotensive haemmorhage.[63] This effect is accompanied by stimulation of other anterior pituitary hormones, including vasopressin and endothelin-1. Secretion of ACTH and β-endorphin to circulating plasma results in an increase of plasma cortisol approximately 5–10 min later.[46,53,60,64]

Calcitonin gene-related and atrial natriuretic peptides
CGRP increases further during this stage of haemorrhage, and plasma levels of ANP reach their nadir value at this time. These observations support the concept that atrial stretch regulates the secretion of this peptide; however, a physiological role for either hormone during hypovolaemia has not yet been discerned.

Endothelial factors
With more severe hypovolaemia plasma levels of endothelin-1 continue to rise. In patients with recurrent vasovagal syncope the effect is particularly pronounced, while it is virtually non-existent in subjects with primary autonomic failure.[52] Thus, it would seem that this hormone is mediated by arterial baroreflexes acting on hypothalamic sites responsible for systemic release, rather than local production, of the hormone. At present the role of NO in causing, or contributing, to this stage of shock has not been determined.

Stage III

In stage III of shock heart rate tends to rise while blood pressure remains extremely low. As this stage terminates in death, cardiovascular reflex regulation cannot be studied during this stage using human subjects. However, limited patient data are available.[10] Recent evidence supports the view that local factors, particularly those of endothelial origin, are important regulators of vascular smooth muscle tone that are responsible for maintaining or exacerbating peripheral vasodilatation. In patients with septic shock, who are unresponsive to infusion of adrenergic agonists, treatment with NO synthase inhibitors N^G-monomethyl-L-arginine (L-NMMA) or N^G-nitro-L-arginine-methylester (L-NAME) improves cardiac output, blood pressure, heart rate and systemic vascular resistance.[65] Similar data from exsanguinated animals suggests that NO may improve blood pressure and survivability from stage III haemorrhagic shock.[66,67] These data await corroboration from human investigations.

Summary

Central hypovolaemia in humans is characterized by three stages, each presenting a unique integrated cardiovascular and endocrine response to the stress. Two stages are easily discriminated in experimental settings: a sympathoexcitatory stage, dominated by the combined effects of neurally and hormonally controlled vasoconstriction, and a sympathoinhibitory stage, dominated by withdrawal of sympathetic activation and increased parasympathetic activity. These stages are readily mimicked in experimental settings using a variety of perturbations, although the haemodynamic descriptors of these stages are not always accurate. It remains the authors' contention that CVP is a poor estimate of the status of CBV, and that this practice could lead to erroneous conclusions in clinical settings. As stage III of hypovolaemic shock is generally observed only in severely ill patients, little information is available to describe this stage. Generally, this stage is characterized by profound vasodilatation, tachycardia and disseminated intravascular coagulation. Current evidence suggests that NO may play an important role mediating these local effects, though the exact role of this paracrine hormone in human hypovolaemic shock remains to be determined.

Acknowledgements

The authors appreciate the helpful suggestions and critique of Benjamin D. Levine, MD, and Jere H. Mitchell, MD.

This work was supported in part by the Presbyterian Health Care System, the Lawson and Rogers Lacy Fund for Cardiovascular Diseases, Simonsen and Weel Corporation, and Lœrdal's Foundation for Acute Medicine.

References

1. Secher NH and Bie P: Bradycardia during reversible haemorrhagic shock – a forgotten observation? *Clinical Physiology*, 1985; **5**, 315–23.
2. Secher NH, Jacobsen J, Friedman DB and Matzen

S: Bradycardia during reversible hypovolaemic shock: associated neural reflex mechanisms and clinical implications. *Clinical and Experimental Pharmacology and Physiology*, 1992; **19,** 733–43.
3. Ebert RV, Stead EA Jr and Gibson JG: Response of subjects to acute blood loss. *Archives of Internal Medicine*, 1941; **68,** 578–90.
4. Poles FC and Boycott M: Syncope in blood donors. *Lancet*, 1942; **2,** 531–5.
5. Barcroft H and Edholm OG: On the vasodilatation in human skeletal muscle during post-haemorrhagic fainting. *Journal of Physiology (London)*, 1945; **104,** 161–75.
6. Wallace J and Sharpey-Schafer EP: Blood changes following controlled haemorrhage in man. *Lancet*, 1941; **2,** 393–5.
7. Barcroft H, Edholm OG, McMichael J and Sharpey-Schafer EP: Posthaemorrhagic fainting. Study by cardiac output and forearm flow. *Lancet*, 1944, **i,** 489–91.
8. Murray RH, Thompson LJ, Bowers JA and Albright CD: Hemodynamic effects of graded hypovolemia and vasodepressor syncope induced by lower body negative pressure. *American Heart Journal*, 1968; **76,** 799–811.
9. Sander-Jensen K, Mehlsen J, Stadeager C, Christensen NJ, Fahrenkurg J, Schwartz TW, Warberg J and Bie P: Increase in vagal activity during hypotensive lower-body negative pressure in humans. *American Journal of Physiology*, 1988; **255,** R149–56.
10. Jacobsen J and Secher NH: Heart rate slowing during haemorrhagic shock. *Clinical Physiology*, 1992; **12,** 659–66.
11. Hinghofer-Szalkay H, Konig EM, Sauseng-Fellegger G and Zambo-Polz C: Biphasic blood volume changes with lower body suction in humans. *American Journal of Physiology*, 1992; **263,** H1270–75.
12. Loeppky JA, Kobayashi Y, Venters MD and Luft UC: Effects of regional hemoconcentration during LBNP on plasma volume determinations. *Aviation, Space, and Environmental Medicine*, 1979; **50,** 763–7.
13. Lightfoot JT, Febles S and Fortney S: Adaptation to repeated lower body negative pressure exposures. *Aviation, Space, and Environmental Medicine*, 1989; **60,** 17–22.
14. Lewis T: Vasovagal syncope and the carotid sinus mechanism. *British Medical Journal*, 1932; **1,** 873–6.
15. Pawelczyk JA, Pawekczyk RA, Matzen S and Secher NH: Thoracic impedance, not central venous pressure, predicts changes in central blood volume during orthostatism. *Federation of American Societies of Experimental Biology Journal*, 1992; **6,** A1771 (abstract).
16. Matzen S, Perko G, Groth S, Friedman DB and Secher NH: Blood volume distribution during head-up tilt induced central hypovolaemia in man. *Clinical Physiology*, 1991; **11,** 411–12.
17. Hagan RD, Diaz FJ and Horvath SM: Plasma volume changes with movement to supine and standing positions. *Journal of Applied Physiology: Respiratory, Environment, and Exercise Physiology*, 1978; **45,** 414–17.
18. Tombridge TL: Effect of posture on hematology results. *American Journal of Clinical Pathology*, 1968; **49,** 491–3.
19. Almquist A, Goldenberg IF, Milstein S, Chen MY, Chen XC, Hansen R, Gornick CC and Benditt DG: Provocation of bradycardia and hypotension by isoproterenol and upright posture in patients with unexplained syncope. *New England Journal of Medicine*, 1989; **320,** 346–51.
20. Cruz JC, Cerretelli P and Farhi LE: Role of ventilation in maintaining cardiac output under positive-pressure breathing. *Journal of Applied Physiology*, 1967; **22,** 900–904.
21. Pawelczyk JA: *The Cardiac Output Response to Continuous Positive Presure Breathing at Rest and During Exercise.* Master's Thesis. The Pennsylvania State University, Philadelphia, PA, 1986.
22. Blomqvist CG and Stone HL: Cardiovascular adjustments to gravitational stress. In Shepherd JT and Abboud FM (eds): *Handbook of Physiology. Section 2: The Cardiovascular System, Volume 3.* Bethesda, MD, American Physiological Society, 1983, 1025–63.
23. Asmussen E: The distribution of the blood between the lower extremities and the rest of the body. *Acta Physiologica Scandinavica*, 1943; **5,** 31–8.
24. Pawelczyk JA, Hanel B, Pawelczyk RA, Warberg J and Secher NH: Leg vasoconstriction during dynamic exercise with reduced cardiac output. *Journal of Applied Physiology*, 1992; **73,** 1838–46.
25. Ebert RV and Stead EA: The effect of the application of tourniquets on the hemodynamics of the circulation. *Journal of Clinical Investigation*, 1940; **68,** 561–7.
26. McMichael J and Sharpey-Schafer EP: Cardiac output in man by a direct Fick method: effect of posture, venous pressure change, atropine, and adrenaline. *British Heart Journal*, 1944; **7,** 33–40
27. Sander-Jensen K, Mehlsen J, Secher NH, Bach FW, Bie P, Giese J, Schwartz TW, Trap-Jensen J and Warberg J: Progressive central hypovolaemia in man – resulting in vasovagal syncope? Haemodynamic and endocrine variables during venous tourniquets of the thighs. *Clinical Physiology*, 1987; **7,** 231–42.
28. Howard P: The physiology of positive acceleration. In Gillis JA (ed.): *A Textbook of Aviation Physiology.* London, Pergamon, 1965, 603–12.
29. Brown GE Jr, Wood EH and Lambert EH: Effects of tetra-ethyl-ammonium chloride on cardiovascular reactions in man to changes in posture and exposure to centrifugal force. *Journal of Applied Physiology*, 1949; **2,** 117–32.

30. Mulvihill-Wilson J, Gaffney FA, Pettinger WA, Blomqvist CG, Anderson S and Graham RM: Hemodynamic and neuroendocrine responses to acute and chronic alpha-receptor blockade with prazosin and phenoxybenzamine. *Circulation*, 1983; **67,** 383–92.
31. Brigden W, Howarth S and Sharpey-Schafer EP: Postural changes in the peripheral blood-flow of normal subjects with observations on vasovagal fainting reactions as a result of tilting, the lordotic posture, pregnancy and spinal anaesthesia. *Clinical Science*, 1950; **9,** 79–90.
32. Lundin S, Kirno K, Wallin BG and Elam M: Effects of epidural anesthesia on sympathetic nerve discharge to the skin. *Acta Anaesthiologica Scandinavica*, 1990; **34,** 492–7.
33. Rordam P, Jensen LP, Schroeder T, Loentzen E and Secher NH: Intraarterial papaverine and leg muscular vascular resistance during *in situ* bypass surgery with high or low epidural anaesthesia. *Acta Anaesthethiologica Scandinavica*, 1993; **37,** 97–101.
34. Arndt JO, Hock A, Stanton-Hicks M and Stühmeier K-D: Peridural anesthesia and distribution of blood in supine humans. *Anesthesiology*, 1985; **63,** 616–23.
35. Kooner JS, Birch R, Frankel HL, Peart WS and Mathias CJ: Hemodynamic and neurohormonal effects of clonidine in patients with preganglionic and postganglionic sympathetic lesions. Evidence for a central sympatholytic action. *Circulation*, 1991; **84,** 75–83.
36. Garty M, Deka-Starosta A, Chang P, Kopin IJ and Goldstein DS: Effects of clonidine on renal sympathetic nerve activity and norepinephrine spillover. *Journal of Pharmacological and Experimental Therapeutics*, 1990; **254,** 1068–75.
37. Kachi T, Iwase S, Mano T, Saito M, Kunimoto M and Sobue I: Effect of L-threo-3,4-dihydroxyphenylserine on muscle sympathetic nerve activities in Shy–Drager syndrome. *Neurology*, 1988; **38,** 1091–4.
38. Schütten HJ, Johannessen AC, Torp-Pedersen C, Sander-Jensen K, Bie P and Warberg J: Central venous pressure – a physiologic stimulus for secretion of atrial natriuretic peptide in humans? *Acta Physiologica Scandinavica*, 1987; **131,** 265–72.
39. Schütten HJ, Kamp-Jensen M, Nielsen SL, Sztuk FJ, Engquist A, Warberg J and Bie P: Inverse relation between central venous pressure and the plasma concentration of atrial natriuretic peptide during positive-pressure breathing. *Acta Physiologica Scandinavica*, 1990; **139,** 389–90.
40. Levine BD, Land LD, Buckey JC, Friedman DB and Blomqvist CG: Ventricular pressure–volume and Frank–Starling relations in endurance athletes: implications for orthostatic tolerance and exercise performance. *Circulation*, 1991; **83,** 1016–23.
41. Dow P: Estimations of cardiac output and central blood volume by dye dilution. *Physiological Reviews*, 1956; **36,** 77–102.
42. Epstein SE, Stampfer M and Beisser GD: Role of the capacitance and resistance vessels in vasovagal syncope. *Circulation* 1968; **37,** 524–33.
43. Buckey JC, Lane LD, Gaffney FA, Watenpaugh DE, Levine BD, Wright SJ and Blomqvist CG: Cardiovascular adaptation to space – SLS-1 results. *American Society for Gravitational and Space Biology Bulletin*, 1992; **6,** 100 (abstract).
44. Schwartz TW: Pancreatic polypeptide: a hormone under vagal control. *Gastroenterology*, 1983; **85,** 1411–25.
45. Sander-Jensen K, Secher NH, Astrup A, Christensen NJ, Giese J, Schwartz TW, Warberg J and Bie P: Hypotension induced by passive head-up tilt: endocrine and circulatory mechanisms. *American Journal of Physiology*, 1986; **25,** R742–8.
46. Matzen S, Secher NH, Knigge U, Bach FW and Warberg J: Effect of diazepam on endocrine and cardiovascular responses to head-up tilt in humans. *Acta Physiologica Scandinavica*, 1993; **148**, 143–51.
47. Matzen S, Schifter S, Radwansky J, Knigge U, Warberg J and Secher NH: Calcitonin gene-related peptide (CGRP) and leg vascular resistance during head-up tilt induced hypovolaemic shock in man. *Acta Physiologica Scandinavica*, 1991; **142,** 313–18.
48. Yndgaard S, Schifter S, Perko G, Matzen S and Secher NH: Calcitonin gene-related peptide (CGRP) during head-up tilt in man. *Acta Physiologica Scandinavica*, 1991; **143,** 129–30.
49. Edwards BS, Zimmerman RS, Schwab TR, Heublein DM and Burnett JC Jr: Atrial stretch, not pressure, is the principal determinant controlling the acute release of atrial natriuretic factor. *Circulation Research*, 1988; **62,** 191–5.
50. Matzen S, Knigge U, Schutten HJ, Warberg J and Secher NH: Atrial natriuretic peptide during head-up tilt induced hypovolemic shock in man. *Acta Physiological Scandinavica*, 1990; **140,** 161–6.
51. Shichiri M, Hirata Y and Ando K: Postural change and volume expansion affect plasma endothelin levels. *Journal of the American Medical Association*, 1990; **263,** 661 (letter).
52. Kaufmann H, Oribe E and Oliver JA: Plasma endothelin during upright tilt: relevance for orthostatic hypotension? *Lancet*, 1991; **338,** 1542–5.
53. Matzen S, Emmeluth C, Milliken M and Secher NH: Plasma endothelin-1 during central hypovolemia in man. *Clinical Physiology*, 1992; **12,** 653–8.
54. Cockcroft JR, Clarke JG and Webb DJ: The effect of intra-arterial endothelin on resting blood flow and sympathetically mediated vasoconstriction in the forearm of man. *British Journal of Clinical Pharmacology*, 1991; **31,** 521–4.
55. Öberg B and Thorén P: Increased activity in left ventricular receptors during hemorrhage or occlu-

sion of caval veins in the cat. A possible cause of vasovagal reaction. *Acta Physiologica Scandinavica*, 1972; **85,** 164–73.
56. Jacobsen J, Søfelt S, Fernandes A, Brocks V, Warberg J and Secher NH: Reduced left ventricular size at the onset of bradycardia during epidural anesthesia. *Acta Anaesthesiologica Scandinavica* 1992; **36,** 831–6.
57. Wallin BG and Sundlöf G: Sympathetic outflow to muscles during vasovagal syncope. *Journal of the Autonomic Nervous System*, 1982; **6,** 287–91.
58. Sanders JS and Ferguson DW: Profound sympathoinhibition complicating hypovolemia in humans. *Annals of Internal Medicine*, 1989; **111,** 439–41.
59. Schadt JC and Ludbrook JM: Hemodynamic and neurohumoral responses to acute hypovolemia in conscious mammals. *American Journal of Physiology*, 1991; **260,** H305–18.
60. Matzen S, Secher NH, Pawelczyk JA, Perko G, Iversen H, Knigge U, Bach FW and Warberg J: Effect of serotonin receptor blockade on endocrine and cardiovascular responses to head-up tilt in humans. *Acta Physiologica Scandinavica*; in press.
61. Schadt JC and Gaddis RR: Renin–angiotensin system and opioids during acute hemorrhage in conscious rabbits. *American Journal of Physiology*, 1990; **258,** R543–51.
62. Wang BC, Flora-Ginter G, Leadley RJ and Goetz KL: Ventricular receptors stimulate vasopressin release during hemorrhage. *American Journal of Physiology*, 1988; **254,** R204–11.
63. Darlington DN, Shinsako J and Dallman MF: Medullary lesions eliminate ACTH responses to hypotensive hemorrhage. *American Journal of Physiology*, 1986; **251,** R106–15.
64. Matzen S, Secher NH, Knigge U, Bach FW and Warberg J: Pituitary–adrenal responses to head-up tilt in humans: effect of H_1- and H_2-receptor blockade. *American Journal of Physiology*, 1992; **263,** R156–63.
65. Petros A, Bennett D and Vallance P: Effect of nitric oxide synthase inhibitors on hypotension in patients with septic shock. *Lancet*, 1991; **338,** 1557–8.
66. Lieberthal W, McGarry AE, Shiels J and Valeri CR: Nitric oxide inhibition in rats improves blood pressure and renal function during hypovolemic shock. *American Journal of Physiology*, 1991; **261,** F868–72.
67. Zingarelli B, Squandrito F, Altavilla D, Calapai G, Calo GM, Saitta A and Caputi AP: Evidence for a role of nitric oxide in hypovolemic hemorrhagic shock. *Journal of Cardiovascular Pharmacology*, 1992; **19,** 982–6.

Part 2
Cardiovascular physiology

4

Autoregulation of blood flow

Niels A Lassen

Autoregulation denotes the tendency for blood flow to remain constant despite variations in perfusion pressure. When arterial blood pressure increases the wall of arteries and arterioles is exposed to increased stretch. The autoregulatory response consists of active contraction of the vessels' smooth muscle cells, an increase in vascular tone overpowering the stretching force and narrowing the lumen. Autoregulation can best be observed when other factors, in particular metabolic and neurogenic factors, remain constant. It is present in isolated organs and must therefore be caused by local factors, whence its name; *auto*regulation meaning *self*-regulation. It has been demonstrated in most tissues but is notably absent in the pulmonary circulation and in the portal circulation of the liver, i.e. regions in which the resistance vessels are not subjected to the relatively strong distending force characteristic of the systemic circulation. This chapter will first discuss briefly the mechanism of autoregulation and then focus on aspects of pathophysiological and clinical relevance.

The mechanism of autoregulation: the myogenic theory

Bayliss published in 1902 his classic paper in which the principle of autoregulation was first put forward.[1] He hypothesized that the reaction was *myogenic*, i.e. caused by a contractile response of the smooth muscle cells in response to the increased stretch resulting from a rise in transmural pressure. The myogenic theory found support in the observations of Fog in the 1930s[2,3] on the diameter of pial arteries measured in anaesthetized cats through a window inserted in the cranium. These studies showed that a sudden rise in blood pressure was followed by a brief pressure-passive dilatation lasting a few seconds followed over the next 20 to 40 seconds by a constriction to a smaller diameter than before the rise in pressure. Meticulous denervation procedures showed that this response was not dependent on the vasomotor nerves.

The myogenic theory has been the subject of many other experimental studies. Johnson and Intaglietta[4] studied the diameter of small arterioles in the mesentery of cats under the condition of zero perfusion pressure obtained by local arterial and venous pressure adjusted to the same level (Fig. 4.1). In this situation a simultaneous rise in both pressures caused a reduction in arteriolar diameter. As the metabolic factor (tissue oxygen demand) was constant as were also neurogenic factors from the central nervous system the autoregulatory response was, by exclusion, considered to be myogenic. The experimental design of Johnson and Intaglietta did not, however, exclude axon reflexes in the local sympathetic nerve to the vessels in the mesentery. This possibility was ruled out in the basically similar studies performed by Meininger and colleagues,[5] in which α-receptor blockade was shown not to inhibit the response.

Convincing support for the myogenic theory has been obtained by measurement of pressure-induced variations of the diameter of isolated arterioles. Kuo *et al.*[6] studied small segments of coronary arterioles cannulated in both ends by glass micropipettes. Arteriolar dilatation and constriction were observed when respectively lowering and increasing the static transmural pressure. The response was found to be independent of the endothelial cell layer, as its mechanical abrasion did not influence the response. Halpern *et al.*[7,8]

obtained similar results in isolated segments of cerebral arterioles, and they could rule out effects of perivascular nerves in the adventitia as they found the autoregulatory response to be preserved when the nerve toxin tetrodotoxin or the α-receptor blocker phentolamine was added to the organ bath.

It can be concluded from the above summarized studies, as well as from the many other studies reviewed by Johnson,[9] that a myogenic mechanism must indeed be involved in the autoregulatory response. Many vessels, in particular venules and lymphatic vessels, show spontaneous oscillations of diameter with a frequency typically of about 6 to 10 per min. This so-called vasomotion is not due to variations in sympathetic tone and it appears to be a purely myogenic response. But it is not a prerequisite for autoregulation, as in most arteriolar networks showing autoregulation vasomotion cannot be detected.[9]

The chemical feedback theory

Even though the contribution of a myogenic mechanism is firmly established, this does not preclude that other factors could simultaneously play a role. In tissues with a high level of oxygen consumption, such as the brain or the myocardium, blood flow subserves, first of all, an adequate supply of oxygen. In both tissues autoregulation is characterized by an amazing constancy of flow, i.e. of oxygen supply. Therefore it is tempting to speculate that the regulation of blood flow by metabolism, a regulation presumed to involve chemical mediators from the tissue affecting the contractile state of the resistance vessels, could contribute to the autoregulatory response.

In this context the study of Meininger *et al.*[5] referred to above is of special relevance. These authors studied the cremaster muscle of rats enclosed in an airtight box with the muscle sticking outside the box and hence being exposed to ambient atmospheric pressure throughout the study. In this situation an increase in box pressure of 10 to 30 mmHg resulted in the same increase in the distending pressure throughout the muscle's circulation. The observed response was a sustained arteriolar constriction and a decrease in flow and in tissue oxygen tension. In this situation, therefore, the myogenic response was independent of and capable of overriding the independent metabolic regulation. In the usual situation, however, when autoregulation is revealed by varying the perfusion pressure, the myogenic and metabolic regu-

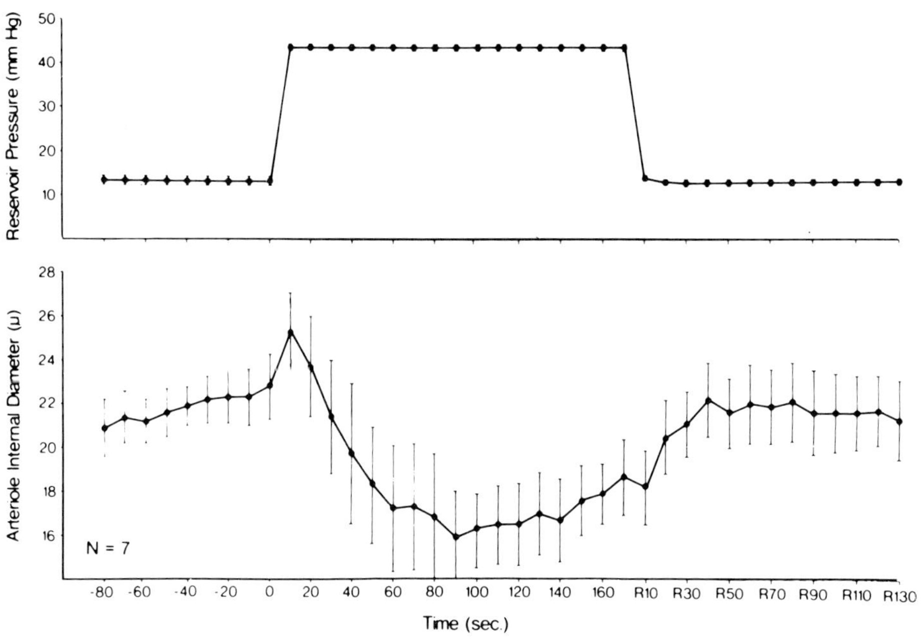

Fig. 4.1. Diameter changes (lower curve) of cat mesentery arteriole diameter when stepwise inducing an increase in distending pressure (upper curve). From Johnson and Intaglietta,[4] with permission; same result as observed by Fog.[2,3]

lation might cooperate in keeping flow constant.

In the kidney the principal role of circulation is not to sustain energy metabolism, but to allow ultrafiltration to proceed as a essential step in the water and electrolyte balance as well as in the elimination of waste products. A chemical feedback from the tubular fluid has recently been shown to be involved in the mechanism of renal autoregulation of flow and glomerular filtration. The renal circulation afforded the first example of autoregulation of organ blood flow in the literature, as already in 1911 Burton-Opitz and Lucas[10] had reported constant flow despite changes in arterial blood pressure. The detailed studies of Selkurt and colleagues from 1946 to 1965 documented the response in detail.[11–13] They stressed that the glomerular filtration rate (GFR) also tended to be constant and they coined the term 'autoregulation' to describe the responses. Renal autoregulation can thus in a way be considered as the prototype of this regulation. Therefore it is particularly interesting that it is in the kidney that current evidence points to a dual mechanism; a chemical feedback and a myogenic response.

Explained by the myogenic mechanism autoregulation means that renal blood flow is the controlled factor; this in its turn determines pressure and flow in the glomeruli and hence GFR. Recent publications strongly suggest, however, that this explanation is inadequate in that the main mechanism of renal autoregulation is the tubuloglomerular feedback mechanism.

The structural basis for this mechanism is the juxtaglomerular apparatus situated where the distal part of the renal tubule makes contact with the vascular pole of the glomerulus from whence it arose. Specifically it is the afferent arteriole, the main determinant in controlling the vascular glomerular pressure, that the distal tubule comes close to. Here its epithelium is changed into a condensed structure, the *macula densa*. The chemical feedback signal is the chloride concentration in the distal tubular fluid. An increase in this concentration is sensed by the macula densa and elicits via unknown (probably chemical) mechanisms afferent arteriolar constriction. This reduces pressure and hence filtration in the glomerulus. As the sodium chloride reabsorption in the proximal part of the tubule continues the concentration drops distal of the site of the macula densa. Now the constrictor signal is attenuated and the afferent arteriole relaxes so that pressure and filtration again increase.

This tubuloglomerular feedback mechanism has been explored by renal physiologists for many years. But the studies of Holstein-Rathlou and Leyssac and their colleagues illustrate the mechanism particularly well.[14–17] They found that this feedback loop tends to be underdampened as it oscillated spontaneously, so that the filtration of a single nephron and also its tubular pressure varies periodically (with about 2 oscillations per min). Since different nephrons do not oscillate in synchrony, total renal blood flow and total GFR are both remarkably constant. The tubuloglomerular feedback implies that GFR, not renal blood flow, is the primary controlled parameter. This concept is indeed more physiologically meaningful than a purely myogenic theory in which no direct control of the essential product (filtration) could be envisaged.

The tubuloglomerular feedback mechanism must be assumed to cooperate with myogenic reactions in causing renal autoregulation. The thesis was discussed here at some length to support in a general sense the idea that, in tissues where the main purpose of circulation is to supply metabolic energy, perhaps a chemical signal related to energy metabolism is involved in autoregulation of flow along with the myogenic mechanism which is in itself 'blind' to the need of the tissue for want of a feedback signal.

Tissue pressure

Tissue pressure influences autoregulation, as this pressure must be subtracted from the arterial pressure in order to estimate the local perfusion pressure. This can be explained by analysing tissue circulation in skin areas exposed to external pressure, the crucial factor in the development of bed sores. If circulation is to continue despite the compression then local venous pressure must increase to a level slightly above local tissue pressure. This shows that with external compression the driving pressure is approximately the pressure difference between local arterial pressure and local tissue pressure. We can also express the effect of tissue pressure by stating that the local transmural pressure difference defines local arterial pressure. In the face of increased tissue pressure it is no longer meaningful to take ambient atmospheric pressure as the pressure of reference. In the following some examples of the role of tissue pressure effects will be presented to illustrate its importance in certain pathophysiological states.

Brain circulation in states with increased intracranial pressure

If artificial cerebrospinal fluid is infused subdurally to raise intracranial pressure, then blood flow is initially maintained at control levels. First, when relatively high pressures of about 600 mmH_2O are reached, flow will start to decrease. Pressures have to reach about 1000 mmH_2O to cause a reduction in flow by about 50 per cent, the level where clear cut symptoms of brain hypoxia develop. Plotting flow as a function of arterial pressure minus intracranial pressure shows the familiar autoregulation curve.

An intracranial space occupying lesion is the primary cause of increased intracranial pressure in most cases. This lesion, be it an oedema, a tumour or a haematoma, will distort the brain and set up *pressure gradients* within the cranial cavity. The result is distortion and local compression of brain tissue, first of all against the rim of the tentorium where typically the temporal lobe's deeper part and the brainstem can become encarcerated. As the brain is not a fluid, but semisolid, local pressures can exceed pressure in the ventricles. However, the two pressures are additive, so that any rise in intracranial pressure increases the local critical compression pressure. This point is discussed in some detail to stress that an intracranial pressure of, say 40 mmHg, is not *per se* a critically high pressure, as it can readily be compensated for by cerebral autoregulation, but such a pressure is, nevertheless, dangerous because it strongly suggests an intracranial mass lesion with local compression, and also because intracranial pressure is not constant but fluctuates, with pressure waves reaching even higher levels developing spontaneously.

Retinal circulation in acute gravitational stress

When the gravitational force is increased in the sitting posture, as can happen in air pilots flying in a curvature (head pointing 'inwards'), a state of temporary blindness, the so-called black-out phenomenon, can develop. It is caused by retinal ischaemia.

Arterial blood pressure at the level of the heart is constant or tends to decrease due to pooling in the lower part of the body (as can be counteracted by inflating a pressure suit). At the level of the eyes and the brain arterial pressure is reduced by the hydrostatic difference, i.e. the distance multiplied by the gravitational force measured in units of standard gravitational force (G units).

It may seem surprising that the tissue first showing ischaemic symptoms is the retina, not the brain. Here it should be recalled that intraocular pressure is normally about 20 mmHg and this pressure does not decrease with acute gravitational stress, while ICP drops to levels close to zero. For this reason low arterial pressure is effectively about 20 mmHg lower in the retina than in the brain cortex. As the two tissues have about the same (high) level of oxygen demand functional failure may, at critical levels of acute gravitational stress, develop only in the eye, not in the brain: the pilot retains consciousness but goes blind!

The compartmental syndromes

In special muscle compartments, notably in the anterior-lateral part of the crus, the fascia over the muscle is quite tight. Swelling of the muscle can cause the local pressure to increase and this in turn decreases the local perfusion pressure, so that a critical reduction in blood flow can result. Priapism should also be considered to be a compartmental syndrome. Here, continued relaxation of the penile resistance keeps the tissue in erection inside the tunica albuginea, and also in this case surgical decompression has sometimes to be resorted to when pharmacological measures are inadequate.

Endocardial perfusion

The inner layers of the myocardium are, as the only tissues in the body, intermittently exposed to very high tissue pressures. This means that the effective perfusion pressure drops to low values during much of the cardiac cycle.

On this basis it is not surprising that a state of reduced *local* arterial pressure, as is the consequence of a coronary occlusion, will first of all render the subendocardial layers ischaemic. Studying autoregulation in the myocardium by selectively varying arterial blood pressure in the left anterior descending coronary artery, Haunsø[18] found that the autoregulatory curve was shifted towards higher pressures in the subendocardial layers compared with the subepicardial layers.

This would appear to explain the high frequency of subendocardial myocardial infarction.

Lower and upper limit of autoregulation

As perfusion pressure is lowered progessively autoregulatory arteriolar dilatation will at first fully compensate, so that blood flow remains constant. But, below a certain threshold of pressure – the *lower limit of autoregulation* – flow starts to drop. This lower limit has been studied in particular in the cerebral circulation,[19,20] but basically the same relation holds for other organs as well. The lower limit of cerebral autoregulation lies at a mean arterial blood pressure of about 70 mmHg in normotensive subjects, while elevated values of 80 to 100 mmHg are found in patients with chronic hypertension. Similar results have been obtained in the myocardium in dogs with chronic renovascular hypertension (Fig. 4.2). Similar results have been obtained in the myocardium in dogs with chronic renovascular hypertension.[21] This shift of the lower limit towards higher pressure levels is probably related to hypertrophy of the arteriolar wall rendering relaxation less effective in widening the lumen.

At pressures below the lower limit cerebral blood flow (CBF) drops progressively, and signs of cerebral ischaemia develop at a pressure threshold of 35 to 40 mmHg in normotensives. This ischaemic threshold is also shifted towards higher levels in hypertensives. In certain types of anaesthesia blood pressure tends to drop, and care must be exercised in limiting this drop in patients with habitual elevated pressure. These considerations also apply to medical treatment of the severest form of arterial hypertension as overzealous pressure reduction to near normal levels may cause permanent ischaemic brain damage.

In the high pressure range autoregulation also has a threshold – the *upper limit of autoregulation*.[22] At arterial pressures beyond this level the arteriolar constriction is unable to withstand the high distending pressure and a forced arteriolar distension occurs.[23,24] This phenomenon begins at local sites, reducing local vascular resistance. Thus, acute hypertension to levels above the upper limit of autoregulation of about 150 mmHg (mean arterial blood pressure) gives rise to focal areas of marked hyperaemia with flows reaching 10-fold the normal level. These local areas become oedematous and the blood–brain barrier becomes protein permeable. This represents in all probability the pathophysiology of the initial stage of acute hypertensive encephalopathy[22] illustrated by the characteristic ophthalmoscopic findings of papill-

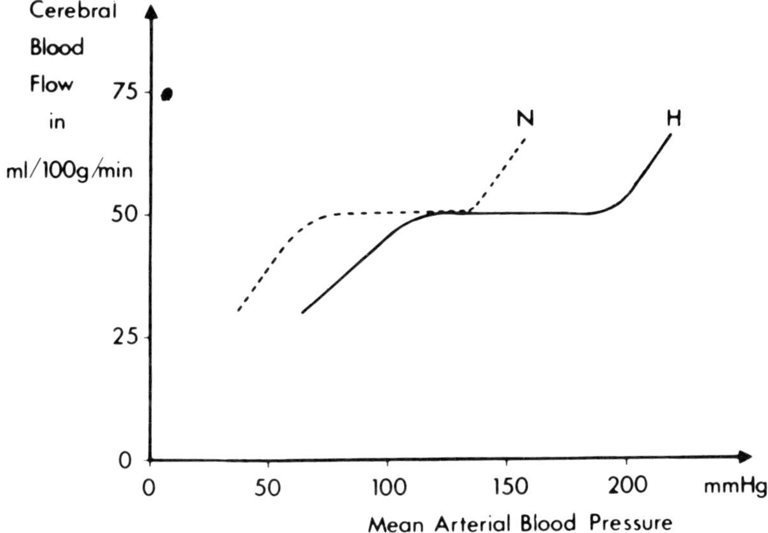

Fig. 4.2. Cerebral blood flow autoregulation; diagrammatic representation of result curves as obtained in the author's laboratory. The lower and upper limits of the autoregulatory plateau are seen as well as the adaptation towards higher levels in chronic hypertension. N, normotensives; H, hypertensives.

oedema and multiple small haemorrhages.

In patients with chronic arterial hypertension the upper limit of autoregulation is also shifted towards higher pressures, the hypertrophied arterioles better withstanding the high distending pressures. This is probably why subacute pressure elevation as seen in glomerulonephritis or in eclampsia of pregnancy risky at pressure elevations, is well tolerated in the chronically hypertensive patient.

Experimental studies have revealed an interaction between the sympathetic tone and the thresholds of cerebral autoregulation. In states with elevated sympathetic tone constricting in particular the larger arteries both the lower and the upper thresholds of autoregulation are shifted towards the right, towards higher pressure levels.[36] This probably also pertains for the ischaemic threshold and may explain why induced hypotension in certain types of anaesthesia (with low or absent sympathetic tone) can be carried to pressure levels, that in other hypotensive states (associated with increased sympathetic tone) will cause brain ischaemia.

Autoregulation of blood flow in disease states

Hyalinosis of the muscular layer of the arterioles are typical findings in long-term diabetes mellitus as well as in long standing chronic arterial hypertension. In both conditions one would expect to find impaired autoregulation. Many long-term diabetics have impaired autoregulation of subcutaneous tissue blood flow and of CBF.[25–27] Autoregulation of GFR is lost in many cases.[28] With regard to chronic arterial hypertension the data in the literature are insufficient. The classic studies of Strandgaard *et al.*[23,24] referred to above are concerned with newly diagnosed hypertensives with rather moderate pressure elevation. Hence the finding of a preserved cerebral autoregulation may not be valid for more severe and, in particular, more chronic cases.

References

1. Bayliss G: On the local reactions of the arterial wall to changes in internal pressure. *Journal of Physiology (London)*, 1902; **28,** 220–31.
2. Fog M: Cerebral circulation. The reaction of the pial arteries to a fall in blood pressure. *Archives of Neurology and Psychiatry*, 1937; **37,** 351–64.
3. Fog M: Cerebral circulation II. Reaction of pial arteries to increase in blood pressure. *Archives of Neurology and Psychiatry*, 1939; **41,** 260–68.
4. Johnson PC and Intaglietta M: Contributions of pressure and flow sensitivity to autoregulation in mesenteric arterioles. *American Journal of Physiology*, 1976; **231,** 1686–98.
5. Meininger GA, Mack CA, Fehr KL and Bohlen HG: Myogenic vasoregulation overrides local metabolic control in resting rat skeletal muscle. *Circulation Research* 1987; **60,** 861–70.
6. Kuo L, Chilian WM and Davis MJ: Coronary arteriolar myogenic response is independent of endothelium. *Circulation Research*, 1990; **66,** 860–66.
7. Halpern W, Mongeon SA and Root DT: Stress, tension, and myogenic aspects of small isolated extraparenchymal rat arteries. In Stephens NL (ed.): *Smooth Muscle Contraction.* New York, Dekker, 1984, 427–55.
8. Halpern W, Osol G and Coy GS: Mechanical behavior of pressurized *in vitro* pre-arteriolar vessels determined with a video system. *Annals of Biomedical Engineering*, 1984; **12,** 463–79.
9. Johnson PC: The myogenic response. In Hamilton WF (ed.): *Handbook of Physiology.* Section 2: *Circulation.* Washington DC, American Physiological Society, 1980, 409–42.
10. Burton-Opitz R and Lucas DR: The blood supply in kidney: the influence of the vagus nerve upon the vascularity of the left organ. *Journal of Experimental Medicine*, 1911; **13**, 308–13.
11. Selkurt EE: The relation of renal blood flow to effective arterial pressure in the intact kidney of the dog. *American Journal of Physiology*, 1946; **147,** 537–49.
12. Selkurt EE: The renal circulation. In Hamilton WF (ed.): *Handbook of Physiology.* Section 2: *Circulation.* Washington DC, American Physiological Society, 1963, 1457–1516.
13. Selkurt EE, Deetjen P and Brechtelsbauer H: Tubular pressure gradients and filtration dynamics during urinary stop flow in the rat. *Pflügers Arch IV. European Journal of Physiology (Berlin)*, 1965; **286,** 19–35.
14. Holstein-Rathlou N-H and Leyssac PP: TGF-mediated oscillations in the proximal intratubular pressure: differences between spontaneously hypertensive rats and Wistar–Kyoto rats. *Acta Physiologica Scandinavica*, 1986; **126,** 333–9.
15. Holstein-Rathlou N-H and Marsh DJ: Oscillations of tubular pressure, flow, and distal chloride concentrations in rat. *American Journal of Physiology*, 1989; **256,** F1007–14.
16. Holstein-Rathlou N-H and Marsh DJ: A dynamic model of the tubuloglomerular feedback system. *American Journal of Physiology* 1990; **258,** F1448–59.
17. Holstein-Rathlou N-H, Wagner AJ and Marsh DJ: Tubuloglomerular feedback dynamics and renal

blood flow autoregulation in rats. *American Journal of Physiology*, 1991; **260,** F53–68.

18. Haunsø S: Lower liomits of blood flow autoregulation in different myocardial layers of the left ventricular free wall of dogs. *Acta Physiologica Scandinavica*, 1981; **112,** 349–50.
19. Lassen NA. Cerebral blood flow and oxygen consumption in man. *Physiological Reviews* 1959; **39,** 183–238.
20. Strandgaard S: Autoregulation of cerebral blood flow in hypertensive patients. The modifying influence of prolonged antihypertensive treatment on the tolerance to acute, drug-induced hypotension. *Circulation*, 1976; **53,** 720–27.
21. Jeremy RW, Fletcher PJ and Thompson J: Coronary pressure–flow relations in hypertensive left ventricular hypertrophy. Comparison of intact autoregulation with physiological and pharmacological vasodilation in the dog. *Circulation Research*, 1989; **65,** 224–36.
22. Lassen NA and Agnoli A: The upper limit of autoregulation of cerebral blood flow – on the pathogenesis of hypertensive encephalopathy. *Scandinavian Journal of Clinical and Laboratory Investigations*, 1973; **30,** 113–16.
23. Strandgaard S, Jones JV, MacKenzie ET and Harper AM: Upper limit of cerebral blood flow autoregulation in the baboon with experimental renovascular hypotension. *Circulation Research*, 1975; **37,** 164–7.
24. Strandgaard S, MacKenzie ET, Sengupta D, Rowan JO, Lassen NA and Harper AM: Upper limit for autoregulation of cerebral blood flow in the baboon. *Circulation Research*, 1974; **34,** 435–40.
25. Kastrup J, Nørgaard T, Parving H-H, Henriksen O and Lassen NA: Impaired autoregulation of blood flow in subcutaneous tissue of long-term Type I (insulin-dependent) diabetic patients with microangiopathy: an index of arteriolar dysfunction. *Diabetologia*, 1985; **28,** 711–17.
26. Bentsen N, Larsen B and Lassen NA: Chronically impaired autoregulation of cerebral blood flow in long-term diabetics. *Stroke*, 1975; **6,** 497–502.
27. Kastrup J, Rørsgård S, Parving H-H and Lassen NA: Impaired autoregulation of cerebral blood flow in long-term Type I (insulin-dependent) diabetic patients with nephropathy and retinopathy. *Clinical Physiology*, 1986; **6,** 549–59.
28. Parving H-H, Kastrup J, Smidt UM, Andersen AR, Feldt-Rasmussen B and Sandahl Christiansen J: Impaired autoregulation of glomerular filtration rate in Type I (insulin-dependent) diabetic patients with nephropathy. *Diabetologia*, 1984; **27,** 547–52.

5

Cardiovascular sensors: the bradycardic phase in hypovolaemic shock

Tage N Jacobsen, Charles M T Jost, Richard L Converse Jr and Ronald G Victor

Introduction

Activation of the sympathetic nervous system, with reflex vasoconstriction and tachycardia, is a major compensatory adjustment during many hypotensive states.[1–4] Indeed, most current medicine textbooks emphasize that sympathetically mediated peripheral vasoconstriction and tachycardia are the classic clinical signs of hypovolaemic shock and suggest that these compensatory adjustments may be lost only in the terminal, irreversible stage of shock.[5–10] In contrast to this traditional teaching, there is increasing experimental evidence – but as yet little clinical recognition[11–13] – that earlier stages of hypovolaemic hypotension also can be accompanied by bradycardia and vasodilatation caused by the reversible, reflex withdrawal of sympathetic drive.[11–17] In the past 20 years our understanding of vasodepressor reaction has been improved greatly by the ability to record sympathetic nerve activity directly not only in experimental animals but also in conscious humans.

This chapter will critically review what is known and what is not known about the cardiovascular sensors that are thought to mediate the autonomic adjustments to haemorrhagic hypotension. The major purpose of this review is to provide a conceptual framework to improve the scientific understanding and clinical recognition of vasodepressor reaction in the setting of hypovolaemic hypotension. The main concept presented here is that activation of inhibitory cardiac afferents is thought to be the primary peripheral reflex mechanism causing vasodepressor reaction in hypovolaemic hypotension. In addition, we will also comment on the complexity of the sympathetic responses to hypotensive haemorrhage and show that these responses are regulated by highly specific reflex pathways that differ greatly not only between different species but even between two organs that are in close proximity.[18]

Activation of inhibitory cardiac afferents as a potential mechanism triggering vasodepressor syncope: the 'ventricular syncope' hypothesis

Normal inverse relation between muscle sympathetic nerve activity and arterial pressure

In 1969 the microneurographic technique for intraneural recordings of sympathetic nerve activity in humans was developed at the University of Uppsala, Sweden, by Hagbarth, Vallbo and colleagues. The details of this technique have been reviewed extensively.[19] Briefly, multiunit recordings of postganglionic sympathetic nerve activity are obtained in unanaesthetized humans by insertion of unipolar microelectrodes into human peripheral nerves. The sympathetic fibres travel in the motor and sensory fascicles, allowing separation of sympathetic traffic targeted to skeletal muscle or to skin. In humans

muscle sympathetic nerve activity (MSNA) is postganglionic, because the conduction velocity is 1 metre per second indicative of unmyelinated C-fibres and is eliminated by ganglionic blockade. The sympathetic nerve activity is predominantly vasoconstrictive because increases are accompanied by regional vasoconstriction and decreases by vasodilatation (Fig. 5.1).[20] Under normal conditions this sympathetic activity is under baroreflex regulation because the activity is locked to the cardiac cycle and is inversely related to blood pressure. The normal inverse relation between MSNA and arterial pressure is also evident during pharmacological manipulations of arterial pressure. (Fig. 5.2).

Studies in experimental animals

Studies in experimental animals have demonstrated that the heart is an important sensory organ containing polymodal afferent, or sensory, nerve endings that are located in the atria, venoatrial junctions, and ventricle.[21–30] When activated by certain chemical and/or mechanical stimuli, these afferent nerve endings evoke a variety of excitatory

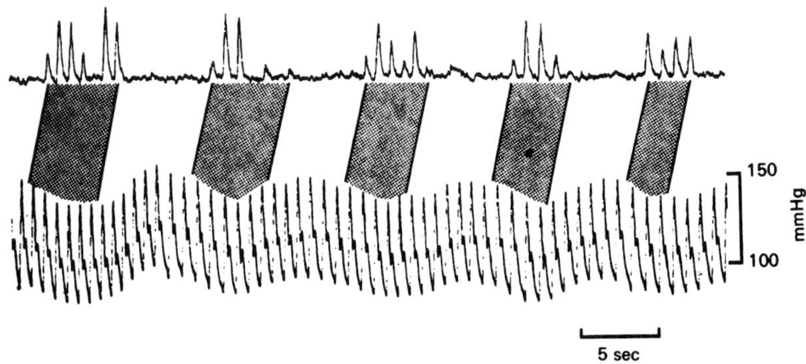

Fig. 5.1. Relation between muscle sympathetic nerve activity and arterial pressure at rest. On this mean voltage display the narrow peaks are spontaneous bursts of sympathetic discharge. Under baseline conditions the sympathetic bursts occur mainly during spontaneous decreases in mean arterial pressure (MAP), and are inhibited during increases in MAP. From Sundlöf and Wallin,[20] with permission.

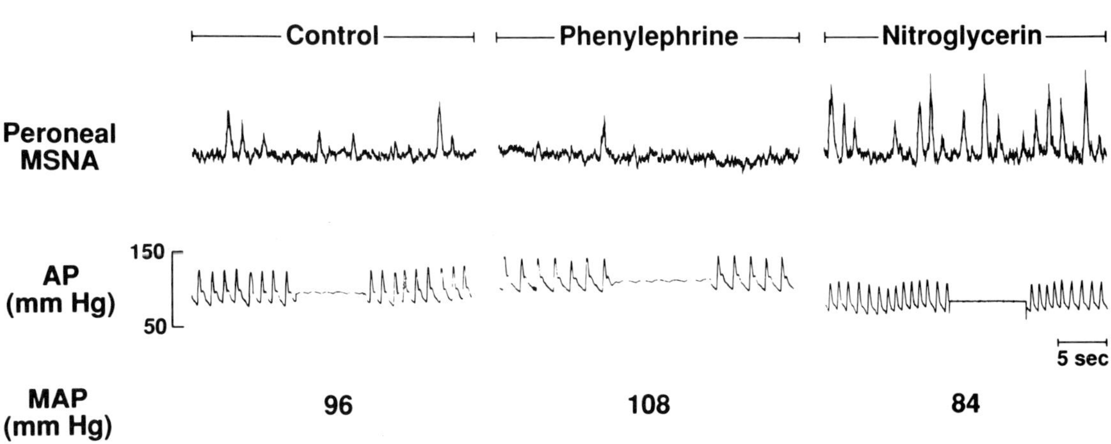

Fig. 5.2. Segments of an original neurogram from one subject showing changes in muscle sympathetic nerve activity (MSNA), phasic arterial pressure (AP) and mean arterial pressure (MAP) during pharmacological alterations in arterial pressure. The sympathetic bursts were almost completely inhibited by an increase in mean arterial pressure of 12 mmHg and were greatly increased both in number and amplitude by a decrease in mean arterial pressure of 12 mmHg. Abstracted from unpublished data from the authors' laboratory.

and inhibitory cardiovascular reflexes.[27,31,32]

Many of the ventricular endings give rise to unmyelinated (C-fibre) vagal afferents that exert a predominantly inhibitory influence on sympathetic vasoconstrictor outflow.[21,26,27] Activation of these afferents with exogenous chemical agents such as veratroidine or nicotine elicits the classic von Bezold–Jarisch reflex, characterized by hypotension, bradycardia, peripheral vasodilatation and gastric relaxation.[31,33,34] Under physiological conditions, ventricular C-fibre afferents are thought to function as mechanoreceptors, i.e. endings that are activated by deformation of their receptive fields.[29] Studies in anaesthetized cats have indicated that the two primary determinants of ventricular mechanoreceptor afferent discharge are ventricular filling pressure and contractility.[24] Thus, ventricular mechanoreceptor discharge normally increases during increases in left ventricular end-diastolic pressure produced by volume expansion and during infusion of positive inotropic agents. Furthermore, this activity decreases during infusion of negative inotropic agents and during mild and moderate reductions in left ventricular end-diastolic pressure produced by non-hypotensive haemorrhage.[26,35–38]

In 1972 Oberg and Thoren[36] found that during more severe (and rapid) reduction in left ventricular end-diastolic pressure produced by hypotensive haemorrhage in cats, ventricular C-fibre discharge did not decrease further but showed a paradoxical burst of activity, which was followed promptly by the sudden onset of bradycardia (Fig. 5.3). In contrast, haemorrhage-induced bradycardia was not preceded by a sudden change in activity of atrial receptor afferents, suggesting that the bradycardia is a reflex arising in the ventricles rather than the atria. The haemorrhage-induced bradycardia indeed was a reflex caused by the activation of C-fibre vagal afferents because it was abolished both by selective cardiac vagal afferent section and by cervical vagal cooling,[35] which selectively impairs conduction in afferent C-fibres while leaving intact conduction in myelinated efferent (motor) vagal fibres.

These observations provided neurophysiological support for the theory, originally advanced in the 1950s by a number of investigators, that during

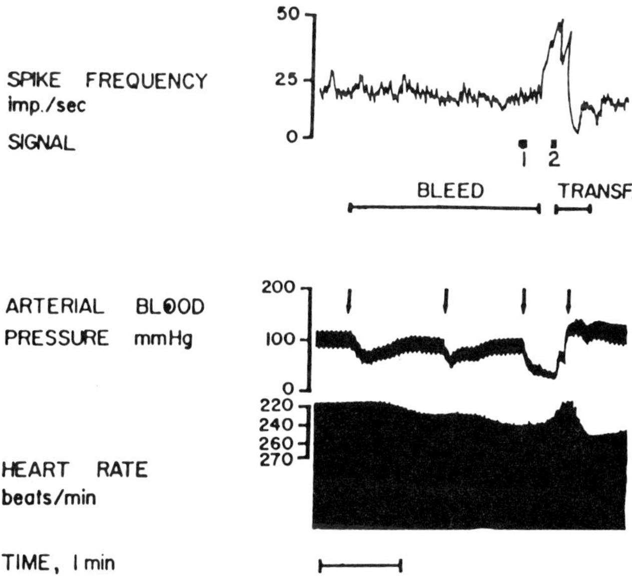

Fig. 5.3. Segments of the original record from one cat showing effects of successive haemorrhages and transfusion on the spike frequency of a single ventricular vagal C-fibre afferent, on arterial pressure and on heart rate. The first two haemorrhages caused ventricular C-fibre afferent activity to decrease slightly and caused small and transient decreases in blood pressure which were partially offset by a compensatory increase in heart rate. In contrast, the third successive haemorrhage caused a sudden explosive increase in C-fibre ventricular afferent activity leading to bradycardia and a profound and sustained decrease in arterial pressure. These responses were reversed by transfusion. Adapted from Oberg,[36] with permission.

severe hypovolaemic hypotension inhibitory ventricular vagal C-fibre afferents are activated by excessive mechanical deformation of their receptive fields when the adrenergically stimulated heart contracts forcefully around an almost empty ventricular chamber (Fig. 5.4).[29,30,39–41]

While there is substantial evidence that this reflex mechanism causes the sudden bradycardia during hypotensive haemorrhage in anaethetized cats,[36–42] there has been much speculation, but as yet no direct proof, that the same mechanism causes the withdrawal of sympathetic vasoconstrictor drive to the peripheral circulation during haemorrhagic hypotension in either experimental animals or humans. In rats haemorrhagic hypotension at first produces small and transient increases in heart rate and RSNA followed by sustained and parallel decreases in RSNA as well as heart rate (and splanchnic sympathetic activity) (Fig. 5.5).[18,43]

These studies also demonstrated that activation of vagal afferents plays a major role in causing this depressor response, the renal sympathetic inhibition being markedly attenuated by cervical vagotomy. However, these experiments: (1) indicate that mechanisms other than vagal afferent activation also contribute to haemorrhage-induced renal sympathoinhibition in the rat as in some experiments the sympathoinhibition was only partially reversed by vagotomy; and (2) do not prove that the left ventricle is the site of origin of this vagal afferent reflex because in rats, unlike cats, mechanical probing has disclosed vagal afferents with receptive fields only in the atria and none in the ventricles.[26,27,44,45] In order to define precisely the receptive fields of the vagal fibres that form the afferent arm of this reflex, single fibre afferent recordings would need to be performed during haemorrhage in rats. Furthermore, there may be chemical, as well as mechanical, factors that trigger this vagal afferent reflex in the rat because subsequent studies have shown that this renal sympathoinhibitory response is abolished by administration of serotonergic antagonists in 'normal' rats and is absent in Brattleboro rats which have a genetic deficiency in vasopressin.[46,47]

Although haemorrhage-induced bradycardia and renal sympathoinhibition now have been demonstrated in a number of mammalian species, there are major interspecies differences in the underlying mechanisms causing these vasodepressor reactions.[2] In conscious dogs and rabbits, for example, progressive haemorrhage also has been shown to cause the same biphasic response in RSNA: the sympathetic activity increases during mild and moderate haemorrhage but then returns to or

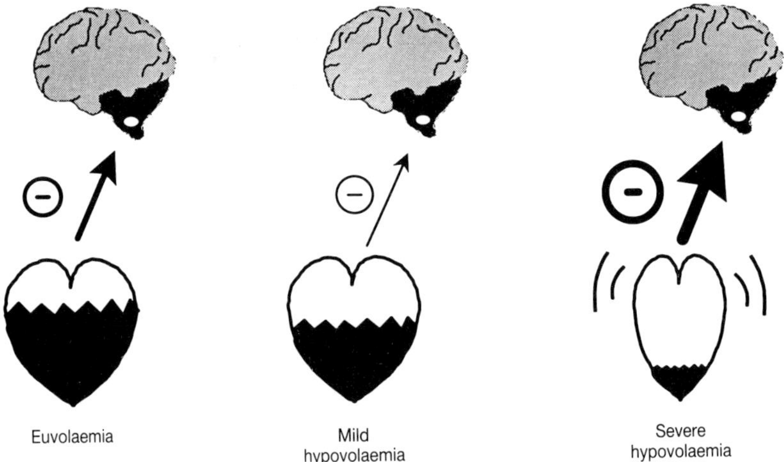

Fig. 5.4. Cartoon illustrating the concept of paradoxical activation of ventricular afferents during hypovolaemic hypotension (the 'ventricular syncope' hypothesis). The thickness of the arrows represents the inhibitory input from the ventricular vagal afferents during progressive reductions in cardiac filling. During euvolaemia, these afferents are thought to exert a tonic inhibitory influence on sympathetic vasomotor outflow. During mild hypovolaemia, as in non-hypotensive haemorrhage, the afferents are unloaded and their inhibitory input is reduced. During severe hypovolaemia, as with hypotensive haemorrhage, the ventricular afferent activity does not decrease further but rather increases paradoxically as the hypercontractile ventricle contracts forcefully around an almost empty ventricular chamber.

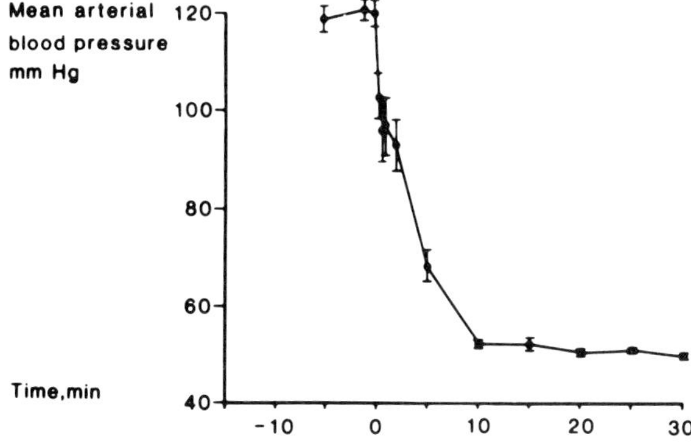

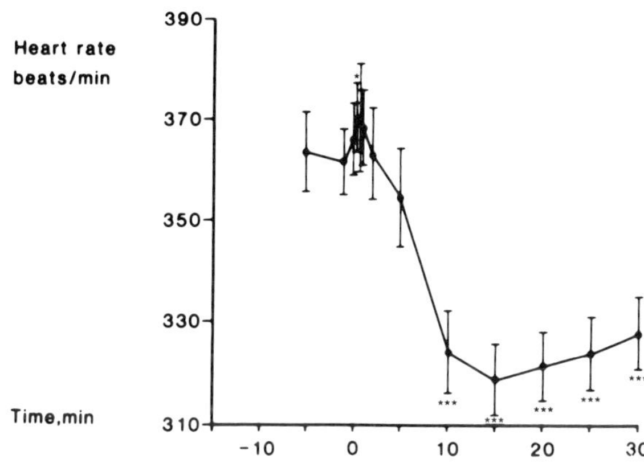

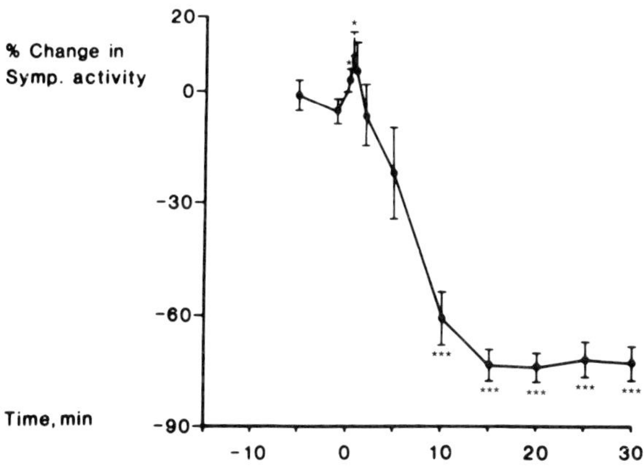

Fig. 5.5. Decreases in mean arterial pressure, heart rate and renal sympathetic nerve activity during severe haemorrhage in chloralose anaesthetized rats. ***, Difference versus prebleeding control ($P < 0.001$). From Skoog *et al.*,[43] with permission.

below baseline levels during severe hypotensive haemorrhage.[48–50] Although activation of vagal afferents clearly is the primary mechanism causing the decreases in RSNA during haemorrhagic hypotension in the rat, vagal afferents do not play a primary role in causing this response in conscious dogs and rabbits because in these species vagotomy has no detectable effect on haemorrhage-induced renal sympathoinhibition.[48] Most of these studies have relied on renal sympathetic activity as the index of sympathetic nerve response to haemorrhage. However, there is recent evidence that regional sympathetic responses to hypotensive haemorrhage are regulated by highly specific reflex pathways that differ greatly not only between the different species but even between sympathetic outflows to different organs that are in close anatomical proximity in the same animal. Thus, in rats haemorrhagic hypotension triggers directionally opposite responses in sympathetic outflow to the kidney and adrenal glands, with renal sympathoinhibition but adrenal sympathoexcitation (Fig. 5.6).[18]

Although a paradoxical increase in ventricular mechanoreceptor discharge is the most widely studied mechanism for the reflex withdrawal of sympathetic outflow during hypovolaemic hypotension,[36] there also is direct experimental evidence in anaesthetized cats that severe carotid sinus hypotension triggers paradoxical increases in carotid baroreceptor discharge (Fig. 5.7).[51]

It is reasonable to speculate that during severe hypotension paradoxical increases in carotid, as well as ventricular, mechanoreceptor discharge are caused by local deformation of the wall of the cardiovascular structures in which the receptors are embedded.[26,51] During hypotension such paradoxical increases in carotid baroreceptor discharge might be further augmented by reflex sympathetic activation. Increases in efferent sympathetic nerve activity and direct application of noradrenaline both have been shown to sensitize arterial baroreceptor discharge.[52,53] However, the functional importance of increased carotid baroreceptor discharge in causing reflex withdrawal of sympathetic vasoconstrictor outflow during hypovolaemic hypotension remains unknown since sinoaortic denervation did not prevent renal sympathoinhibition during severe haemorrhage in either anaesthetized rats or conscious dogs.[18,48]

Taken together, these observations from animal experiments suggest that multiple, complex, and

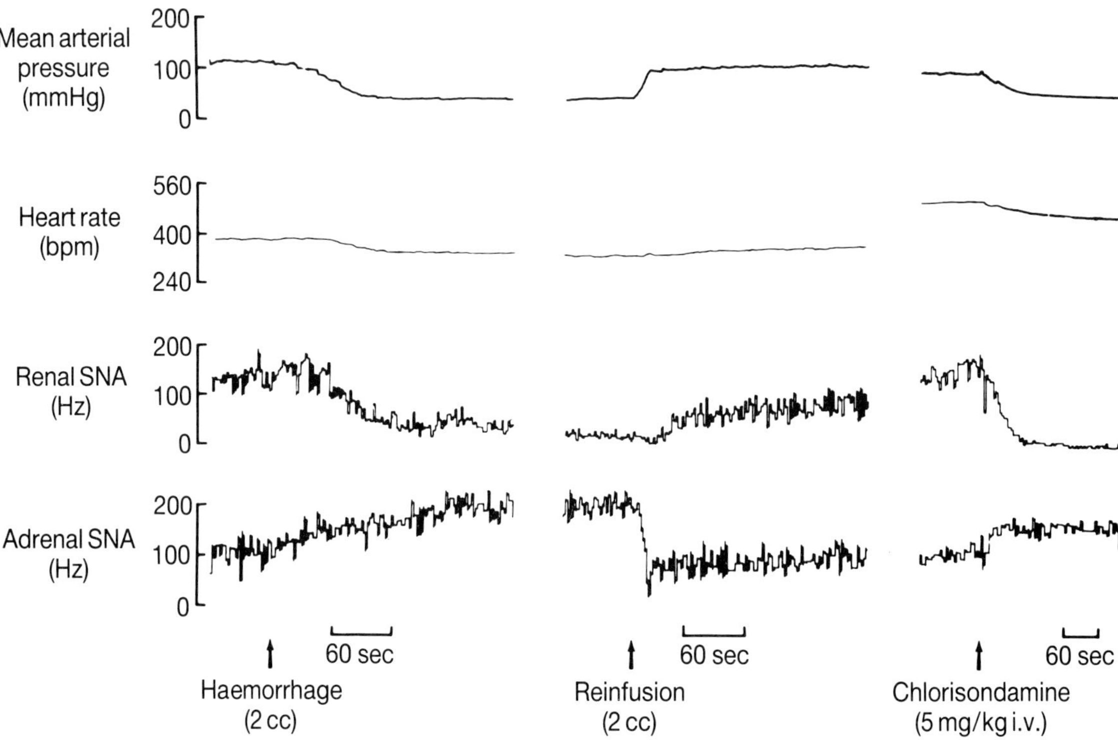

Fig. 5.6. Segments of an illustrative record from a rat showing response of mean arterial pressure, heart rate, and renal and adrenal sympathetic nerve activity (SNA) (displayed as a time frequency histogram) during hypotensive haemorrhage, reinfusion of blood and ganglionic blockade with chlorisondamine. Haemorrhagic hypotension decreased renal SNA and heart rate but simultaneously increased adrenal SNA. These variables returned to control after transfusion. Ganglionic blockade abolished SNA in the postganglionic renal nerve but did not decrease thereafter and tended to increase SNA in the adrenal nerve, which is mainly preganglionic. From Victor *et al.*,[18] with permission.

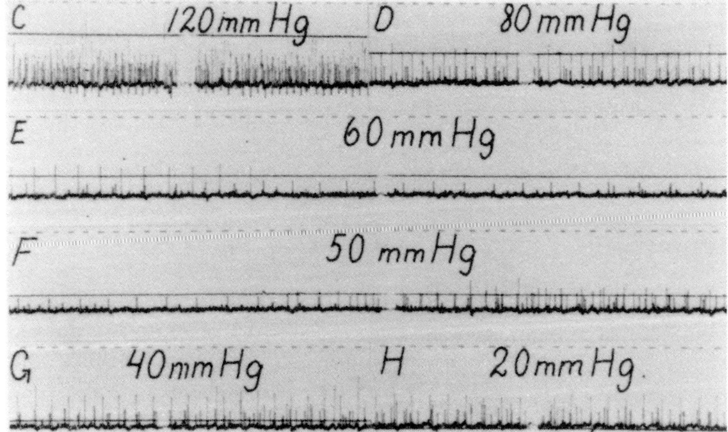

Fig. 5.7. Segments of an original record showing effects of progressive reductions in carotid sinus pressure on single fibre carotid baroreceptor discharge in the cat. The discharge frequency of this fibre decreased progressively (almost to zero) as carotid sinus pressure was reduced progressively from 120 to 50 mmHg. As carotid sinus pressure was reduced below 50 mmHg, however, baroreceptor discharge did not decrease further but rather showed an abrupt, 'paradoxical' increase in activity. From Landgren,[51] with permission.

perhaps some as yet undefined, mechanisms are likely to be involved in the regulation of sympathetic outflow during severe hypotensive haemorrhage and that considerable caution should be taken in extrapolating these experimental data directly to humans.

Studies in humans

In the past 50 years, however, there have been a number of reports indicating that hypovolaemic hypotension can trigger relative bradycardia in the clinical, as well as in the experimental, setting. Hypotension with an inappropriately 'normal' heart rate has been reported in haemorrhagic shock in World War II air-raid casualties;[54,55] in obstetric patients with acute intraperitoneal bleeding;[14] in patients presenting to the emergency room with severe but reversible hypovolaemic shock[12,13,56] due to trauma and other causes; and in patients experiencing hypovolaemic hypotension during major abdominal surgery.[57] In a study of 20 consecutive patients presenting to the Rigshospitalet in Copenhagen, Denmark, with haemorrhagic shock, the average heart rate was 73 beats/min even though the average blood pressure was 81/55 mmHg.[56] Furthermore, the heart rate increased to 102 beats/min during transfusion.

Thus, in contrast to the traditional teaching, these important studies strongly suggest that relative bradycardia: (1) is more common than previously recognized in patients with haemorrhagic hypotension; and (2) is rapidly reversed with volume expansion, suggesting that the bradycardia is caused mainly by a reflex rather than by irreversible damage to neural or cardiovascular tissues (i.e. that the shock has not yet reached the irreversible stage).

Although sympathetic nerve activity has not yet been recorded in humans during haemorrhagic hypotension, direct measurements of MSNA have documented acute sympathoinhibition (with bradycardia and classic vasovagal symptoms) in humans during upright tilt,[58] infusion of nitroprusside (Fig. 5.8)[58] and haemodialysis,[17] which are three examples of hypotension with relative hypovolaemia.

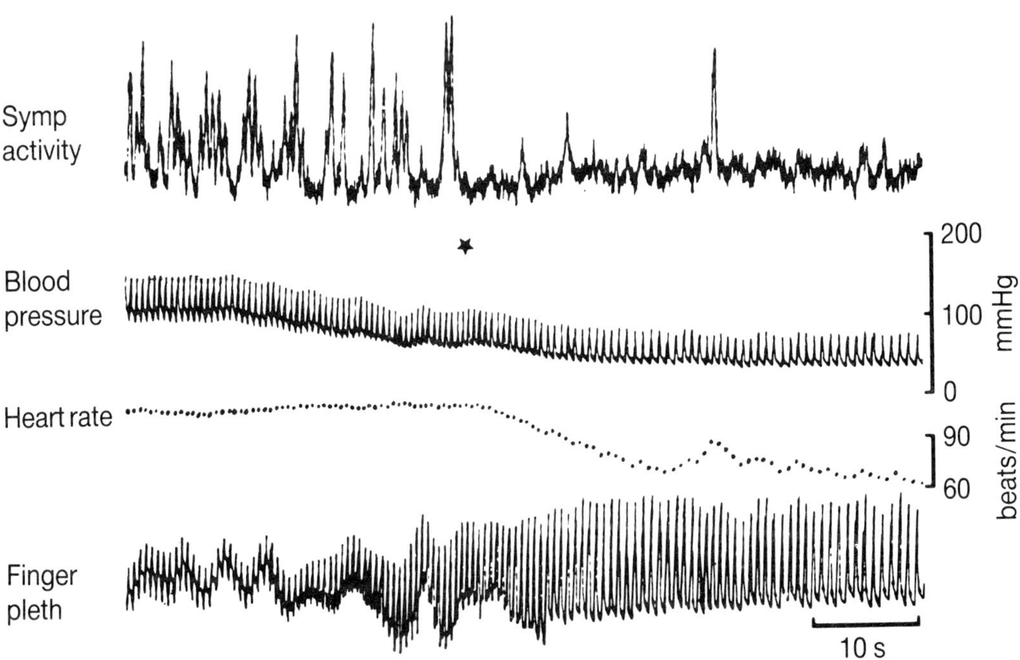

Fig. 5.8. Decreases in muscle sympathetic nerve activity, blood pressure, heart rate and finger blood flow (pulse plethysmogram) during vasovagal syncope (*) evoked by intravenous infusion of nitroprusside. From Wallin and Sundlöf,[58] with permission.

Because nitroprusside is a mixed vasodilator decreasing both preload and afterload, many authors have suggested that the vasodepressor reactions during decreases in preload produced by upright tilt, nitroprusside, haemodialysis or haemorrhage all are caused by the same mechanism; paradoxical withdrawal of sympathetic activity due to increased mechanical stimulation of ventricular afferents, i.e. 'ventricular' or 'neurocardiogenic' syncope.[30,59] While the data from haemorrhage experiments in animals make this an attractive hypothesis, at present the experimental evidence to support this in humans is at best circumstantial.

We recently had an unexpected opportunity to test this hypothesis in a patient who had undergone cardiac transplantation, an operation that causes both efferent and afferent denervation of the ventricles. During this operation the ventricular afferents are severed, but afferents from the remnant atria, venoatrial junctions, pulmonary veins and arterial baroreceptors are left intact. While recording MSNA (in the peroneal nerve) in an attempt to assess arterial baroreflex function with intravenous infusion of nitroprusside, classic vasovagal symptoms suddenly developed in the patient.[60] These symptoms occurred immediately following the peak increases in sympathetic nerve activity and heart rate produced by the nitroprusside and were accompanied by the abrupt cessation of the sympathetic discharge and a slowing of the innervated remnant atrial heart rate (Fig. 5.9).

This latter study documents that vasodilator-induced hypovolaemic hypotension can precipitate a classic vasodepressor syncope in a patient with transplantation-induced ventricular denervation. The failure of cardiac transplantation to prevent sympathetic inhibition and classic vasovagal syn-

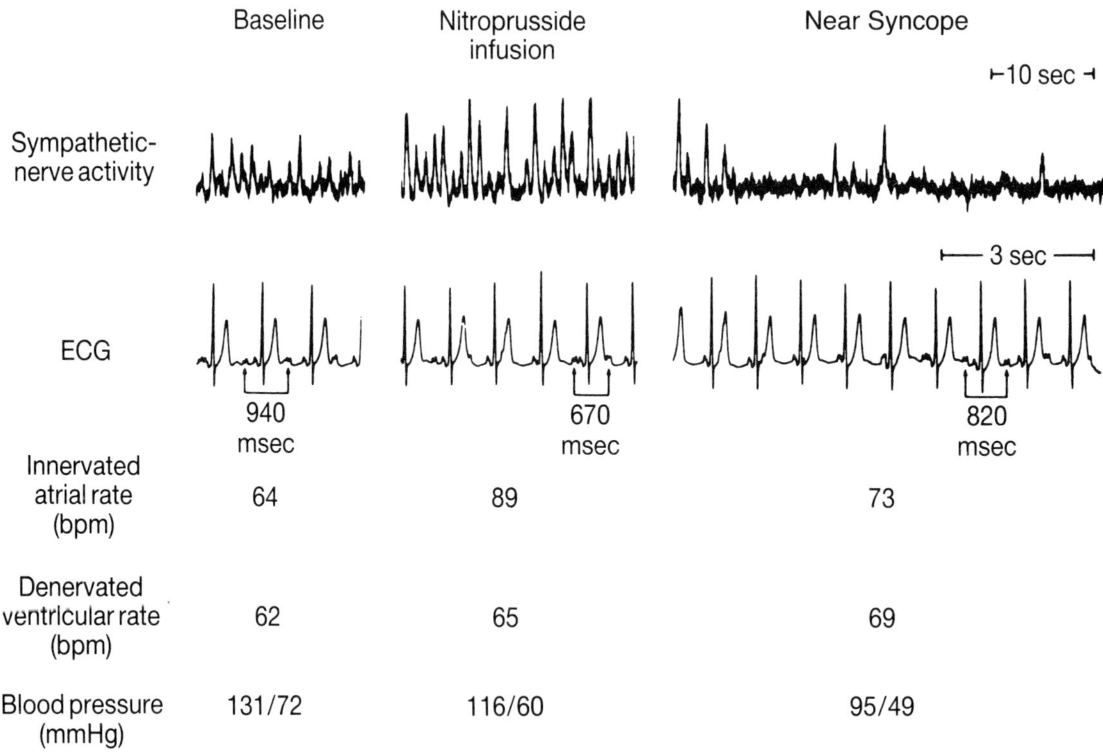

Fig. 5.9. Segments of the original record in a 41-year-old heart transplant recipient 11 months after transplantation, showing the mean voltage neurogram of muscle sympathetic nerve activity and the electrocardiogram (ECG) at baseline, during the infusion of nitroprusside and during a near syncope episode immediately following completion of the infusion. All measurements were performed with the patient supine. The numbers shown in brackets below the electrocardiogram represent the P–P intervals of the innervated atrial remnant in milliseconds. In contrast to the clear decrease in the rate of the innervated atrial remnant, the rate of the transplanted, denervated ventricle did not decrease during the near syncopal episode. Reprinted by permission of the *New England Journal of Medicine* (**322**; 603, 1990).[60]

cope after the infusion of a vasodilator therefore indicates that ventricular mechanoreceptor activation is not the only mechanism that can trigger sympathetic inhibition during hypovolaemic hypotension and is consistent with animal data indicating that multiple, redundant, and perhaps as yet unidentified, mechanisms may be involved. In conscious dogs, for example, haemorrhagic hypotension-induced sympathoinhibition also is not prevented by cardiac denervation.[48] It is important to emphasize, however, that these findings in a heart transplant recipient certainly do not exclude the possibility that ventricular afferent activation is one of the important mechanisms triggering hypovolaemia-induced vasovagal reaction in humans with intact cardiac innervation.

For example, ventricular mechanoreceptor-induced vasovagal syncope has been proposed recently as a common cause of otherwise unexplained syncope in patients with normal electrophysiological testing.[59,61,62] These investigators based their initial conclusion on the finding that upright tilt together with intravenous infusion of isoproterenol provoked acute hypotension with bradycardia in 9 of 11 patients with a history of recurrent syncope but did so in only 2 of 18 subjects with no such history. The investigators hypothesized that the combination of decreased preload and ventricular dimension (produced by upright tilt) and increased cardiac contractility (produced by isoproterenol) increased the activity of ventricular mechanoreceptors, triggering reflex bradycardia and peripheral vasodilatation. A subsequent study by Shalev *et al.*[63] provided some echocardiographic support for the assumption that the isoproterenol tilt test does indeed produce a vigorous myocardial contraction together with a decrease in left ventricular end-diastolic dimension, and further reported that prevention of the increased contractility with cardiac β-adrenergic receptor blockade (metoprolol) prevented vasovagal syncope in three of five patients during tilting alone and in four of four patients during tilting plus isoproterenol.

While provocative, these data should be interpreted cautiously because of the small numbers of subjects, failure to control for emotional factors and other flaws in experimental design – a major oversight in these studies is that the test–retest reproducibility of the isoproterenol tilt test to repeatedly provoke vasovagal syncope in a given patient has never been reported.[64] Because emotional factors are likely to contribute greatly to the development of vasovagal syncope during tilt testing in habitual fainters, the metoprolol data cannot be interpreted meaningfully until further studies determine whether the vasovagal reaction does or does not habituate when a given patient is tested repeatedly. Furthermore, it is unclear whether the echocardiographic changes were the cause or the consequence of the syncope, since a small hypercontractile ventricle would be the inevitable consequence of sudden severe decreases in preload and afterload.

In a different clinical setting, regular haemodialysis, we recently reported that the sudden onset of severe hypotension was immediately preceded by echocardiographic evidence of left ventricular cavity obliteration (Fig. 5.10), raising the possibility (but certainly not proving) that ventricular mechanoreceptor activation might be one important cause of dialysis-induced hypotension.[17]

The neurocirculatory responses from the same patient are shown in Fig. 5.11. During the first two-thirds of the haemodialysis session, the patient's baroreceptor reflexes seemed to function normally. A modest fall in mean arterial pressure (from 116 to 100 mmHg) was accompanied by the appropriate brisk reflex increase in MSNA, heart rate and vascular resistance. With the abrupt onset of severe hypotension, however, normal baroreflex function was replaced by a sudden appearance of an 'inappropriate' vasodepressor reaction. As mean arterial pressure fell further from 100 to 60 mmHg, sympathetic activity, heart rate and vascular resistance did not increase further but rather decreased 'paradoxically' to or below baseline levels. These inhibitory autonomic responses were followed by the development of classic signs and symptoms of vasovagal syncope.

To further examine the underlying mechanism(s) triggering this vasodepressor reaction, we performed additional experiments in which we dissected the dialysis procedure into its component parts, ultrafiltration alone (the isosmotic removal of plasma water) and dialysis alone (the removal of uraemic toxins and electrolytes). In a subset of haemodialysis patients we found that dialysis alone had no effect on arterial pressure and calf vascular resistance whereas ultrafiltration alone reproduced the decreases in blood pressure and vascular resistance caused by the normal haemodialysis procedure. These findings strengthen the conclusion that volume removal is the key stimulus triggering the paradoxical withdrawal of reflex vasoconstriction, which we believe is one important cause of

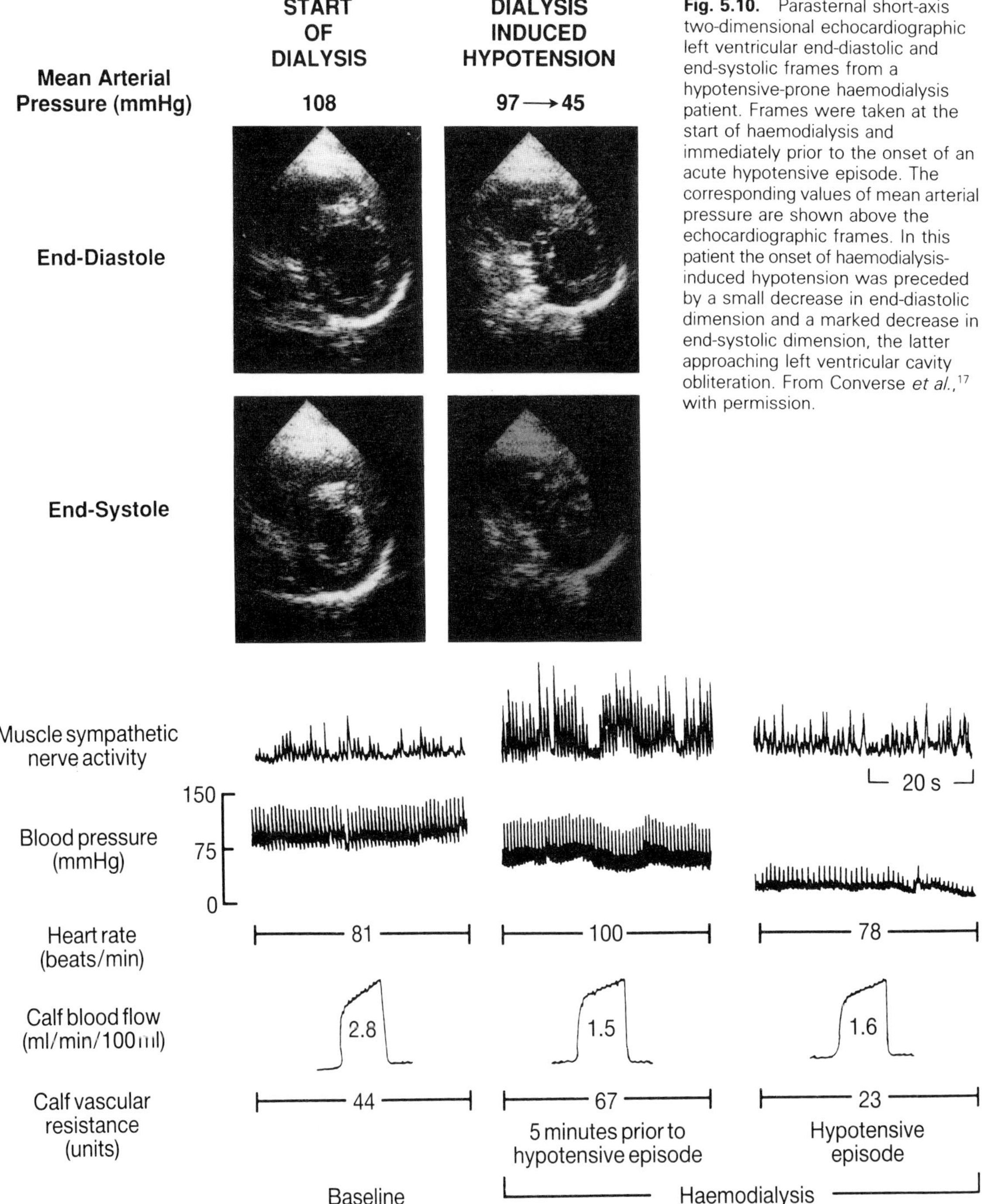

Fig. 5.10. Parasternal short-axis two-dimensional echocardiographic left ventricular end-diastolic and end-systolic frames from a hypotensive-prone haemodialysis patient. Frames were taken at the start of haemodialysis and immediately prior to the onset of an acute hypotensive episode. The corresponding values of mean arterial pressure are shown above the echocardiographic frames. In this patient the onset of haemodialysis-induced hypotension was preceded by a small decrease in end-diastolic dimension and a marked decrease in end-systolic dimension, the latter approaching left ventricular cavity obliteration. From Converse *et al.*,[17] with permission.

Fig. 5.11. Segments of an original record from one hypotensive-prone patient showing the mean voltage neurogram of sympathetic nerve activity, the blood pressure tracing and plethysmographic tracings of calf blood flow at baseline and during haemodialysis. Haemodialysis initially caused increases in sympathetic nerve activity and decreases in calf blood flow accompanied by moderate decreases in blood pressure and increases in heart rate. With further haemodialysis, an abrupt fall in blood pressure was accompanied by abrupt decreases in sympathetic nerve activity, heart rate and vascular resistance. From Converse *et al.*,[17] with permission.

hypotension during haemodialysis. These findings, however, again provide only circumstantial evidence in support of, and do not prove, the 'ventricular mechanoreceptor' hypothesis.

Summary and conclusions

Most current textbooks of internal medicine and cardiology emphasize that activation of the sympathetic nervous system produces many of the classic clinical signs of hypovolaemic shock, including peripheral vasoconstriction and tachycardia. Although some textbooks suggest that acidaemia and hypoxaemia may attenuate the ability of the cardiovascular system to respond appropriately to increased sympathetic neural drive during the decompensated stage of hypovolaemic shock. In contrast to this traditional teaching, the wealth of experimental animal and human data reviewed in this chapter demonstrate that, regardless of the precise underlying mechanism(s), sympathetic inhibition can occur in a much earlier stage of hypovolaemic hypotension than previously thought and that such sympathoinhibition is often reversible.

Acknowledgement

This chapter was supported by National Heart, Lung and Blood Institute Grant RO-1 HL44010.

References

1. Bedford EA and Jackson HC: The epinephrine content of the blood in conditions of low blood pressure and 'shock'. *Proceedings of the Society for Experimental Biology and Medicine*, 1916; **13,** 85–7.
2. Vatner SF: Effects of hemorrhage on regional blood flow distribution in dogs and primates. *Journal of Clinical Investigation*, 1974; **54,** 225–35.
3. Abboud FM: Shock. In Wyngaarden JB, Smith LM and Bennett JC (eds): *Cecil Textbook of Medicine*. Philadelphia, PA, WB Saunders Co., 1985, 211–25.
4. Vissing SF, Scherrer U and Victor RG: Relation between sympathetic outflow and vascular resistance in the calf during perturbations in central venous pressure. Evidence for cardiopulmonary afferent regulation of calf vascular resistance in humans. *Circulation Research*, 1989; **65,** 1710–17.
5. Wiel MH, von Planta M and Rackow EC: Acute circulatory failure (shock). In Braunwald E (ed.): *Heart Disease. A Textbook of Cardiovascular Medicine*, 4th edn. Philadelphia, PA, WB Saunders Co., 1991: 569–84.
6. Guyton AC: *Textbook of Medical Physiology*, 8th edn. Philadelphia, PA, WB Saunders Co., 1991, 263–71.
7. Hurst JW, Schlant RC, Rackley CE, Sonnenblick EH and Wenger NK: *The Heart*, 7th edn, New York, NY, McGraw-Hill, 1990, 442–61.
8. West JB; *Physiological Basis of Medical Practice*, 12th edn, Baltimore, MD, Williams and Wilkins, 1991, 318–31.
9. Parrillo JH: Shock. In Wilson JD, Braunwald E, Isselbacher KJ, Petersdorf RG, Martin JB, Fauci AS and Root RK (eds): *Harrison's Principles of Internal Medicine*, 12th edn, New York, NY, McGraw-Hill, 1991, 232–7.
10. Ferguson DW: Shock. In Wyngaarden JB, Smith LH and Bennet JC (eds): *Cecil Textbook of Medicine*, 19th edn. Philadelphia PA, WB Saunders Co., 1991, 207–28.
11. Secher NH, Jensen KS and Werner C: Bradycardia during hypovolemic shock, clinical observations of heart rate and blood pressure. *Acta Physiologica Scandinavica*, 1984; **121,** 49A (abstract).
12. Secher NH, Sander-Jensen K, Werner C and Warberg J: Bradycardia during severe but reversible hypovolemic shock in man. *Circulatory Shock*, 1984; **14,** 267–74.
13. Secher NH and Bie P: Bradycardia during reversible hemorrhagic shock – a forgotten observation? *Clinical Physiology*, 1985; **5,** 315–23.
14. Jansen RPS: Relative bradycardia: a sign of acute intraperitoneal bleeding. *Australian and New Zealand Journal of Obstetrics and Gynaecology*, 1978; **18,** 206–8.
15. Ludbrook J: Vasodilator responses to acute blood loss. *Australian and New Zealand Journal of Surgery*, 1987; **57,** 511–13.
16. van Lieshout JJ, Wieling W, Karemaker JM and Eckberg DL: The vasovagal response. *Clinical Science*, 1991; **81,** 575–85.
17. Converse RL Jr, Jacobsen TN, Jost CMT, Toto RD, Grayburn PA, Obregon TM, Fouad-Tarazi F and Victor RG: Paradoxical withdrawal of reflex vasoconstriction as a cause of hemodialysis-induced hypotension. *Journal of Clinical Investigation*, 1992; **90,** 1657–65.
18. Victor RG, Thoren P, Morgan DA and Mark AL: Differential control of adrenal and renal sympathetic nerve activity during hemorrhagic hypotension in rats. *Circulation Research*, 1989; **64,** 686–94.
19. Vallbo AB, Hagbarth K-E, Torebjörk HE and Wallin BG: Somatosensory, proprioceptive, and sympathetic activity in human peripheral nerves. *Physiology Review*, 1979; **59,** 919–57.
20. Sundlöf G and Wallin BG: Human muscle nerve sympathetic activity at rest. Relationship to blood

pressure and age. *Journal of Physiology (London)*, 1978; **274,** 621–37.
21. Coleridge HM, Coleridge JCG and Kidd C: Cardiac receptors in the dog, with particular reference to two types of afferent ending in the ventricular wall. *Journal of Physiology (London)*, 1964; **174,** 323–9.
22. Oberg B and Thoren P: Studies on left ventricular receptors. Signalling in non-medullate vagal afferents. *Acta Physiologica Scandinavica*, 1972; **85,** 145–63.
23. Thoren PN: Activation of left ventricular receptors with nonmedullated vagal afferent fibers during occlusion of a coronary artery in the cat. *American Journal of Cardiology*, 1976; **37,** 1046–51.
24. Thoren PN: Characteristics of left ventricular receptors with nonmedullated vagal afferents in cats. *Circulation Research*, 1977; **40,** 415–21.
25. Coleridge JCG and Coleridge HM: Afferent C-fiber and cardiorespiratory chemoreflexes. *American Review of Respiratory Disease*, 1977; **115,** 251–60.
26. Thoren P: Role of cardiac vagal C-fibers in cardiovascular control. *Reviews of Physiology, Biochemistry and Pharmacology*, 1979; **86,** 1–94.
27. Thoren P, Noresson E and Ricksten S-E: Cardiac receptors with vagal non-medullated vagal afferents in the rat. *Acta Physiologica Scandinavica*, 1979; **105,** 295–303.
28. Coleridge HM and Coleridge JCG: Cardiovascular afferents involved in regulation of peripheral vessels. *Annual Review of Physiology*, 1980; **42,** 413–27.
29. Bishop VS, Malliani A and Thoren P: Cardiac mechanoreceptors. In Shepherd JT and Abboud FM (eds): *Handbook of Physiology, Section 2: The Cardiovascular System, Volume 3.* Bethesda, MD, American Physiological Society, 1983, 497–545.
30. Abboud FM: Ventricular syncope: is the heart a sensory organ? *New England Journal of Medicine*, 1989; **320,** 390–92.
31. Jarish A and Zotterman Y: Depressor reflexes from the heart. *Acta Physiologica Scandinavica*, 1949; **16,** 31–51.
32. Oberg B and White S: Circulatory effects of interruption and stimulation of cardiac vagal afferents. *Acta Physiologica Scandinavica*, 1970; **80,** 383–94.
33. von Bezold A and Hirt L: Uber die physiologischen wirkungen des essigsauren veratrins. *Unters Physiologische Laboratorium Wurzburg*, 1867; **1,** 73–156.
34. Abrahamsson H and Thoren P: Vomiting and reflex vagal relaxation of the stomach elicited from heart receptors in the cat. *Acta Physiological Scandinavica*, 1973; **88,** 433–9.
35. Oberg B and White S: The role for vagal cardiac nerves and arterial baroreceptors in the circulatory adjustment to hemorrhage in the cat. *Acta Physiologica Scandinavica*, 1970; **80,** 395–403.
36. Oberg B and Thoren P: Increased activity in left ventricular receptors during hemorrhage or occlusion of caval veins in the cat. A possible cause of the vasovagal reaction. *Acta Physiologica Scandinavica*, 1972; **85,** 164–73.
37. Longhurst JC: Cardiac receptors: their function in health and disease. *Progress in Cardiovascular Diseases*, 1984; **27,** 201–22.
38. Hainsworth R: Reflexes from the heart. *Physiological Reviews*, 1991; **71,** 617–58.
39. Henry JP: *Studies of the Physiology of Negative Acceleration. An Approach to the Problem of Protection.* Air Force Technical Report H 5953, USAF Air Material Command WPAF Base, OH, Oct. 1950.
40. Sharpey-Shafer EP: Emergencies in general practice. Syncope. *British Medical Journal*, 1956; **1,** 506–9.
41. Mark AL and Mancia G: Cardiopulmonary baroreflexes in humans. In Shepherd JT and Abboud FM (eds): *Handbook of Physiology. Section 2: The Cardiovascular System, Volume 3.* Bethesda, MD, American Physiological Society, 1983, 795–813.
42. Oberg B and Thoren P: Increased activity in vagal cardiac afferents correlated to the appearance of reflex bradycardia during severe hemorrhage in cats. *Acta Physiologica Scandinavica*, 1970; **80,** 22–3A (communication).
43. Skoog P, Mansson J and Thorén P: Changes in renal sympathetic outflow during hypotensive haemorrhage in rats. *Acta Physiologica Scandinavica*, 1985; **125,** 655–60.
44. Thoren P: Reflex bradycardia elicited from left ventricular receptors during acute severe hypoxia in cats. *Acta Physiologica Scandinavica*, 1973; **87,** 103–12.
45. Thoren P: Evidence for a depressor reflex elicited from left ventricular receptors during occlusion of one coronary artery in the cat. *Acta Physiologica Scandinavica*, 1973; **88,** 23–34.
46. Morgan DA, Thoren P, Wilczynski EA, Victor RG and Mark AL: Serotonergic mechanisms mediate renal sympathoinhibition during severe hemorrhage in rats. *American Journal of Physiology*, 1988; **255,** H496–502.
47. Peuler JD, Schmid PG, Morgan DA and Mark AL: Inhibition of renal sympathetic activity and heart rate by vasopressin in hemorrhaged diabetes insipidus rats. *American Journal of Physiology*, 1990; **258,** H706–12.
48. Morita H and Vatner S: Effects of hemorrhage on renal nerve activity in conscious dogs. *Circulation Research*, 1985; **57,** 788–93.
49. Morita H, Manders WT and Vatner SF: Opiate receptor mediated decrease in renal activity during hemorrhage in conscious rabbits. *Circulation*, 1985; **72,** 244 (abstract).
50. Morita H, Nishida Y, Motochigawa H, Uemura N, Hosomi H and Vatner SF: Opiate receptor mediated decrease in renal nerve activity during hypotensive hemorrhage in conscious rabbits. *Circulation Research*, 1988; **63,** 165–72.
51. Landgren S: On the excitation mechanism of the

carotid baroreceptors. *Acta Physiologica Scandinavica*, 1952; **24,** 1–34.

52. Felder RB, Heesch CM and Thames MD: Reflex modulation of carotid sinus baroreceptor activity in the dog. *American Journal of Physiology*, 1983; **244,** H437–43.
53. Munch PA, Thoren PN and Brown AM: Dual effects of norepinephrine and mechanisms of baroreceptors stimulation. *Circulation Research*, 1987; **61,** 409–19.
54. Grant RT and Reeve EB: Clinical observations on aid-raid casualties. *British Medical Journal*, 1941; **ii,** 293–7; 329–32.
55. McMichael J: Clinical aspects of shock. *Journal of the American Medical Association*, 1944; **124,** 275–81.
56. Sander-Jensen K, Secher NH, Bie P, Warberg J and Schwartz TW: Vagal slowing of the heart during hemorrhage: observations from 20 consecutive hypotensive patients. *British Medical Journal*, 1986; **292,** 364–6.
57. Rørsgaard S and Secher NH: Slowing of the heart during hypotension in major abdominal surgery. *Acta Anaesthesiologica Scandinavica*, 1986; 507–10.
58. Wallin BG and Sundlöf G: Sympathetic outflow to muscles during vasovagal syncope. *Journal of the Autonomic Nervous System*, 1982; **6,** 287–91.
59. Almquist A, Goldenberg IF, Milstein S, Chen M-Y, Chen X, Hansen R, Gornick CG and Benditt DG: Provocation of bradycardia and hypotension by isoproterenol and upright posture in patients with unexplained syncope. *New England Journal of Medicine*, 1989; **320,** 346–51.
60. Scherrer U, Vissing SF, Morgan BJ, Hanson P and Victor RG: Vasovagal syncope after infusion of a vasodilator in a heart-transplant recipient. *New England Journal of Medicine*, 1990; **322,** 602–4.
61. Milstein S, Buetokofer J, Lesser J, Goldenberg IF, Benditt DG, Gornick C and Reyes JW: Cardiac asystole: a manifestation of neurally mediated hypotension bradycardia. *Journal of the American College of Cardiology*, 1989; **14,** 1626–32.
62. Chen M-Y, Goldenberg IF, Milstein S, Buetikofer J, Almqvist A, Lesser J and Benditt DG: Cardiac electrophysiologic and hemodynamic correlates of neurally mediated syncope. *American Journal of Cardiology*, 1989; **63,** 66–72.
63. Shalev Y, Gal R, Tchou PJ, Anderson AA, Avitall B, Akhtar M and Jozayeri MR: Echocardiographic demonstration of decreased left ventricular dimensions and vigorous myocardial contraction during syncope induced by head-up tilt. *Journal of the American College of Cardiology*, 1991; **18,** 746–51.
64. Rea RF: Neurally mediated hypotension and bradycardia: which nerves? how mediated? *Journal of the American College of Cardiology*, 1989; **14,** 1633–4.

6

Cardiovascular regulation during hypovolaemic shock – central integration

Emrys Kirkman and Roderick A Little

The aim of this chapter is to review aspects of the central nervous organization of the cardiovascular response to acute hypovolaemia, where possible identifying neurotransmitters involved in these central nervous pathways, and hence suggesting pharmacological agents that could be used to modify the response.

Acute circulatory hypovolaemia is the consequence of haemorrhage or a loss of circulatory fluid into the tissues, often as a result of trauma, and is therefore frequently accompanied by tissue damage or 'injury'. In the context of this chapter, the term 'injury' will be used to denote tissue damage and the associated activation of afferent nociceptive fibres, and does not itself involve the loss of circulating fluid. There is evidence that the cardiovascular response to hypovolaemia can be modified by the response to 'injury'. However, relatively little is known of the central nervous pathways specifically involved in the responses to either hypovolaemia or 'injury'. Fortunately, there is a wealth of knowledge regarding the pathways of individual cardiovascular reflexes which together may generate the responses to hypovolaemia and 'injury'. It is therefore pertinent to summarize briefly the cardiovascular responses to hypovolaemia and its component reflexes, before discussing the relevant central nervous pathways and how the response may be modulated by concomitant 'injury'. Finally, the clinical implications of this information will be discussed.

The cardiovascular response to hypovolaemia

One of the most studied causes of acute circulatory hypovolaemia is haemorrhage, both real[1,2] and simulated.[3,4] The cardiovascular response to haemorrhage has been reviewed extensively elsewhere[5] (see also this volume), and will therefore be the subject of only a brief summary in this chapter.

A progressive 'simple' haemorrhage (loss of blood in the absence of major tissue damage, e.g. rupture of varices) produces a biphasic pattern of response (see Fig. 3.2, p. 26). In the initial stages there is a progressive increase in heart rate and vascular resistance which can maintain arterial blood pressure close to prehaemorrhage levels following blood losses of up to 10–15 per cent of the blood volume in a young, otherwise healthy, individual.[1,6] However, as the severity of haemorrhage increases and exceeds 20 per cent of the blood volume, a very different pattern of response becomes apparent, namely a marked bradycardia and peripheral vasodilatation accompanied by a precipitous fall in blood pressure, which may lead to syncope (see Fig. 3.2, p. 26).[1] Since the elucidation of the mechanisms (and central nervous pathways) of these responses to blood loss have involved investigations on animals, it should be stressed that the finer details of the response appear to vary depending on species studied, and the choice of anaesthetic agent, if any.[5] The pattern of response seen in the conscious rat clearly resembles that seen in humans (Fig. 6.1a), with heart rate during severe

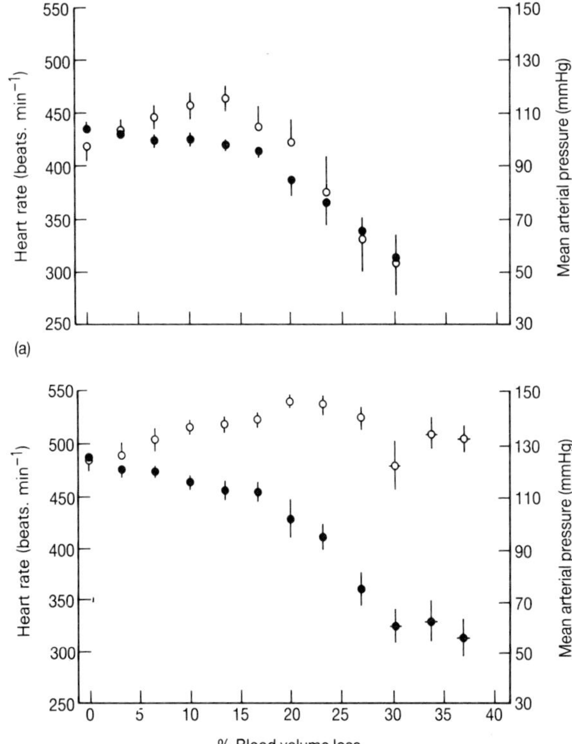

Fig. 6.1. The effects of (a) progressive 'simple' haemorrhage and (b) haemorrhage in the presence of bilateral hind-limb ischaemia on heart rate (○) and mean arterial blood pressure (●) in the conscious rat. Values are expressed as means ±SE.

haemorrhage falling below prehaemorrhage values. By contrast, severe hypovolaemia in the conscious rabbit does not generally yield a frank bradycardia, with heart rate falling below the maximum levels seen during the early response, but remaining above prehaemorrhage levels.[7] Despite the modest effect on heart rate, severe hypovolaemia does result in a marked reduction in vascular resistance and hence hypotension in the conscious rabbit, as in humans.[7]

The function of the two stages of the response to hypovolaemia appears to be protective. Stage 1 (response to mild or moderate blood loss) maintains arterial blood pressure, and, due to a selective pattern of increased vascular resistance, preserves blood flow and hence oxygen delivery to those organs most critically dependent on it, i.e. brain and myocardium, at the expense of less dependent organs, e.g. skeletal muscle.[8] The second, bradycardic, stage limits the haemorrhage-induced reduction in end-systolic blood volume,[9] and may reduce cardiac work at a time when coronary perfusion may be in danger of becoming compromised, thus limiting the possibility of ischaemic damage to the heart.[10]

Reflexes involved in the response to haemorrhage

In explaining the biphasic response to blood loss three reflexes need to be considered; the arterial baroreceptor reflex, a reflex originating from the heart (the 'cardiac' reflex), and the arterial chemoreceptor reflex.

The arterial baroreceptor reflex

This reflex is thought to be responsible for the maintenance of arterial blood pressure following the loss of 10–15 per cent of the blood volume. The baroreceptor reflex normally minimizes moment-to-moment variations in blood pressure around a given 'set-point', which itself can be altered.[11] The baroreceptor endings are located mainly in the aortic arch and carotid sinus.[8] The baroreceptors respond to the degree of stretch of the arterial wall produced by the intraluminal pressure, rather than to the intraluminal pressure itself,[12] and display a 'rate sensitivity' that allows them to respond to the rate of change of arterial blood pressure as well as to its absolute level.[13] Consequently, they can respond to a change in pulse pressure as well as changes in mean pressure.

Thus, as pulse pressure diminishes during haemorrhage there is a decrease in baroreceptor afferent activity, even in the absence of a fall in *mean* arterial pressure. This change in baroreceptor afferent activity is signalled to the brain via the vagus nerve (from the aortic arch baroreceptors) and the sinus nerve, a branch of the glossopharyngeal nerve (from the carotid sinus baroreceptors[8,11]). The efferent limb of the baroreceptor reflex is carried in the vagus and sympathetic nerves to the heart, and in the sympathetic vasoconstrictor nerves to the blood vessels.[8] When the baroreceptors are unloaded following a haemorrhage there is a resultant reflex withdrawal of vagal–cardiac and an enhancement of sympatho–cardiac activity, leading to a tachycardia, and an increase in the activity of the sympathetic vasoconstrictor fibres leading to increased total peripheral resistance. It should be emphasized that activation of the sympathetic supply to the various vascular beds is not uniform, with some experiencing a more intense vasoconstriction than others.[8] As a consequence of these haemodynamic changes, any haemorrhage-induced falls in arterial blood pressure are minimized or prevented in the face of losses of up to 10–15 per cent of the blood volume, and blood flow is maintained to tissues critically dependent on oxygen delivery (e.g. brain) at the expense of other organs (e.g. skeletal muscle) where oxygen delivery is less critical, at least in the short-term.

However, as blood loss exceeds 20 per cent of the blood volume, blood pressure falls dramatically (Fig. 6.1a and Fig. 3.2, see p. 26). This is not due to a sudden failure of the baroreceptor reflex,[15] or the imminent demise of the heart, but rather is due to the activation of a second reflex – that elicited by activation of cardiac afferents.

The 'cardiac' reflex

Following a severe haemorrhage (>20 per cent of the blood volume) it has been postulated that mechanosensitive receptor endings located in the ventricular myocardium are stimulated by deformations of the ventricular wall as the heart contracts vigorously around an incompletely filled chamber.[16] The receptor endings form part of a heterogeneous population of receptors consisting of purely mechano-, purely chemo- and mixed mechano/chemosensitive endings.[17] The efferent pathway from these ventricular receptors is carried in C-fibres in the vagus.[17] Stimulation of these cardiac vagal afferent C-fibres by either mechanical or chemical means (e.g. prostaglandin E_2(PGE_2), 5-HT or phenylbiguanide[18]) leads to a profound reflex bradycardia, hypotension and reduction in skeletal muscle and renal vascular resistance,[19,20] a pattern of response reminiscent of that seen during severe hypovolaemia. The bradycardia is due to increased vagal efferent activity to the heart, while the reduction in vascular resistance is due to a withdrawal of sympathetic vasoconstrictor tone.[19,20] Evidence supporting the role of this 'cardiac' reflex in the response to severe haemorrhage is provided by the observation that instillation of procaine into the pericardial sac so as to block the afferent pathway can prevent the reduction in renal sympathetic vasoconstrictor activity normally seen during severe central hypovolaemia.[7,21] Furthermore, sectioning the cervical vagi can reverse the bradycardia in experimental animals, and both the bradycardia and fall in blood pressure are attenuated markedly in animals that are deficient in afferent C-fibres.[2] It therefore seems likely that the depressor reflex associated with a severe haemorrhage originates from the heart itself, and the afferent pathway is carried in cardiac vagal C-fibres. However, some recent studies shed doubt on the precise nature of the afferent pathway,[22–24] and suggest that the chemosensitive (5-HT sensitive) vagal afferent C-fibres may not play a role in the response to severe haemorrhage, at least in the rabbit (see p. 63).[23,24]

Since the efferent limb mediating the cardioinhibitory component of this reflex is carried in the vagus nerve (see above), it is not surprising that the bradycardia can be prevented by treatment with atropine in both humans[1,25] and experimental animals.[2] However, caution must be exercised before undertaking such a treatment, since there are indications that blocking this bradycardia may be deleterious (see pp. 70–71), unless there is very severe bradycardia or asystole.

The arterial chemoreceptor reflex

The third reflex of importance in the cardiovascular response to haemorrhage is the arterial chemoreceptor reflex. The arterial chemoreceptors are found in the carotid and aortic bodies, close to the carotid sinus and aortic arch, respectively. They respond to changes in oxygen tension, a fall in oxygen tension increasing chemoreceptor afferent activity. In addition, increases in carbon dioxide tension and falls in arterial blood pH increase the sensitivity of the arterial chemoreceptors to hypoxia.[26] Stimulation of arterial chemoreceptors produces an increase in respiration,[14] while the primary cardiovascular effects are a vagally mediated bradycardia and a vasoconstriction in, for example, skeletal muscle, which is due to increased sympathetic vasoconstrictor tone.[27] This pattern of response is subsequently modified by the increased respiratory activity, which tends to inhibit both the vagal activity to the heart and the sympathetic vasoconstrictor activity.[28]

Following a severe haemorrhage the arterial chemoreceptors are activated as a result of a reduction in blood flow through the carotid and aortic bodies secondary to the fall in arterial blood pressure, and to sympathetic vasoconstriction in the bodies themselves[29,30] mediated by the local release of both noradrenaline and its cotransmitter neuropeptide Y.[31] Therefore, during the hypotensive stage of a severe haemorrhage stimulation of the arterial chemoreceptors may prevent arterial blood pressure from falling even further,[32] and may be responsible for the increase in respiration noted following severe haemorrhage.[33] Since an increase in respiratory activity has been shown to reduce the reflex bradycardia produced by stimulation of cardiac C-fibre afferents,[20] it is possible that the enhanced respiratory activity seen following a severe haemorrhage may attenuate the bradycardia seen under these circumstances. This interaction between the respiratory and cardiovascular responses to chemoreceptor stimulation may also have further implications for the treatment of injured patients. For example, procedures such as intubation which inhibit respiratory activity can unmask a dangerous bradycardia.[34] The role of the chemoreceptors in helping to maintain blood pressure will, of course, be increased in the injured patient with thoracic injuries that may impair pulmonary function.

Central nervous pathways involved in the cardiovascular response to haemorrhage

The central nervous pathway of the baroreceptor reflex has been studied extensively, and is the subject of numerous reviews.[28,35] Consequently, this chapter will provide only a brief summary of some of the central nervous pathways involved in this reflex.

The baroreceptor afferent fibres terminate exclusively within the nucleus of the tractus solitarius (NTS) in the brainstem.[28] As described earlier, the efferent limb of the baroreceptor reflex is carried in both the parasympathetic nerves (vagi) to the heart and the sympathetic supply to the heart and peripheral vasculature. The cell bodies of the vagal cardiac preganglionic motor neurones are located in the nucleus ambiguus and dorsal vagal motor nucleus.[36,37] The sympathetic preganglionic cell bodies are found in the intermediolateral columns of the thoracic and upper lumbar segments of the spinal cord.[38]

Control of vagal efferent activity

The baroreceptor afferents are thought to influence vagal efferent activity via two main pathways; a short latency pathway that is complete within the medulla, i.e. a segmental pathway traversing from the NTS to the nucleus ambiguus, and a longer latency pathway that ascends to relay in the anterior hypothalamus before descending to the nucleus ambiguus (Fig. 6.2a).[28] Activation of either of these pathways, following stimulation of the baroreceptors, leads to excitation of the vagal cardiac preganglionic motor neurones within the nucleus ambiguus[28] and consequently a bradycardia.

The arterial chemoreceptor afferents also terminate within the NTS.[28,39] From the NTS there is a secondary, excitatory projection that activates both the vagal cardiac preganglionic motor neurones and the inspiratory neurones within the nucleus ambiguus (Fig. 6.2b). Additionally, the arterial chemoreceptors may influence neurones within the vagal nuclei via a direct (primary afferent) projection.[39] The inspiratory neurones (which project to the spinal cord and activate the motor neurones which cause contraction of the diaphragm[40,41]) send a cholinergic inhibitory collateral onto the vagal cardiac preganglionic motor neurone.[42] This, coupled with a second inhibitory output originating from lung stretch afferent fibres,[27] which are activated when the lungs inflate during inspiration, attenuates or even reverses the increase in vagal efferent activity to the heart. However, when the arterial chemoreceptor-induced respiratory stimulation is prevented, e.g. during intubation, then the bradycardia becomes apparent.[34]

The central nervous pathway of the reflex elicited by activation of the cardiac C-fibre afferents has been studied less extensively. Nevertheless, the afferent fibres appear to terminate within the NTS[43] and, via a secondary pathway, lead to excitation of vagal efferent fibres to the heart.

Control of sympathetic efferent activity

The cell bodies of the sympathetic preganglionic neurones (which cause vasoconstriction) are found in the intermediolateral column of the spinal cord. They are influenced by nervous pathways descending from the brain. One such pathway, which is a major source of excitatory drive to the sympathetic preganglionic neurones, originates in the nucleus paragigantocellularis lateralis in the rostral ventrolateral medulla (RVLM; Fig. 6.3).[44,45] This pathway, probably by releasing the excitatory amino acid glutamate within the intermediolateral cell column,[46] contributes towards the maintenance of resting sympathetic tone, and hence arterial blood pressure. Activation of the baroreceptor

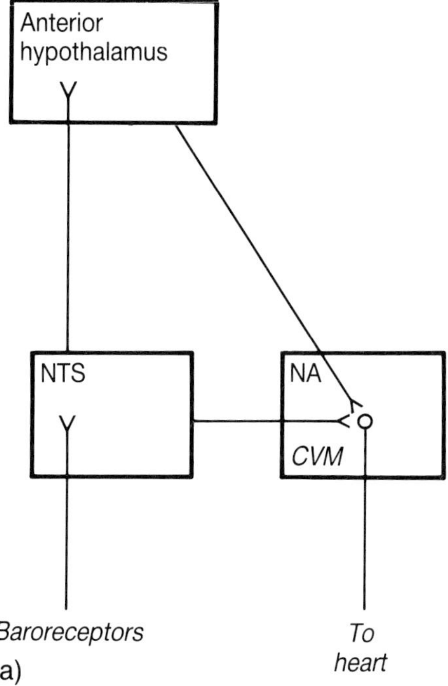

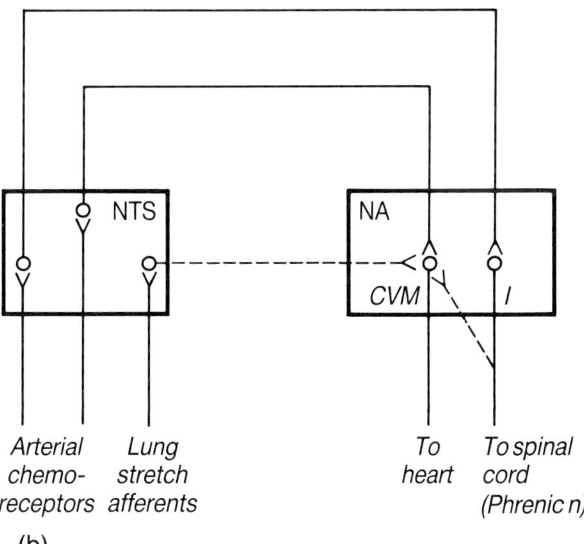

Fig. 6.2. (a) Schematic diagram indicating two pathways whereby the baroreceptors can influence vagal efferent activity to the heart and (b) pathways whereby activation of the arterial chemoreceptors leads to excitation of vagal cardiac and inspiratory neurones, while stimulation of the lung stretch receptors leads to inhibition of the vagal cardiac neurones. —, Excitatory pathways; ---, inhibitory pathways; NTS, nucleus tractus solitarius; NA, nucleus ambiguus; CVM, vagal cardiac preganglionic motorneurone; I, inspiratory neurone.

afferents leads to an inhibition of these sympatho-excitatory cells within the RVLM[47] via a pathway which originates in the NTS and relays in the caudal ventrolateral medulla (CVLM;[35] Fig. 6.3). There is evidence to suggest that this pathway involves both excitatory amino acids acting at *N*-methyl-D-aspartate (NMDA) and non-NMDA receptors in the CVLM,[48] and the inhibitory amino acid γ-aminobutyric acid (GABA) within the RVLM.[35] Unfortunately, pharmacological interference with these amino acid neurotransmitters is unlikely to be useful clinically since they are major transmitters in a large number of other (unrelated) control systems.

In addition to releasing the excitatory amino acid glutamate within the intermediolateral cell column to maintain sympathetic tone (see above), it has been suggested that individual RVLM neurones may also release a number of other neurotransmitters that can influence the sympathetic vasomotor activity.[49] A recent study has suggested the exciting possibility that events, e.g. haemorrhage, could cause an alteration in the synthesis, and hence possibly the relative proportion of the various cotransmitters released within the spinal cord by these RVLM neurones.[50] Thus, it may be possible that haemorrhage can modulate the effects of this neuronal pathway merely by altering the relative proportions of transmitters and cotransmitters released by its terminations.

The central nervous pathways mediating the

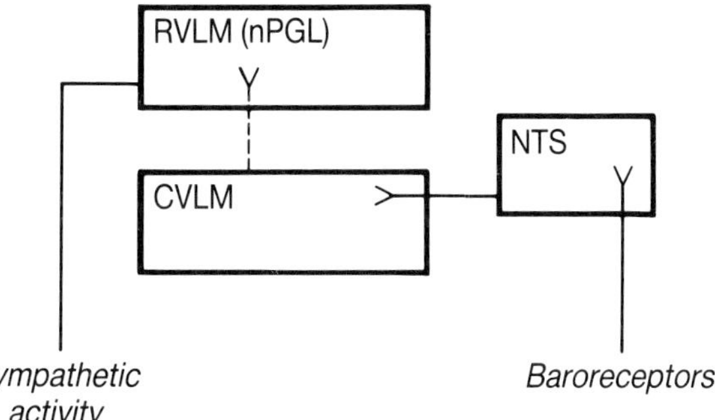

Fig. 6.3. Schematic diagram indicating a pathway whereby the baroreceptors can influence sympathetic efferent activity to the heart and blood vessels. —, Excitatory pathways; ---, inhibitory pathways; NTS, nucleus tractus solitarius; CVLM, caudal ventrolateral medulla; RVLM, rostral ventrolateral medulla; nPGL, nucleus paragigantocellularis lateralis. *Note*: This represents a simplified account, for fuller details see Seller.[35]

sympathoinhibition associated with severe hypovolaemia have been studied less extensively. The primary afferent fibres (the cardiac vagal C-fibres; see p. 63) terminate within the NTS (see pp. 64–5). The secondary projection appears to ascend to suprapontine levels before descending again to the medulla,[51] producing a sympathoinhibitory effect involving the activation of δ-opioid receptors.[7] This pathway could be a potential target for pharmacological interference in the traumatized patient (see below).

Neurotransmitters involved in the cardiovascular response to blood loss

The endogenous opioids

There is a strong body of evidence suggesting that the endogenous opioid system may be involved in the response to severe hypovolaemia. Most of the evidence suggests a role for the opioid system in the sympathoinhibitory response. However, there is also some, albeit weaker, evidence suggesting their role in the bradycardic response. Thus, the opioid antagonist naloxone, when given intravenously, was shown to attenuate the reduction in sympathetic efferent activity and the associated hypotension, and possibly the bradycardia which accompanies severe hypovolaemia.[21,52] Naloxone, in this case, is thought to exert its effect via an antagonist action at δ-opiate receptors within the medulla.[7,53,54] It should be stressed here that although the administration of naxolone, or of a more specific δ-opioid receptor antagonist (ICI 174864), clearly blocked the sympathoinhibition,[53,23] the effects of δ-antagonism on the bradycardia were less clear. This may be due to the relatively small bradycardic response to severe hypovolaemia even in the absence of δ-antagonism in these studies, which were conducted on rabbits. Nevertheless the trend is apparent (Fig. 2 in Evans and Ludbrook[23]). Since δ-opioid receptor antagonism appears to block *both* the vagal and the sympathetic component of the response to severe hypovolaemia, it is likely that the endogenous opioids are important early in the reflex pathway, before the two limbs diverge. One likely area is the NTS,[54] which contains a dense population of δ-opioid receptors.[55,56]

In addition to the δ-opioid receptors, the μ- and the κ-receptors also appear to be capable of modifying the response to severe hypovolaemia. Thus, μ- and κ-receptor *agonists* can also prevent the reflex sympathoinhibition (and possibly the bradycardia) seen during severe hypovolaemia.[23,53,54] However, it is unlikely that the μ-opioid receptor participates in the normal 'physiological' response to severe haemorrhage,[54] although the use of μ-receptor agonists, e.g. the anaesthetics fentanyl and alfentanyl,[5] may provide a pharmacological means of inhibiting the depressor effect of a severe haemorrhage. Whether this would be beneficial or detrimental (bearing in mind the potential protective effects of this depressor reflex, and the consequences of blocking it; see pp. 63 and 70–71) remains to be seen.

The studies of the role of central opioid receptors in the response to severe hypovolaemia also raise another important question:

What is the precise nature of the afferent pathway involved in the 'cardiac' reflex?

It has long been argued that the afferent pathway is carried in the cardiac vagal C-fibres, which arise from a heterogenous population of receptors in the ventricular myocardium, some responding purely to mechanical, some to chemical, but the majority to both stimuli (see p. 63). No distinction has been made between the physiological responses to these various receptors, or indeed their reflex pathways.[17] However, Evans and Ludbrook[23] showed in the rabbit that whereas the depressor response to severe hypovolaemia could be inhibited by antagonizing δ-opioid receptors or stimulating μ-receptors within the medulla, the depressor response seen when the cardiac ventricular receptors were stimulated chemically with the 5-HT_3 receptor agonist phenylbiguanide could not, indicating that different central nervous pathways were used by the two responses. Evans and Ludbrook[23] concluded that the cardiac afferents responsible for initiating the depressor response associated with severe hypovolaemia were unlikely to correspond to the phenylbiguanide (5-HT, chemosensitive) receptors, at least in the rabbit. It is therefore possible that they have uncovered a neurochemical difference in the reflex arcs initiated, respectively, by the two populations of receptors. However, this explanation is likely to be an oversimplification since it does not account for the majority of ventricular receptors that respond to both mechanical and chemical stimuli. Clearly this requires further investigation.

5-Hydroxytryptamine

Despite the absence of a peripheral role for 5-HT

in the response to severe hypovolaemia, it does appear to play a role within the central nervous system. Blockade of the 5-HT system, either with p-chlorophenylalanine (PCPA, which blocks the synthesis of 5-HT) or with the 5-HT receptor antagonist methysergide, specifically prevents or reverses both the sympathoinhibitory and the bradycardic response to severe haemorrhage, while leaving baroreflex control intact.[57] Although the 5-HT 'blocking' agents were given intravenously, their sites of action are likely to be central in this case, since any effects of 5-HT on the ventricular receptors (largely discounted in the response to hypovolaemia; see p. 66) is mediated via 5-HT_3 receptors,[58] where methysergide has little activity.[59] It is impossible to determine the central site(s) at which the 5-HT antagonists attenuate the response to severe hypovolaemia from these studies. However, the picture becomes very complicated with recent reports that 5-HT *agonists* can also produce a similar effect (cited by Evans and Ludbrook[60]), presumably at a different central nervous site.

The parabrachial nuclei and the caudal ventrolateral periaqueductal grey

More rostrally in the brainstem, cells within the ventrolateral parts of the parabrachial nuclei and the Kolliker–Fuse nucleus provide a major projection to the ventrolateral medulla (Fig. 6.4).[61] These areas are of particular interest since they receive a projection from the NTS,[62] and hence are likely to receive haemodynamic information. Recent studies by Ward[63] have shown that cells in this region respond to haemorrhage. Three patterns of response could be found that were related to the anatomical location of the cells within the parabrachial and Kolliker–Fuse nuclei:[63]

(a) The first group of neurones exhibited an increase in activity following haemorrhage, which was not reversed immediately during reinfusion, i.e. the neurones appeared to show a *memory* of the blood loss. Ward[63] suggested that these cells may therefore be responding to the neuroendocrine as well as the haemodynamic changes induced by blood loss.

(b) A second group of neurones exhibited an increased activity during haemorrhage, which was reversed by reinfusion. These cells are thought to signal changes in blood *volume* rather than pressure.

(c) The final group of cells showed a reduction in activity during haemorrhage, which was reversed on reinfusion, i.e. a mirror image of the activity in (b). This last group of cells may receive an input from other areas within the parabrachial nuclei since they do not receive directly any cardiovascular afferent information.

Ward[63] concludes by stating that although the specific functions of these parabrachial neurones are obscure at present, they may play a critical role in the control of neuroendocrine and sympathetic responses to blood loss (Fig. 6.4).

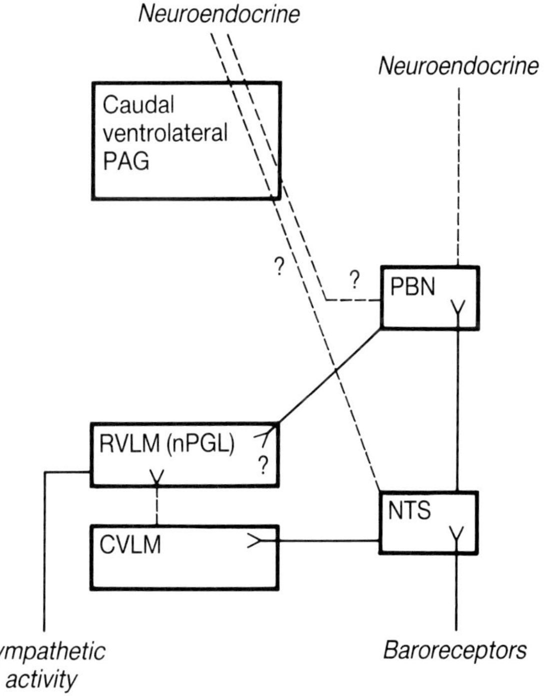

Fig. 6.4. Schematic diagram indicating some of the central nervous pathways involved in an integrated cardiovascular and neuroendocrine response to haemorrhage. —, Excitatory pathways; ---, inhibitory pathways; ?, putative pathways which may be excitatory or inhibitory; Baroreceptors, arterial baroreceptors (and other cardiovascular receptors, e.g. atrial low pressure baroreceptors); NTS, nucleus tractus solitarius; PBN, parabrachial and Kolliker–Fuse nuclei; PAG, periaqueductal grey; CVLM, caudal ventrolateral medulla; RVLM, rostral ventrolateral medulla; nPGL, nucleus paragigantocellularis lateralis.

Finally, the caudal ventrolateral periaqueductal grey may also play a role in the cardiovascular response to haemorrhage, since lesions in this area impair markedly the ability to respond to a mild haemorrhage.[64] This region may contain cell bodies or fibres of passage transmitting information from the NTS and parabrachial nuclei to the lateral hypothalamus (Fig. 6.4), and may therefore be involved in both the cardiovascular and neuroendocrine responses to haemorrhage.[64]

Thus, a number of central nervous pathways can be identified as being of importance in the cardiovascular response to blood loss. The functions of some of these pathways are relatively clear, while others require further investigation.

The cardiovascular response to combined haemorrhage and tissue injury

In direct contrast to haemorrhage, tissue injury/ischaemia produces an increase in arterial blood pressure accompanied by a tachycardia.[65–67] The increase in arterial blood pressure that accompanies 'injury' is largely mediated by an increase in sympathetic outflow to the vasculature and a consequent increase in total peripheral resistance.[68] The 'injury'-induced pressor response is accompanied by a tachycardia, rather than the bradycardia that would be expected were the baroreceptor reflex functioning normally (see above). This pattern of response is possible because there is a concomitant reduction in the sensitivity and a rightward resetting (i.e. towards a higher arterial blood pressure) of the baroreflex following 'injury'.[69] The reduction in baroreceptor reflex sensitivity in humans is evident within 3 hours of 'injury' of moderate severity (e.g. fracture of a long bone) and is persistent such that only partial recovery has occurred at 14 days after 'injury'.[70] Predictably, the cardiovascular changes elicited by a progressive haemorrhage are altered markedly by the presence of concomitant tissue 'injury'.[2] The initial tachycardia following a loss of 10–15 per cent blood volume is reduced as a consequence of an injury-induced diminished baroreflex sensitivity. However, this does not lead to hypotension, quite the contrary, since the response to 'injury' itself produces a tachycardia and increased vascular resistance (see above). Furthermore, the vagal bradycardia following severe blood loss is prevented (Fig. 6.1). This attenuation of the heart rate changes normally associated with severe blood loss seems to offer some degree of protection against the hypotensive effects of a severe haemorrhage.[2] However, this protection may be more apparent than real, since animals subjected to haemorrhage and concomitant 'injury' demonstrate a lower survival rate compared with animals subjected to haemorrhage alone (see pp. 70–71).[71]

The mechanism of the attenuation of the response to haemorrhage by that to 'injury' is at least partly the result of an interaction between the central nervous pathways involved in the two responses.

Central nervous pathways organizing the cardiovascular response to 'injury' and their interaction with those involved in the response to hypovolaemia

The afferent pathway of the response to 'injury' appears to run in somatic (including nociceptive) fibres arising in the damaged tissues. Afferent information then ascends in the spinal cord (probably via the spinothalamic tract) to the brain.[69] Activity in these somatic afferent fibres may be capable of modulating the response to hypovolaemia at a number of central nervous loci: the NTS (the primary relay station for the arterial baroreflex and the cardiac vagal C-fibre afferents); the nucleus ambiguus and dorsal vagal motor nucleus (vagal outflow involved in the baroreflex and the 'cardiac' reflex); and the RVLM (sympathetic outflow, again involved in the baroreflex and the 'cardiac' reflex). Thus, it has recently been shown that activation of somatic afferent Aδ-fibres can lead to inhibition of baroreflex sensitive neurones within the NTS via a GABA-ergic mechanism.[72] Furthermore, activity in somatic nociceptive afferent fibres may induce a long lasting inhibition of vagal cardiac preganglionic motorneurones in the nucleus ambiguus[73] and attenuate the vagally mediated bradycardia evoked during stimulation of either the NTS[73] or cardiac vagal C-fibre afferents (Kirkman and Little, unpublished data). Finally, activity in the somatic afferent fibres can modulate sympathoexcitatory neurones in the RVLM (see below).

The precise mechanism whereby the response to 'injury' modifies cardiovascular control is unknown since very little is known regarding the central nervous pathways involved in the response to injury. Fortunately there is an extensive literature relating to the central nervous pathways which mediate a related response, namely the visceral alerting response of the defence reaction.

The link between the response to 'injury' and the defence reaction

There are a number of marked similarities between the response to 'injury' and the visceral alerting response of the defence reaction.[74]

Activation of the visceral alerting response produces a simultaneous increase in heart rate and blood pressure and an attenuation of the baroreceptor reflex, similar to the changes induced by 'injury' (see above). Furthermore, the *dorsal* periaqueductal grey (PAG, an area known to integrate the defence reaction[75]) has been shown to display increased neuronal activity following 'injury',[76] while lesions of this area in the rat prevent the reduction in baroreflex sensitivity normally elicited by 'injury'.[77] Therefore, it has been suggested that the response to 'injury' may be mediated via the defence reaction.[74]

Pathways involved in integrating the visceral alerting response of the defence reaction

The visceral alerting response of the defence reaction can be induced by electrical stimulation at a number of sites including an area in the hypothalamus ventral to the fornix, and in the dorsomedial PAG.[78] Of these areas, only the dorsomedial PAG appears capable of fully integrating the defence reaction,[75] whereas the region in the hypothalamus identified by electrical stimulation[78] may contain fibres of passage from a number of more rostral sites in the hypothalamus which together can integrate the defence reaction.[79]

In common with the response to 'injury' (see above), activity within the 'defence pathways' can modify cardiovascular reflexes at a number of loci – the NTS, the vagal nuclei and areas controlling sympathetic efferent activity. For reasons of clarity the effects of the 'defence pathways' on the NTS and vagal cardiac outflow will be discussed separately from the modulation of sympathetic control in the following sections, although it must be stressed that these areas are intimately linked.

Modulation at the NTS and vagal motor nuclei

When the baroreceptors are stimulated, activity in the vagal cardiac motorneurones (in the nucleus ambiguus; see pp. 64–5) is increased via two main excitatory pathways: from the NTS there is both a 'segmental' pathway within the medulla and a pathway ascending to relay in the anterior hypothalamus before descending again to the vagal nuclei (see above: Fig. 6.2a). Activity in the 'defence pathways' can inhibit vagal efferent activity by at least three mechanisms. First, there are inhibitory GABA-ergic projections from the defence areas onto the vagal cardiac motorneurones.[80] Second, activation of the defence reaction can cause an inhibition within the NTS,[81,82] where GABA has recently been shown to act as an inhibitory transmitter[83] (bearing a marked similarity to the effects of 'injury'; see pp. 68–9). Third, activation of the defence reaction can lead to an excitation of inspiratory neurones within the nucleus ambiguus,[28] which again will inhibit the vagal cardiac preganglionic motorneurones (see pp. 64–5). These pathways are summarized in Fig. 6.5. The inhibition by the defence reaction may not be restricted to an attenuation of baroreflex-elicited vagal efferent activity, but may also affect vagal activity generated by other reflexes, e.g. by activation of cardiac C-fibre afferents, which are implicated in the response to severe hypovolaemia (see p. 63).

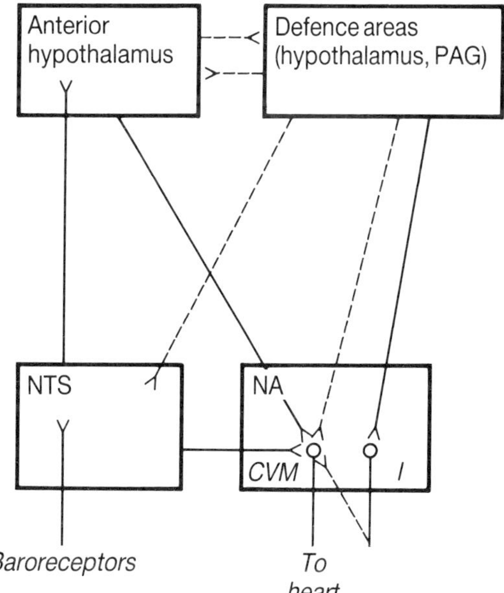

Fig. 6.5. Schematic diagram indicating some of the pathways whereby activity in the defence areas (stimulated following injury?) can modify the baroreflex control of vagal efferent activity to the heart. —, Excitatory pathways; – – –, inhibitory pathways; PAG, periaqueductal grey; NTS, nucleus tractus solitarius; NA, nucleus ambiguus; CVM, cardiac vagal motorneurone; I, inspiratory neurone. *Source*: Spyer.[28]

Modulation of sympathetic efferent activity

The increase in arterial blood pressure during the visceral alerting response is mediated in part by a sympathetically induced increase in total peripheral resistance, which would counteract the reflex sympathoinhibition associated with severe hypovolaemia. The increase in total peripheral resistance during the defence reaction is not the result of an indiscriminate vasoconstriction, but rather is due to a highly organized pattern involving increased resistance in vascular beds such as the renal and mesenteric and a reduction in skeletal muscle vascular resistance. There is sufficient differentiation within the PAG to organize these changes, since it contains groups of cells that are viscerotopically organized with respect to their control over various vascular beds.[84]

The efferent pathways mediating these cardiovascular effects relay in the nucleus paragigantocellularis lateralis in the RVLM.[85–87] The RVLM appears to integrate the efferent activity of a number of cardiovascular reflexes and response patterns[88,89] since it receives input from a number of sites that are known to be involved in cardiovascular and somatosensory control. Of particular interest in the context of this chapter are the hypothalamic and PAG defence areas, the lateral hypothalamus, the NTS, the CVLM and the nucleus parabrachialis (NPB; see pp. 67–8),[89–91] many of which converge onto the same neurone in the RVLM.[89] The RVLM, in turn, sends an efferent excitatory output to the intermediolateral column (sympathetic preganglionic motorneurones). In animals such as the cat the cardiovascular sympathoexcitatory drive originates from a specialized subnucleus, the sub-retrofacial nucleus (sub-RFN),[92] where the neurones are arranged topographically according to the type of vascular bed that they control[93] and receive an equally well organized projection from equivalent areas within the PAG (see above).[84]

Clearly, activation of the visceral alerting response of the defence reaction, possibly as a result of peripheral 'injury', can modify the activity of the sympathoexcitatory neurones within the RVLM. There is enough scope for integration within the RVLM to allow an interaction between the sympathoexcitatory effects of 'injury' and the sympathoinhibitory effects of severe hypovolaemia. Interestingly, activation of 5-HT receptors within the RVLM can reduce the activity of the sympathoexcitatory neurones,[94,95] and hence possibly attenuate the vasoconstrictor effects of the defence reaction, and possibly 'injury'. Conversely, 5-HT antagonism can reverse the sympathoinhibitory effects of severe hypovolaemia (see p. 67). It is tempting to speculate that this may be mediated at the same site, although a point elsewhere (possibly earlier) on the reflex, must also be involved since 5-HT antagonism can reverse both the vasodilator and the bradycardia even during severe hypovolaemia (see p. 67).

Finally, it has been shown that the activity of the tonically active sympathoexcitatory cells within the RVLM can be modulated by activity in somatic afferent fibres from skin and muscle.[96] Interestingly, the sympathoexcitatory cells are inhibited by group III and IV muscle afferent fibres,[96] which is somewhat surprising since these muscle afferents have been implicated in the response to 'injury'.[69] One possible explanation is that whereas these effects of cutaneous and muscle afferents were studied on barosensitive units in the RVLM, other non-barosensitive units may not behave in the same way.

Clinical implications

From the preceding sections it is apparent that the cardiovascular response to haemorrhage and 'injury' is organized by a variety of highly ordered central nervous pathways, and that a number of pharmacological agents may modify the response to hypovolaemia. Thus, it may be possible to attenuate the depressor response to severe haemorrhage using either μ-opioid agonists, e.g. the anaesthetic agents fentanyl or alfentanyl,[5] or by using serotonergic antagonists active at the 5-HT_1 receptor subtype (see pp. 66–7). In addition to these opioid and serotonergic agents, it appears that a number of general anaesthetic agents can potentially modify the response to acute hypovolaemia. Some of these agents, e.g. the barbiturates, are known to attenuate the baroreceptor reflex,[68] while others, e.g. propofol, may leave the baroreceptor reflex relatively intact while attenuating selectively the response to stimulation of the cardiac C-fibre afferents.[97]

Before choosing to modify pharmacologically the cardiovascular response to severe hypovolaemia, it is important to ascertain whether the treatment is likely to be beneficial or detrimental. Caution must be employed before advocating the use of such treatment, or indeed using pharmacological agents that may block the response to severe hypovolaemia as a 'side effect', since the depressor response to severe hypovolaemia may be protective (see pp. 62–4). Consequently, administration of atropine to block the bradycardia associated with severe haemorrhage may increase mortality and morbidity.[98] Similarly, blockade of the depressor response to a severe haemorrhage by concomitant tissue 'injury' (see pp. 68–70) appears to be deleterious. Recent studies have demonstrated that superimposition of somatic afferent nerve activity (to simulate 'injury'), or a real injury, upon haemorrhage protects against the hypotensive effects of blood loss but leads to greater falls in cardiac index and systemic oxygen delivery than those produced by an equivalent 'simple' haemorrhage (Fig. 6.6).[99] In the case of severe hypovolaemia the logical treatment would therefore appear to be a restoration of intravascular volume and hence a reduction in the activation of the 'cardiac' reflex, whereupon the haemodynamic disturbances should correct themselves.

Finally, some anaesthetic agents, e.g. the barbiturates, attenuate the cardiovascular response to 'injury' while others, e.g. propofol, leave the response largely intact,[77] which again has implications for the nature of the secondary problems faced by the injured individual (see above).

These considerations are highly speculative, and should be taken simply to indicate that caution must be exercised before adopting a treatment that merely blocks one aspect of the response to hypovolaemia. Clearly, this area demands further study.

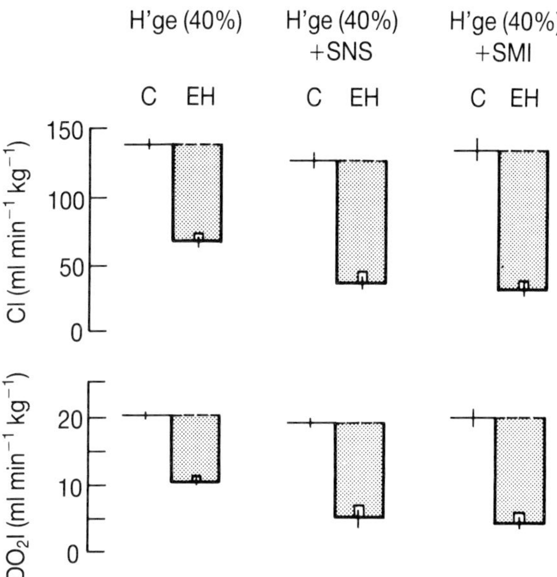

Fig. 6.6. Effects of somatic afferent nerve stimulation (SNS) and skeletal muscle injury (SMI) on the changes in cardiac output (CI, expressed as cardiac index) and oxygen delivery index (DO_2I) produced by a haemorrhage (H'ge) of 40 per cent of estimated blood volume in pigs anaesthetized with isoflurane. C, control, EH, end haemorrhage.

Conclusions

The organization of the central nervous pathways involved in the cardiovascular response to haemorrhage and 'injury', i.e. trauma, are very complicated. A better understanding of how these central pathways function and interact, together with a knowledge of the neurotransmitters and pharmacological receptors involved, is needed to further both our understanding of how agents, e.g. the opioid and serotonergic agents, may modify the responses and to allow the development of new treatment regimes. However, before these new regimes are used, it is important to determine which of the responses to trauma are beneficial and which are detrimental to the victim. Only then will we be able to decide which aspects of the response to modify, and which to leave alone.

References

1. Barcroft H, Edholm OG, McMichael J and Sharpey-Schafer EP: Posthaemorrhagic fainting. Study by cardiac output and forearm flow. *Lancet*, 1944; **i,** 489–91.
2. Little RA, Marshall HW and Kirkman E: Attenuation of the acute cardiovascular responses to haemorrhage by tissue injury in the conscious rat. *Quarterly Journal of Experimental Physiology*, 1989; **74,** 825–33.
3. Ludbrook J, Potocnik SJ and Woods RL: Simulation of acute haemorrhage in unanaesthetized rabbits. *Clinical and Experimental Pharmacology and Physiology*, 1988; **15,** 575–85.
4. Brown E, Goei JS, Greenfield ADM and Plassaras GC: Circulatory responses to simulated gravitational shifts of blood in man induced by exposure of the body below the iliac crests to subatmospheric pressure. *Journal of Physiology*, 1966; **183,** 607–27.
5. Schadt JC and Ludbrook J: Hemodynamic and

neurohumoral responses to acute hypovolemia in conscious mammals. *American Journal of Physiology*, 1991; **260,** H305–18.
6. Secher NH and Bie P: Bradycardia during reversible haemorrhagic shock – a forgotten observation? *Clinical Physiology*, 1985; **5,** 315–23.
7. Evans RG, Ludbrook J and Potocnik SJ: Intracisternal naloxone and cardiac nerve blockade prevent vasodilatation during simulated haemorrhage in awake rabbits. *Journal of Physiology*, 1989; **409,** 1–14.
8. Kirchheim H: Systemic arterial baroreceptor reflexes. *Physiological Reviews*, 1976; **56,** 100–77.
9. Sander-Jensen K, Marving J, Secher NH, Hansen IL, Giese J, Warberg J and Bie P: Does the decrease in heart rate prevent a detrimental decrease of the end-systolic volume during central hypovolemia in man? *Angiology*, 1990; **41,** 687–95.
10. Kirkman E and Little RA: The pathophysiology of trauma and shock. In Kox WJ and Gamble J (eds): *Ballière's Clinical Anaesthesiology, Fluid Resuscitation*, Volume 2(3). London, Ballière Tindall, 1988, 467–82.
11. Cowley AW, Liard JF and Guyton AC: Role of baroreceptor reflex in daily control of arterial blood pressure and other variables in dogs. *Circulation Research*, 1973; **32,** 564–76.
12. Angell-James JE: The effects of changes of extramural, 'intrathoracic', pressure on aortic-arch baroreceptors. *Journal of Physiology*, 1971; **214,** 89–103.
13. Angell-James JE and Daly M de B: Comparison of the reflex vasomotor responses to separate and combined stimulation of the carotid sinus and aortic arch baroreceptors by pulsatile and non-pulsatile pressures in the dog. *Journal of Physiology*, 1970; **209,** 257–93.
14. Heymans C and Neil E: *Reflexogenic Areas of the Cardiovascular System*. London, Churchill, 1958.
15. Little RA, Randall PE, Redfern WS, Stoner HB and Marshall HW: Components of injury (haemorrhage and tissue ischaemia) affecting cardiovascular reflexes in man and rat. *Quarterly Journal of Experimental Physiology*, 1984; **69,** 753–62.
16. Öberg B and Thorén P: Increased activity in left ventricular receptors during hemorrhage or occlusion of caval veins in the cat. A possible cause of the vasovagal reaction. *Acta Physiologica Scandinavica*, 1972; **85,** 164–73.
17. Coleridge JCG and Coleridge HM: Chemoreflex regulation of the heart. In Berne RM (ed.): *Handbook of Physiology. Section 2. Volume 1.* Bethesda, MD, American Physiological Society, 1979, 653.
18. Baker DG, Coleridge HM and Coleridge JCG: Vagal afferent C-fibres from the ventricle. In Hainsworth R, Kidd C and Lindern RJ (eds): *Cardiac Receptors*. Cambridge, Cambridge University Press, 1979, 117–37.
19. Öberg B and Thorén P: Circulatory response to stimulation of left ventricular receptors in the cat. *Acta Physiologica Scandinavica*, 1973; **88,** 8–22.
20. Daly M de B, Kirkman E and Wood LM: Cardiovascular responses to stimulation of cardiac receptors in the cat and their modification by changes in respiration. *Journal of Physiology*, 1988; **407,** 349–62.
21. Burke SL and Dorward PK: Influence of endogenous opiates and cardiac afferents on renal nerve activity during haemorrhage in conscious rabbits. *Journal of Physiology*, 1988; **402,** 9–27.
22. Al-Timman JKA and Hainsworth R: Reflex vascular responses to changes in left ventricular pressures, heart rate and inotropic state in dogs. *Experimental Physiology*, 1992; **77,** 445–69.
23. Evans RG and Ludbrook J: Chemosensitive cardiopulmonary afferents and the haemodynamic response to simulated haemorrhage in conscious rabbits. *British Journal of Pharmacology*, 1991; **102,** 553–9.
24. Ludbrook J and Evans RG: Cardiac chemoreceptors: pharmacological curiosities or physiological tools? *Clinical and Experimental Pharmacology and Physiology*, 1991; **18,** 101–5.
25. Lewis T: Vasovagal syncope and the carotid sinus mechanism. *British Medical Journal*, 1932; **i,** 873–6.
26. Biscoe TJ, Purves MJ and Sampson SR: The frequency of nerve impulses in single carotid body chemoreceptor afferent fibres recorded *in vivo* with intact circulation. *Journal of Physiology*, 1970; **208,** 121–31.
27. Daly M de B: Peripheral arterial chemoreceptors and the cardiovascular system. In Acker H and O'Regan RG (eds): *Physiology of the Peripheral Arterial Chemoreceptors*. Amsterdam, Elsevier Science, 1983, 325–93.
28. Spyer KM: Central control of the cardiovascular system. *Recent Advances in Physiology*, 1984; **10,** 163–200.
29. Daly M de B, Lambertsen CJ and Schweitzer A: Observations on the volume of blood flow and oxygen utilization of the carotid body in the cat. *Journal of Physiology*, 1954; **125,** 67–89.
30. Acker H and O'Regan RG: The effects of stimulation of autonomic nerves on carotid body blood flow in the cat. *Journal of Physiology*, 1981; **315,** 99–110.
31. Potter EK and McCloskey DI: Excitation of carotid body chemoreceptors by neuropeptide-Y. *Respiratory Physiology*, 1987; **67,** 357–65.
32. Kenney RA and Neil E: The contribution of aortic chemoceptor mechanisms to the maintenance of arterial blood pressure of cats and dogs after haemorrhage. *Journal of Physiology*, 1951; **112,** 223–8.
33. D'Silva JL, Gill D and Mendel D: The effects of acute haemorrhage on respiration in the cat. *Journal of Physiology*, 1966; **187,** 369–77.
34. Angell-James JE and Daly M de B: Some aspects of

upper respiratory tract reflexes. *Acta Otolaryngologica*, 1975; **79,** 242–52.

35. Seller H: Central baroreceptor reflex pathways. In Kirchheim HR and Persson PB (eds): *Baroreceptor Reflexes: Integrative Functions and Clinical Aspects*. Berlin, Springer-Verlag, 1991, 45.
36. McAllen RM and Spyer KM: The location of cardiac vagal preganglionic motorneurones projecting to the heart and lungs. *Journal of Physiology*, 1978; **282,** 353–64.
37. Jordan D, Khalid MEM, Schneiderman N and Spyer KM: The location and properties of preganglionic vagal cardiomotor neurones in rabbit. *Pflügers Archiv. European Journal of Physiology (Berlin)*, 1982; **395,** 244–50.
38. Henry JL and Calaresu FR: Topography and numerical distribution of neurons of the thoracolumbar intermediolateral nucleus in the cat. *Journal of Comparative Neurology*, 1972; **144,** 205–14.
39. Finley JCW and Katz DM: The arterial organization of carotid body afferent projections to the brainstem of the rat. *Brain Research*, 1992; **572,** 101–16.
40. Cohen MI, Piercey MF, Gootman PM and Wolotsky P: Synaptic connections between medullary inspiratory neurons and phrenic motoneurons as revealed by cross correlation. *Brain Research*, 1974; **81,** 319–24.
41. Ellenberger HH and Feldman JL: Monosynaptic transmission of respiratory drive to phrenic motoneurons from brainstem bulbospinal neurons in rats. *Journal of Comparative Neurology*, 1988; **269,** 47–57.
42. Garcia M, Jordan D and Spyer KM: Studies on the properties of cardiac vagal neurones. *Neuroscience Letters*, 1978; **suppl. 1**, S16.
43. Bennett JA, Goodchild CS, Kidd C and McWilliam PN: Neurones in the brain stem of the cat excited by vagal afferent fibres from the heart and lungs. *Journal of Physiology*, 1985; **369,** 1–15.
44. Ross CA, Ruggiero DA, Joh TH, Park DH and Reis DJ: Rostral ventrolateral medulla: selective projections to the thoracic autonomic cell column from the region containing C_1 adrenaline neurons. *Journal of Comparative Neurology*, 1984; **228,** 168–85.
45. Brown DL and Guyenet PG: Cardiovascular neurons of brain stem with projections to spinal cord. *American Journal of Physiology*, 1984; **247,** R1009–16.
46. Morrison SF, Callaway J, Milner TA and Reis DJ: Rostral ventrolateral medulla: a source of the glutamatergic innervation of the sympathetic intermediolateral nucleus. *Brain Research*, 1991; **562,** 126–35.
47. Dembowsky K and McAllen RM: Baroreceptor inhibition of subretrofacial neurons: evidence from intracellular recordings in the cat. *Neuroscience Letters*, 1990; **111,** 139–43.
48. Jung R, Bruce EN and Katona PG: Cardiorespiratory responses to glutamatergic antagonists in the caudal ventrolateral medulla of rats. *Brain Research*, 1991; **564,** 286–95.
49. Chalmers JP and Pilowsky PM: Brainstem and bulbospinal neurotransmitter systems in the control of blood pressure. *Journal of Hypertension*, 1991; **9,** 675–94.
50. McAllen RM, Badoer E, Shafton AD, Oldfield BJ and McKinley MJ: Haemorrhage induces c-*fos* immunoreactivity in spinally projecting neurones of the cat subretrofacial nucleus. *Brain Research*, 1992; **575,** 329–32.
51. Evans RG, Ludbrook J, Woods RL and Casley D: Influence of higher brain centres and vasopressin on the haemodynamic response to acute central hypovolaemia in rabbits. *Journal of the Autonomic Nervous System*, 1991; **35,** 1–14.
52. Ludbrook J and Rutter PC: Effect of naloxone on haemodynamic responses to acute blood loss in unanaesthetized rabbits. *Journal of Physiology*, 1988; **400,** 1–14.
53. Evans RG, Ludbrook J and van Leeuwen AF: Role of central opiate receptor subtypes in the circulatory responses of awake rabbits to graded caval occlusions. *Journal of Physiology*, 1989; **419,** 15–31.
54. Evans RG and Ludbrook J: Effects of μ-opioid receptor agonists on circulatory responses to simulated haemorrhage in conscious rabbits. *British Journal of Pharmacology*, 1990; **100,** 421–6.
55. Dashwood MR, Muddle JR and Spyer KM: Opiate receptor subtypes in the nucleus tractus solitarii of the cat: the effect of vagal section. *European Journal of Pharmacology*, 1988; **155,** 85–92.
56. May CN, Dashwood MR, Whitehead CJ and Mathias CJ: Differential cardiovascular and respiratory responses to central administration of selective opioid agonists in conscious rabbits: correlation with receptor distribution. *British Journal of Pharmacology*, 1989; **98,** 903–13.
57. Morgan DA, Thorén P, Wilczynski EA, Victor RG and Mark AL: Serotonergic mechanisms mediate renal sympathoinhibition during severe hemorrhage in rats. *American Journal of Physiology*, 1988; **255,** H496–502.
58. Kay IS and Armstrong DJ: Phenylbiguanide not phenyldiguanide is used to evoke the pulmonary chemoreflex in anaesthetized rabbits. *Experimental Physiology*, 1990; **75,** 383–9.
59. Peroutka SJ: 5-Hydroxytryptamine receptor sub types: molecular, biochemical and physiological characterization. *Trends in Neuroscience*, 1988; **11,** 496–500.
60. Evans RG and Ludbrook J: Opioid mechanisms in trauma. In Cooper G, Dudley HAF, Gann D, Little RA and Maynard RL (eds): *Scientific Foundations of Trauma*. Oxford, Butterworth Heinemann, in press.
61. Fulwiler CE and Saper CB: Subnuclear organization of the efferent connections of the parabrachial nucleus in the rat. *Brain Research*, 1984; **319,** 229–59.
62. Loewy AD and Burton H: Nuclei of the solitary tract:

efferent projections to the lower brain stem and spinal cord of the cat. *Journal of Comparative Neurology*, 1978; **181,** 421–49.

63. Ward DG: Neurons in the parabrachial nuclei respond to hemorrhage. *Brain Research*, 1989; **491,** 80–92.
64. Ward DG and Darlington DN: Lesions of the caudal periaqueductal gray prevent compensation of arterial pressure during haemorrhage. *Brain Research*, 1987; **407,** 369–75.
65. Alam M and Smirk FH: Observations in man upon a blood pressure raising reflex arising from the voluntary muscles. *Journal of Physiology*, 1937; **89,** 372–83.
66. Alam M and Smirk FH: Observations in man on a pulse accelerating reflex from the voluntary muscles of the legs. *Journal of Physiology*, 1938; **92,** 167–77.
67. Howard JM, Artz CP and Stahl RR: Hypertensive response to injury. *Annals of Surgery*, 1955; **141,** 327–36.
68. Redfern WS: *Effects of Limb Ischaemia on the Cardiac Component of the Baroreceptor Reflex in the Unanaesthetized Rat – Afferent, Central and Efferent Mechanisms*. PhD Thesis, University of Manchester, Manchester, 1981.
69. Redfern WS, Little RA, Stoner HB and Marshall HW: Effect of limb ischaemia on blood pressure and the blood pressure–heart rate reflex in the rat. *Quarterly Journal of Experimental Physiology*, 1984; **69,** 763–79.
70. Anderson ID, Little RA and Irving MH: An effect of trauma on human cardiovascular control: baroreflex suppression. *Journal of Trauma*, 1990; **30,** 974–81.
71. Overman RR and Wang SC: The contributory role of the afferent nervous factor in experimental shock: sublethal hemorrhage and sciatic nerve stimulation. *American Journal of Physiology*, 1947; **148,** 289–95.
72. McMahon SE, McWilliam PN, Robertson J and Kaye JC: Inhibition of carotid sinus baroreceptor neurones in the nucleus tractus solitarius of the anaesthetized cat by electrical stimulation of hindlimb afferent fibres. *Journal of Physiology*, 1992; **452,** 224P.
73. Wang Q, Guo X-Q and Li P: The inhibitory effects of somatic input on the excitatory responses of vagal cardiomotor neurones to stimulation of the nucleus tractus solitarius in rabbits. *Brain Research*, 1988; **439,** 350–53.
74. Quest JA and Gebber GL: Modulation of baroreceptor reflexes by somatic afferent nerve stimulation. *American Journal of Physiology*, 1972; **222,** 1251–9.
75. Hilton SM and Redfern WS: A search for brain stem cell groups integrating the defence reaction in the rat. *Journal of Physiology*, 1986; **378,** 213–28.
76. Jones RO: *The Identification of the Brain Areas Involved in the Interaction between Peripheral Injuries and Baroreceptor Reflex Activity in the Rat*. PhD Thesis, University of Manchester, Manchester, 1989.
77. Jones RO, Kirkman E and Little RA: The involvement of the midbrain periaqueductal grey in the cardiovascular response to injury in the conscious and anaesthetized rat. *Experimental Physiology*, 1990; **75,** 483–95.
78. Yardley CP and Hilton SM: The hypothalamic and brainstem areas from which the cardiovascular and behavioural components of the defence reaction are elicited in the rat. *Journal of the Autonomic Nervous System*, 1986; **15,** 227–44.
79. Lovick TA: Projections from the diencephalon and mesencephalon to nucleus paragigantocellularis lateralis in the cat. *Neuroscience*, 1985; **14,** 853–61.
80. Jordan D, Khalid MEM, Schneiderman N and Spyer KM: The inhibitory control of vagal cardiomotor neurones. *Journal of Physiology*, 1980; **301,** 54–5P.
81. McAllen RM: Inhibition of the baroreceptor input to the medulla by stimulation of the hypothalamic defence area. *Journal of Physiology*, 1976; **257,** 45–6P.
82. Mifflin SW, Spyer KM and Withington-Wray DJ: Baroreceptor inputs to the nucleus tractus solitarius in the cat: modulation by the hypothalamus. *Journal of Physiology*, 1988; **399,** 369–87.
83. Bennett JA, McWilliam PN and Shepheard SL: A gamma-aminobutyric-acid-mediated inhibition of neurones in the nucleus tractus solitarius of the cat. *Journal of Physiology*, 1987; **392,** 417–30.
84. Carrive P, Bandler R and Dampney RA: Viscerotopic control of regional vascular beds by discrete groups of neurons within the midbrain periaqueductal gray. *Brain Research*, 1989; **493,** 385–90.
85. Hilton SM, Marshall JM and Timms RJ: Ventral medullary relay neurones in the pathway from the defence areas of the cat and their effect on blood pressure. *Journal of Physiology*, 1983; **345,** 149–66.
86. Lovick TA: Ventrolateral medullary lesions block the antinociceptive and cardiovascular responses elicited by stimulating the dorsal periaqueductal grey matter in rats. *Pain*, 1985; **21,** 241–52.
87. Lovick TA: Analgesia and the cardiovascular changes evoked by stimulating neurones in the ventrolateral medulla in rats. *Pain*, 1986; **25,** 259–68.
88. Lovick TA: Differential control of cardiac and vasomotor activity by neurones in nucleus paragigantocellularis lateralis in the cat. *Journal of Physiology*, 1987; **389,** 23–35.
89. Lovick TA: Convergent afferent inputs to neurones in nucleus paragigantocellularis lateralis in the cat. *Brain Research*, 1988; **456,** 183–7.
90. Andrezik JA, Chan-Palay V and Palay SL: The nucleus paragigantocellularis lateralis in the rat. Demonstration of afferents by the retrograde transport of horseradish peroxidase. *Anatomy and Embryology*, 1981; **161,** 373–90.
91. Lovick TA: Projections from brainstem nuclei to the nucleus paragigantocellularis lateralis in the cat.

Journal of the Autonomic Nervous System, 1986; **16,** 1–11.
92. Siddall PJ and Dampney RA: Relationship between cardiovascular neurones and descending antinociceptive pathways in the rostral ventrolateral medulla of the cat. *Pain*, 1989; **37,** 347–55.
93. McAllen RM and Dampney RA: Vasomotor neurons in the rostral ventrolateral medulla are organized topographically with respect to type of vascular bed but not body region. *Neuroscience Letters*, 1990; **110,** 91–6.
94. Lovick TA: Cardiovascular response to 5HT in the ventrolateral medulla of the rat. *Journal of the Autonomic Nervous System*, 1989; **28,** 35–41.
95. Lovick TA: Effect of 5HT in the ventrolateral medulla on the pressor response and analgesia evoked by stimulation of the dorsal periaqueductal grey matter in anaesthetized rats. *Journal of Physiology*, 1989; **418,** 84P.
96. Terui N, Saeki Y and Kumada M: Confluence of barosensory and nonbarosensory inputs at neurons in the ventrolateral medulla in rabbits. *Canadian Journal of Physiology and Pharmacology*, 1987; **65,** 1584–90.
97. Kirkman E, Marshall HW and Little RA: Modulation by anaesthetic agents of the reflex cardioinhibitory responses to activation of the baroreflex and the cardiopulmonary C-fibre afferents in the rat. *British Journal of Pharmacology*, 1992; **105,** 31P.
98. Barriot P, Riou B and Buffat J-J: Pre-hospital management of severe haemorrhagic shock. In Vincent JL (ed.): *Update in Intensive Care and Emergency Medicine 3*. Berlin, Springer-Verlag, 1987, 377–84.
99. Rady M, Little RA, Edwards JD, Kirkman E and Faithfull S: The effect of nociceptive stimulation on the changes in hemodynamics and oxygen transport induced by hemorrhage in anesthetized pigs. *Journal of Trauma*, 1991; **31,** 617–21.

7

Cardiovascular regulation: efferent autonomic pathways and mechanisms

Murray Esler, John Ludbrook and B Gunnar Wallin

Introduction

We have tried to achieve two goals in writing this chapter. One was to give the reader up to date information about the gross and microscopical anatomy of the vagal and sympathetic efferent pathways that are involved in the regulation of the heart and blood vessels, and an indication of how these pathways function in terms of putative transmitter mechanisms. The second goal was to describe how the functions of these efferent pathways can be studied in humans, and to give some of the results of studies in persons exposed to acute central hypovolaemia or suffering from vasovagal syncope.

Structure and function of autonomic cardiovascular pathways

Gross anatomy

The general outline of the anatomical pathways followed by preganglionic cardiac vagal, and pre- and postganglionic cardiac and vascular sympathetic, neurones to reach their target organs has been known for many years from gross anatomical dissection and from degeneration studies (Figs 7.1 and 7.2).[1] The cardiac parasympathetic motoneurones are located in the medulla oblongata. Their preganglionic axons leave the medulla in the vagus nerves and enter the superior, middle and inferior cardiac branches of the vagus. These branches join with postganglionic sympathetic axons (see below) to form the two divisions of the cardiac plexus. The parasympathetic preganglionic axons synapse in cardiac miniganglia, most of which are located subendocardially over the posterior walls of the atria, especially the right atrium.[2] The postganglionic axons are distributed to the sinoatrial pacemaker, the ventricular conducting system, and probably to the ventricular myocardium. It seems that right and left vagi are fairly equally represented at each of these sites.

The organization of the cardiovascular elements of the sympathetic nervous system is more complex (Fig. 7.1).[1] The sympathetic cardiovascular motoneurones are located in the intermediolateral cell columns of the thoracolumbar regions of the spinal cord. Their axons leave the spinal cord in the T_1 to L_2 ventral roots to reach the paravertebral chain of sympathetic ganglia via white rami communicantes. They then take one of three courses.

(a) Those destined for blood vessels in skin and skeletal muscle travel up or down the paravertebral sympathetic chain for a short distance before synapsing in paravertebral ganglia. The postganglionic axons enter spinal nerves via grey rami communicantes, are distributed in peripheral nerves, and only in the last few centimetres of their course do they leave these to reach blood vessels.

(b) The preganglionic axons directed towards the blood vessels of the abdominal viscera usually pass through the paravertebral sympathetic chain, without making synapses, to enter one of the three thoracic splanchnic nerves: greater (T_5–T_9), lesser (T_{10}–T_{11}) or least (T_{12}). They

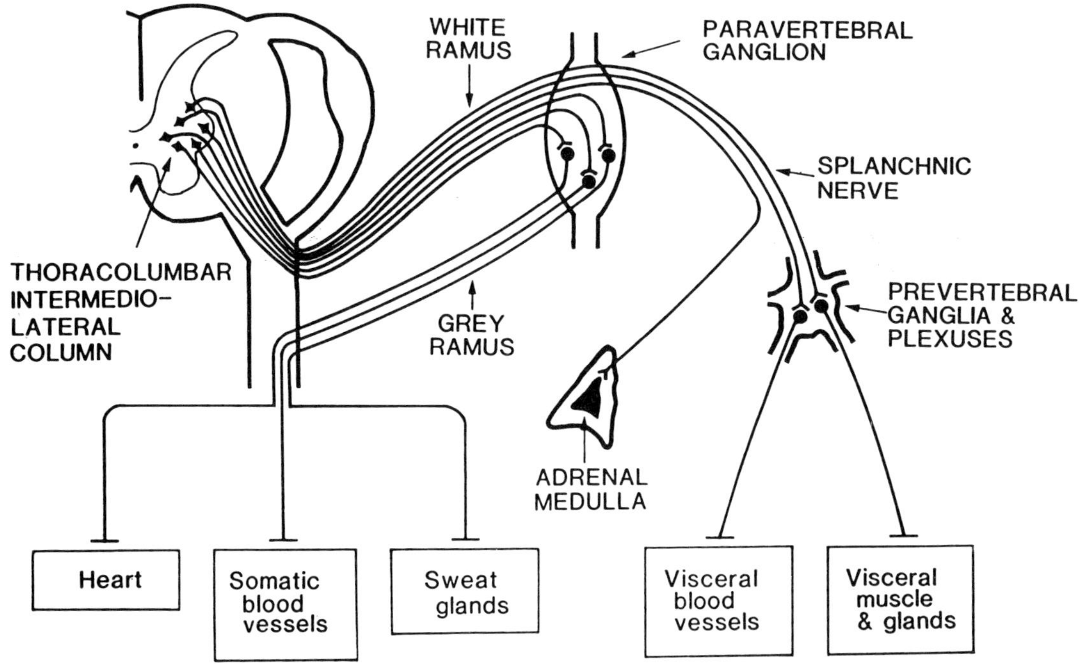

Fig. 7.1. General organization of the sympathetic nervous system. From Ludbrook and McLachlan,[1] with permission.

synapse in one of the prevertebral ganglia or ganglionic plexuses located round the origins of the visceral branches of the abdominal aorta (for example, coeliac, renal, superior and inferior mesenteric). Sympathetic preganglionic axons directed towards the pelvic viscera also pass through the paravertebral chain to synapse in the superior or inferior hypogastric plexuses. The postganglionic axons reach their targets by travelling along the abdominal and pelvic visceral arteries.

(c) The cardiac preganglionic axons synapse in the three cervical and first five or six thoracic paravertebral ganglia. The postganglionic axons join the two divisions of the cardiac plexus where they mingle with vagal preganglionic axons (see above). The upper division consists of the superior, middle and inferior cardiac nerves which receive sympathetic contributions from the three cervical ganglia and parasympathetic contributions from the superior and middle cardiac branches of the vagus nerve. The lower division comprises postganglionic sympathetic axons from the thoracic paravertebral ganglia and preganglionic parasympathetic fibres from the inferior cardiac branches of the vagus. The sympathetic postganglionic axons terminate in the sinoatrial pacemaker, the conducting system of the ventricles and on myocardial cells, especially those in the ventricles. The sinoatrial node is supplied chiefly from the right sympathetic chain, and the atrioventricular node the ventricular conduction system and myocardium from the left side.[3]

Techniques for identifying microscopic and functional connections

The study of the microstructural and functional connections of the neurones that are responsible for the regulation of heart rate and the diameter of blood vessels has been revolutionized by the introduction of new techniques during the last decade or so. Before then, the identification of neurone pools that, for instance, give rise to vagal preganglionic axons, relied on degeneration techniques. But now the structural interrelation of neurones can be identified by marker substances such as horseradish peroxidase, latex microspheres and plant lectins that travel in an retrograde or antegrade fashion after microinjection into axons or cell bodies, and recently by neurotropic viruses that

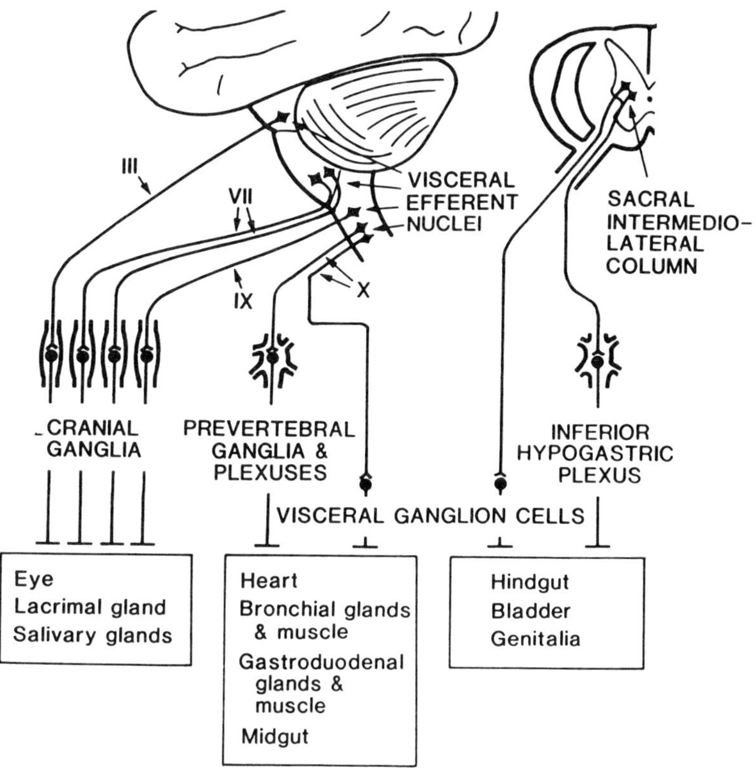

Fig. 7.2. General organization of the parasympathetic nervous system. From Ludbrook and McLachlan,[1] with permission.

can cross several synapses in a retrograde direction. It has also been possible to identify functional connections of neurones, originally by electrical stimulation of small neurone pools (which also stimulated fibres of passage) and now by the much more selective method of microinjecting excitatory amino acids such as l-glutamate or inhibitory amino acids such as glycine or GABA. Electrical recordings can be made from single neurones thought to be involved in cardiovascular control, originally extracellularly but now, in a few cases, intracellularly. An exciting new technique is to make use of the protein Fos, a product of the proto-oncogene c-*fos* which is expressed when neurones are strongly activated, to detect neurone pools that are excited by physiological disturbances in conscious animals. The transmitters produced by cardiovascular neurones can be identified by histochemical or immunohistochemical techniques, and the specific receptor sites at which they may act by autoradiography. The transmitter mechanisms that do or may operate at synapses in cardiac or vascular autonomic pathways can be identified by a variety of techniques, from classic, gross neuropharmacological experiments to intracellular recordings in association with intra- or extracellular microinjection of putative neurotransmitters. Obviously, few of these techniques can be applied to humans so the information gained from them that will be presented below refers chiefly to cats, rats and rabbits. However, there is little reason to believe that humans are different, except in such details as specific peptide neuropeptide neurotransmitters or neuromodulators (for which there do appear to be species differences).

Origins within the central nervous system

Studies in a variety of mammals place the cell bodies of cardiac vagal axons in the nucleus ambiguus and dorsal vagal motor nucleus, both of which lie within the medulla oblongata and are the most important components of what is sometimes called the vagal complex.[4–6] The distribution of the cardiac motoneurones between these two nuclei varies among species, and it has been suggested that there has been a phylogenetic ventral migration of cardiac vagal neurones from the dorsal vagal nucleus to the nucleus ambiguus.[2] The cardiac vagal cell bodies give rise chiefly to myelinated axons that are classified as B-fibres on the basis of conduction velocity, though there is some evidence that vagal unmyelinated axons with different functional properties may also be directed to the heart.[7] These cardiac preganglionic axons leave the medulla in the Xth cranial nerve. Vagal preganglionic axons directed to the coronary and bronchial vasculature are also included in the vagus nerves.

The site of origin of input to sympathetic cardiovascular neurones has attracted an enormous amount of interest over the past 10–15 years. It is now clear that the RVLM is the main source of excitation of sympathetic cardiovascular preganglionic neurones in the intermediolateral cell columns of the spinal cord.[8–14] Chemical inhibition or electrical destruction of the RVLM bilaterally causes blood pressure to fall to levels that are similar to those after cervical spinal cord transection. Conversely, chemical excitation of the RVLM neurones causes a large rise in blood pressure. There is now very good evidence that the neurones responsible for most of the tonic sympathetic vasonstrictor drive are located in a small area of the RVLM, sometimes called the sub-RFN.[12,13] These neurones project directly to, and synapse with, preganglionic sympathetic neurones in the thoracolumbar spinal cord (as well as to other sites), and they receive projections from important relay stations for cardiovascular reflexes such as the NTS, hypothalamus and CVLM (Fig. 7.3). There is growing evidence of a viscerotopic segregation of neurones within the sub-RFN according to whether they are directed to muscle, skin or kidney.[12,13,15]

There are still a number of uncertainties about the sub-RFN. It has not yet been decided whether its neurones act as the primary pacemakers that generate tonic sympathetic vasoconstrictor drive or whether they are driven from elsewhere in the brainstem (for instance, from neural networks in the medullary reticular formation).[10] Neither has it been established what transmitter or transmitters are utilized by the neurones of the sub-RFN.[13,14] Within the RVLM are neurones containing amines such as serotonin (5-HT), adrenaline and acetylcholine (ACh); amino acids such as glutamate; and neuropeptides such as substance P, neuropeptide Y, galanin, neuropeptide K, neurotensin, somatostatin, glucagon and enkephalin. It remains to be established which of these transmitters are important in driving the sympathetic preganglionic neurones (though glutamate is the front-running candidate), and whether the viscerotopic localiz-

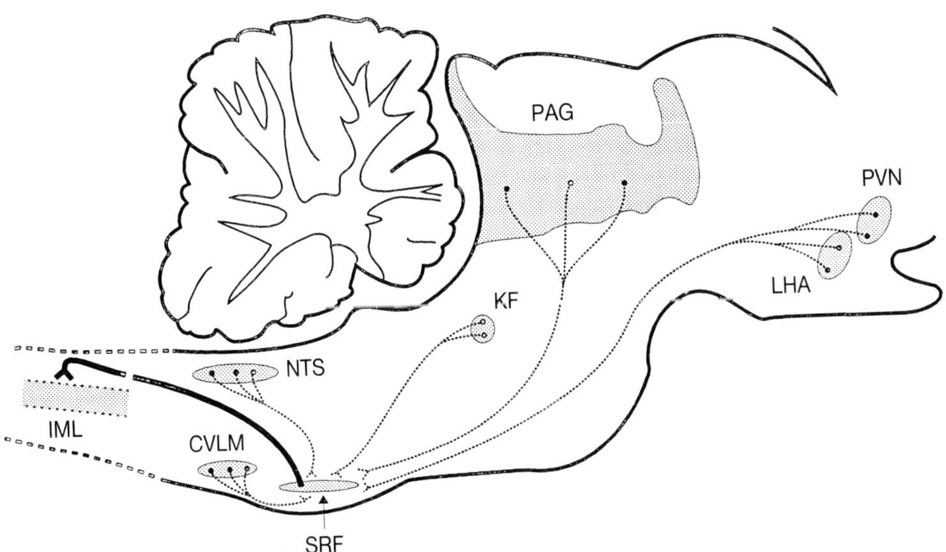

Fig. 7.3. The main connections of the sub-retrofacial (SRF) nucleus. ....., Input; —, output; CVLM, caudal ventrolateral medulla; IML, intermediolateral cell column; KF, Kölliker–Fuse nucleus; LHA, lateral hypothalamic area; NTS, nucleus tractus solitarii; PAG, periaqueductal grey; PVN, paraventricular nucleus. From Dampney,[12] with permission.

ation of neurones in the sub-RFN corresponds to neurones that utilize different neurotransmitters and neuromodulators.

Cardiovascular sympathetic drive is tonically restrained, especially by input to the central nervous system from the arterial baroreceptors. It is known that the first synapse of the baroreceptor afferents is in the NTS, but it is not certain by what route baroreceptor input inhibits the cardiovascular sympathetic drive that originates in the sub-RFN. It has been recognized for some time that neurones within the CVLM exert a tonic inhibitory influence on cardiovascular sympathetic drive.[8,9,14] There is growing evidence, both neuroanatomical and neurophysiological, that the CVLM is an important (if not the all-important) relay station between baroreceptor input and the RVLM.[14,16–19]

Spinal preganglionic neurones

Sympathetic

These are located in the intermediolateral cell column between the T_1 and L_2 segments of the spinal cord. There is also good evidence of viscerotopic localization at this level, so that it is possible to distinguish, structurally or functionally, groups of neurones that project to the heart, skeletal muscle, skin and the viscera; and to some extent it is possible to distinguish cardiovascular neurones from others by their microscopic appearance and lateral position.[20,21] Cardiovascular sympathetic preganglionic neurones receive direct input from bulbar neurones (NTS, RVLM, CVLM, A_5 and caudal raphe nuclei), suprabulbar neurones (hypothalamic, paraventricular) and spinal interneurones.[14,22,23]

The synaptic endings on sympathetic preganglionic neurones, or within the intermediolateral cell column more generally, contain a bewildering array of amines (noradrenaline, adrenaline, 5-HT, dopamine), amino acids (glutamate, GABA, glycine) and peptides (substance P, vasopressin and oxytocin; but also metenkephalin, thyrotropin-releasing hormone (TRH), neurophysin, somatostatin, cholecystokinin, corticotropin-releasing factor (CRF) and neurotensin!).[14,22,24] A variety of binding sites (for instance, α_2-adrenoceptor, 5-HT and substance P) have also been demonstrated on preganglionic neurones by autoradiography.[22] When applied by microiontophoresis, noradrenaline, adrenaline and dopamine inhibit the firing of preganglionic neurones by acting at α_2-adrenoceptors, but there is also evidence that noradrenaline can excite these neurones by acting at α_1-adrenoceptors.[14,22] The situation is just as confused with respect to 5-HT which, when applied microiontophoretically, excites some preganglionic neurones and inhibits others.[25] There is somewhat more consistency with respect to amino acid neurotransmitters. Glutamate consistently excites, and GABA (and perhaps glycine) consistently inhibits, the firing of preganglionic neurones, so it has been suggested that glutamate and GABA are respectively the main excitatory and inhibitory transmitters for descending bulbospinal pathways.[22,26] Microiontophoretically applied substance P excites preganglionic neurones, though with a much slower time-course than glutamine.[22] Arginine vasopressin (AVP) has been variously reported to inhibit or excite preganglionic neurones, and it is not clear whether this is the excitatory neurotransmitter for the descending paraventriculo–spinal pathway.[22] What role, if any, is played by the many other neuropeptides that have been identified in the intermediolateral cell column is not known. In summary, the opportunities for integration of cardiovascular and somatosensory reflexes at the beginning of the final common pathway for cardiovascular sympathetic drive are almost boundless. Just which pathways and which neurotransmitters and neuromodulators are actually involved is still unclear, but the matter is the subject of feverish investigation.

Parasympathetic

The preganglionic cell bodies lie in the sacral (S_1–S_4) intermediolateral cell column (Fig. 7.2). A minority are directed at blood vessels, especially those of the male and female genital tract.

Autonomic ganglia

In both cardiac vagal and sympathetic ganglia and in the adrenal medulla ACh, acting at neuronal-type nicotinic cholinoceptors, has been known for a long time to be the principal neurotransmitter. Transmission is blocked by a variety of quaternary ammonium compounds, such as hexamethonium, mecamylamine and trimetaphan. However, there is electrophysiological evidence that other excitatory transmitter mechanisms, such as muscarinic cholinergic and peptidergic, also play a role.[21] The former has been implicated in chemoreflex pathways to sympathetic postganglionic neurones and adrenal chromaffin cells.

Neuroeffector mechanisms on blood vessels

Sympathetic

Until recently noradrenaline, acting at α_1-adrenoceptors on blood vessels and at β_1-adrenoceptors in the heart, was regarded as the sole excitatory transmitter mechanism at sympathetic neuroeffector junctions. Now there are seen to be at least two difficulties with this simple scheme. The first is that though there are α_1-adrenoceptors on vascular smooth muscle, and activation of them by exogenous noradrenaline results in contraction, there are serious doubts that they constitute part of the neuroeffector mechanism.[27,28] Instead, there are rival hypotheses which suppose either that: (1) neurally released noradrenaline acts at non-α_1-adrenoceptors (sometimes described as γ-receptors); or (2) neurally released adenosine triphosphate (ATP) acts on P_2-receptors. The second difficulty is that there is now a massive literature on non-adrenergic mechanisms in which neurotransmitters or neuromodulators (purines, neuropeptide Y, opioids, CGRP) have been implicated. Neuropeptide Y in particular (and in some species galanin) has been shown to be costored and coreleased with noradrenaline in blood vessels and the heart and to potentiate the vasoconstrictor and cardioacceleratory actions of noradrenaline.[29–31]

A controversy has surrounded the question of whether there are sympathetic vasodilator neurones in humans. There is good evidence for a sympathetic cholinergic vasodilator mechanism to skeletal muscle in laboratory animals, especially cats and dogs, but there have been doubts whether a similar mechanism exists in primates, especially humans.[32,33] There were several reports in the 1950s and 1960s that the vasodilatation taking place in human forearm muscle in response to emotional stimuli could be much reduced by systemic or intra-arterial infusion of atropine, and persisted after α-adrenoceptor blockade.[34] One report suggested that sympathetic cholinergic vasodilatation occurred during the syncopal (decompensatory) phase of acute central hypovolaemia.[35] But the explanation of these phenomena on the basis of a sympathetic cholinergic vasodilator mechanism was rather discounted when it proved impossible to find cholinesterase around sympathetic terminals in the vasculature of skeletal muscle of primates, including humans.[32] However, new evidence has now been adduced that supports the possibility of sympathetic cholinergic vasodilatation in human skeletal muscle, this time in non-exercising muscles during static exercise of other muscle groups and resulting from central command.[36] Though the notion that there is a sympathetic cholinergic vasodilator mechanism in human skeletal muscle, activated by emotional stimuli, central command to exercise and perhaps by input from cardiac afferents in severe hypovolaemia, is an attractive one it has to be said that it has not been proven beyond reasonable doubt.[37]

There is better evidence for a sympathetic vasodilator mechanism in human skin.[34] It is necessary to postulate an active dilator mechanism to account for the repeated observation that the increase in forearm skin blood flow that results from elevation of central body temperature is greater than that which results from sympathetic blockade.[34] However, the association of the onset of sweating with a great increase in skin blood flow, and the absence of this increase in subjects with congenital absence of sweat glands,[38] seems to link this phenomenon with the undisputed sympathetic cholinergic excitation of sweat glands. Recently, vasodilatation of the skin of the human foot in response to stimulation of the lumbar sympathetic chain during operation under epidural anaesthesia has been reported, and ascribed to sympathetic vasodilator or sudomotor fibres.[39] There is a structural substrate for supposing that the mechanism may be cholinergic since cholinesterase is present within the specialized arteriovenous anastomoses (AVAs) of human acral skin.[40]

Apart from the classical mammalian peripheral autonomic neurotransmitters (noradrenaline and ACh), some 20 other putative neurotransmitters and neuromodulators acting on blood vessels have been proposed, on the basis that they are found in prejunctional nerve terminals and that they are vasoactive when applied to blood vessels.[29,31,37] These are lumped together as non-adrenergic, non-cholinergic (NANC) transmitters. The difficulty is to decide: (1) that they genuinely act as neurotransmitters or neuromodulators in the intact organism; and (2) that they do so in humans. The most promising candidates are ATP (mesenteric vasoconstrictor), serotonin (5-HT, cerebral vasodilator), neuropeptide Y (vasoconstrictor in many systemic vessels), and dopamine (vasodilator at AVAs in acral skin).

Parasympathetic

These mechanisms are not of great scientific interest in the context of blood loss and shock, but may be of personal interest to investigators. Suffice to say that there is debate whether vasoactive intestinal peptide (VIP) or NO is the transmitter responsible for tumescence of erectile tissue in the genital tract.[41]

Cardiac neuroeffector mechanisms

It has been the doctrine that the principal vagal transmitter mechanism to the heart is ACh, acting at muscarinic cholinergic receptors; and that the principal sympathetic mechanism in mammals is neurally released noradrenaline (and circulating adrenaline), acting at β_1-adrenoceptors. But it has recently been suggested that this simple doctrine may be untrue. Hirst *et al.*[28] have argued that vagally released ACh acts on a subset of muscarinic receptors that are distinct from the classical sort. And they have doubted that sympathetically released noradrenaline acts on the cardiac pacemaker through conventional β_1-adrenoceptors. In addition, there are a number of transmitters that are colocalized with noradrenaline or ACh in cardiac autonomic nerve terminals,[42] and peptide neuromodulators seem to come into play at least in the regulation of heart rate. Neuropeptide Y (or in some species galanin) has been demonstrated to contribute to the cardioacceleration resulting from sympathetic stimulation.[30] As well, there are clear cut interactions between the vagal and sympathetic control of heart rate, of a mutually inhibitory nature and occurring at prejunctional sites. Sympathetic attenuation of the bradycardic effects of vagal stimulation has been shown to be due to a presynaptic action of neuropeptide Y at vagal nerve endings,[30] and possibly also to an action of noradrenaline at vagal prejunctional α_1-adrenoceptors.[43] Vagal attenuation of the cardioacceleratory effects of sympathetic nerve stimulation appears to be due to activation of muscarinic cholinergic receptors on prejunctional sympathetic fibres.[43]

Sympathetic and parasympathetic postganglionic axons not only end in the sinoatrial pacemaker and conducting system of the heart, but also in the myocardium (notably the ventricles). The innervation is dense in the case of the sympathetic, and there is little dispute that the activation of β_1-adrenoceptors on myocardial cells, whether by sympathetic stimulation or by circulating catecholamines, increases myocardial contractility. It is not nearly so certain, however, that increased cardiac vagal drive reduces myocardial contractility under physiological conditions, chiefly because of the difficulty of separating chronotropic from inotropic effects when measuring contractility.[44,45]

Humoral and neurohumoral cardiovascular effector mechanisms

Adrenal medullary hormones

The adrenal chromaffin cells are the homologues of sympathetic postganglionic neurones. Their granules contain adrenaline and noradrenaline in varying proportions according to species. They also contain a variety of neuropeptides (neuropeptide Y, opioids). These substances are coreleased into the bloodstream with catecholamines in response to increased adrenal nerve drive. The ACh released from the sympathetic preganglionic nerve terminals has been regarded as acting at neuronal-type nicotinic cholinoceptors on the chromaffin cells, but there is evidence that muscarinic cholinoceptors may also be involved, at least in some species and by way of some reflex pathways, in adrenaline release.[46]

Arginine vasopressin

The largest store of this neuropeptide is in the neurones of the supraoptic and paraventricular nuclei of the hypothalamus, which project to blood vessels within the posterior lobe of the pituitary gland. In conformity with the dual function of AVP as a water regulating (antidiuretic) hormone and a pressor substance, these neurones receive connections from cerebral osmoreceptors and from afferent cardiovascular pathways. A clear connection has been established between incoming arterial and cardiac baroreceptor afferents, the NTS, the A_1 (noradrenergic) neurone pool of the medulla oblongata and the AVP-containing cells of the supraoptic nucleus.[47,48] There is also evidence that AVP can act as a neurotransmitter or neuromodulator within the central nervous system. From the point of view of cardiovascular control the most important question is whether and how circulating AVP can modulate heart rate or vascular smooth muscle tone. It appears to be able to do so by at least two mechanisms:

(a) a direct vasoconstrictor action, argued on the basis that in haemorrhage or acute central hypovolaemia the plasma concentrations of AVP are high enough to vasoconstrict blood vessels, or that the vasopressin V_1 (vascular) antagonist can be shown to attenuate the vasoconstriction observed under hypovolaemic conditions.[49]
(b) though AVP cannot cross the blood–brain barrier, it can act on the brain through specific circumventricular organs such as the area postrema. There is evidence that it can modulate cardiovascular functions by this mechanism.[50]

Angiotensin II

This is produced by the sequence:

Angiotensinogen → Angiotensin I → Angiotensin II
⇑ Renin ⇑ AI converting enzyme

in which plasma angiotensinogen is converted successively to AI and AII. The largest store of renin is found in the juxtaglomerular apparatus of the kidney, but it has been identified in a great many tissues, including the central nervous system.

It is uncertain whether renal renin is released as a direct result of sympathetic drive to the kidney. Experiments in conscious animals suggest that it may be controlled by an intrarenal barostat mechanism which senses directly a fall in afferent arteriolar pressure (see Chapter 10). Neither is it quite certain that plasma AII can reach levels that have a direct vasoconstrictor action, even in profound hypovolaemia (see Chapter 2). However, there is evidence that it can modulate central regulation of cardiovascular functions through the area postrema.[49]

Measuring efferent autonomic drive to the heart and blood vessels in humans

General

Biochemical methods, in particular the measurement of urinary excretion and plasma concentration of the sympathetic neurotransmitter noradrenaline, have been applied extensively for almost 40 years to quantify total sympathetic nervous system activity in laboratory experiments and in clinical investigations. All rely on the proportionality that usually exists between rates of sympathetic nerve firing and the rate of diffusion of noradrenaline into the plasma after its release.[51] However, global measures of sympathetic function neglect the fact that the sympathetic nervous system exhibits regional differentiation. Thus, in some reflex responses and some disease states certain sympathetic outflows may be activated while others are unchanged or inhibited. Examples are the relatively selective excitation of cardiac sympathetic outflow by experimental mental stress, and the preferential increase of RSNA when dietary sodium is restricted.[51] In order to provide a comprehensive analysis of sympathetic nervous function, regional patterns of sympathetic activity need to be delineated.

Sympathetic function

Each of the various elements in sympathetic nervous control of the cardiovascular system has provided a basis for tests of regional sympathetic nervous function. Similar methods have been used to study sympathetic nervous function in laboratory research on experimental animals and in clinical research on human volunteers or patients, as set out below.

(a) Electrophysiological recordings can be made of multiunit or single fibre sympathetic discharge rates in anaesthetized or awake animals. The clinical counterpart is clinical microneurography, in which multiunit sympathetic firing rates can be measured in accessible subcutaneous nerves which carry sympathetic efferent fibres to skin or skeletal muscle.[52]
(b) Biochemical techniques, typically utilizing radiotracer methodology, can be employed to measure the rates of tissue noradrenaline turnover and of organ-specific noradrenaline spillover to plasma.[51,53,54]
(c) Power spectral analysis can be used to study spontaneous circulatory rhythms.[55] This technique is particularly suited to clinical research. Using sophisticated mathematical partitioning, the individual, superimposed rhythms that produce cyclical variations in heart rate or arterial pressure can be separated and quantified. Heart rate variability is largely attributable to the influence of the autonomic

nervous system. High frequency (~0.3 Hz) and low frequency (~0.1. Hz) components of heart rate variability can be delineated. Low frequency variability derives in part from the cardiac sympathetic nerves and is reduced by β-adrenoceptor blockade.[55] The high frequency component is linked to respiration, is associated in particular with vagal drive and is abolished by atropinization.

(d) Pharmacological autonomic blockade can be used to quantify, by subtraction, the prevailing level of neural cardiovascular drive.[56] The method utilizes the change in measured cardiovascular variables such as vascular resistance, arterial pressure and heart rate after pharmacological autonomic blockade to gauge the overall neurogenic component in vascular tone or the contributions of vagal and sympathetic drive to heart rate.

The information provided about sympathetic function by these last two techniques is indirect. The circulatory variables measured are influenced not only by the rate of sympathetic nerve firing, but also by the responsiveness of the cardiovascular effectors. Electrophysiological techniques for measuring sympathetic nerve discharge rates, and biochemical methods for assessing neurotransmitter release rates, test sympathetic function more directly.

Vagal function

Tests of parasympathetic regulation of the circulation are less well developed than tests of sympathetic function, but they are also less pertinent, except in the case of the heart. There, the influence of the vagus on heart rate and on the electrical stability of the myocardium is of particular importance. There are no clinical tests based on neurotransmitter (ACh) release since the survival of ACh in the synaptic space and in the circulation is so brief because of the powerful actions of fixed and circulating cholinesterases. Neither are there electrophysiological techniques that are clinically applicable.

Pharmacological blockade of the actions of ACh with atropine can be used to estimate vagal tone, from the changes produced in heart rate and cardiac output.[56] Atropinization has also been used to estimate the extent to which vagal withdrawal contributes to the increase in heart rate resulting from stimuli such as exercise, assumption of the upright posture, and mental stress. As we indicated earlier, vagal control of heart rate can be evaluated by spectral analysis of the variation in heart rate,[55,57] since the high frequency component at about 0.3 Hz which is associated with respiratory rhythms is under vagal influence. Tests of arterial baroreflex sensitivity in humans also depend mainly on vagal function. Baroreceptor–heart rate curves can be constructed that relate heart rate to changes in systemic blood pressure induced by intravenous injection of vasoactive drugs or to changes in carotid sinus transmural pressure induced by enclosing the neck in a variable-pressure chamber.[57,58]

Sympathetic microneurography in humans

Although it is possible to record activity in single sympathetic fibres, most microneurographic measurements of sympathetic activity are made from several fibres (multiunit recording).[52,59] The impulses occur in synchronized bursts separated by more or less complete neural silence. The average firing rate in single sympathetic fibres is usually <1–2 Hz, but the instantaneous firing frequencies within each burst vary considerably, and high instantaneous rates can be reached even when the average frequency is low. Since some blood vessels respond poorly to frequencies of <1 Hz, this irregularity of discharge may have physiological importance.

There are clear differences between the patterns of skin and muscle sympathetic activity both at rest and in response to various manoeuvres, indicating that the sympathetic outflow to different tissues is controlled differentially. But there is a remarkable concordance between resting sympathetic traffic directed to different muscles, and also between sympathetic traffic in different nerves directed to the skin of the hands and feet. These findings are consistent with the notion that there are distinct groups of sympathetic preganglionic neurones, each of which is subjected to its own, fairly homogeneous, supraspinal drive. Thus the old concept that the sympathetic drive to blood vessels is global and homogeneous is no longer tenable.

Skin sympathetic activity

Sympathetic activity in skin nerves usually consists of a mixture of vasoconstrictor and sudomotor impulses, but the relative proportions of these and the strength of their activity may vary according to which area of skin a particular nerve is directed.

The skin is a thermoregulatory organ, and in the nerves to the hands and feet changes of environmental temperature lead to selective activation of either vasoconstrictor or sudomotor fibres, with suppression of activity in the other.[52,59] There is little evidence that arterial baroreflexes influence the sympathetic outflow to skin, but respiratory stimuli or stimuli causing arousal or emotional reactions usually evoke clear increases in sympathetic activity. Depending on the subject's thermal state, the increased sympathetic activity may lead to either an increase or a decrease of skin blood flow.[60] This shows that skin sympathetic activity includes impulses causing vasodilation, but it is not clear whether these are carried by specific vasodilator fibres or whether the increase in blood flow is secondary to activation of sweat glands by sudomotor fibres.

Muscle sympathetic nerve activity

Sympathetic traffic in muscle nerves is dominated by vasoconstrictor impulses. In a given subject the strength of the activity at rest is similar in different muscle nerves and it is remarkably constant over many months.[52,59] There are, however, consistent and sometimes large differences among individual subjects. These differences may, to a large extent, determined genetically,[75] but there is also some association with age and heart rate.[52] The strength of MSNA decreases during synchronized sleep,[61,62] but arousal or mental stress lasting less than a minute has no effect. When stress is of longer duration, however, sympathetic activity increases in the peroneal nerve in the leg but remains unchanged in the radial nerve in the arm.[59] Thus, the differentiation of sympathetic activity may extend also to the anatomical location of muscles.

The bursts of MSNA occur predominantly during reductions of blood pressure, and the fluctuations of activity are intimately related to variations in the level of diastolic blood pressure.[52] But only a weak relation, or none, has been found between mean levels of sympathetic activity and blood pressure in normotensive subjects.[63]

Reflexes that affect MSNA can be evoked from several receptor fields. The influence of arterial baroreceptors is complex. In the case of carotid baroreceptors, the effects of dynamic stimulation are much more efficient than those of static stimulation.[59] In contrast, static stimulation of aortic baroreceptors causes sustained changes in muscle sympathetic activity.[64] Unloading of cardiopulmonary receptors causes a marked static increase in MSNA,[52] and an acute increase of CBV leads to a sustained reduction.[65] These findings suggest that the effects of postural change on muscle sympathetic activity originate to a large extent from cardiopulmonary baroreceptors, whereas the influence of arterial baroreceptors is less important. Stimulation of arterial or central chemoreceptors by hypoxia and hypercapnia increases muscle sympathetic activity,[66,67] though if there is a simultaneous increase in ventilation the effect may be blunted, presumably because of input from pulmonary stretch receptors. If intramuscular chemoreceptors are stimulated during isometric handgrip, sympathetic activity increases in the non-contracting arm and leg muscles.[59] But there is recent evidence that when a leg muscle is weakly contracted, sympathetic traffic to that muscle decreases.[68]

MSNA is also influenced by several hormones. Insulin-induced hypoglycaemia,[59] as well as infusion of 2-deoxy-D-glucose,[69] causes an increase. The underlying mechanisms are complex but glucopenia of the central nervous system may contribute. An increase in activity is also observed during and after intravenous infusions of adrenaline.[70]

Clinical studies

Microneurography has been used to analyse sympathetic drive in a variety of clinical settings. It has been used in drug studies, for instance to investigate the effects of anaesthetic regimens; and to clarify pathophysiological mechanisms, for instance in patients with hypertension or heart failure. During acute vasovagal syncope[71,72] and in long lasting vasodepressor attacks[73] the syncopal reaction was associated with sudden cessation of MSNA (Fig. 7.4). Although activation of vasodilator fibres cannot be excluded, the results show that withdrawal of sympathetic vasoconstrictor drive is an important cause of the fall in blood pressure that precedes syncope. The mechanism behind the sympathetic withdrawal probably varies. It is likely that in some cases syncope is due to a central mechanism (emotional syncope), and in other cases to a reflex effect from arterial or cardiopulmonary baroreceptors (postural or hypovolaemic syncope). A special type of syncope, also associated with cessation of MSNA, can accompany glossopharyngeal neuralgia.[59] In this rare

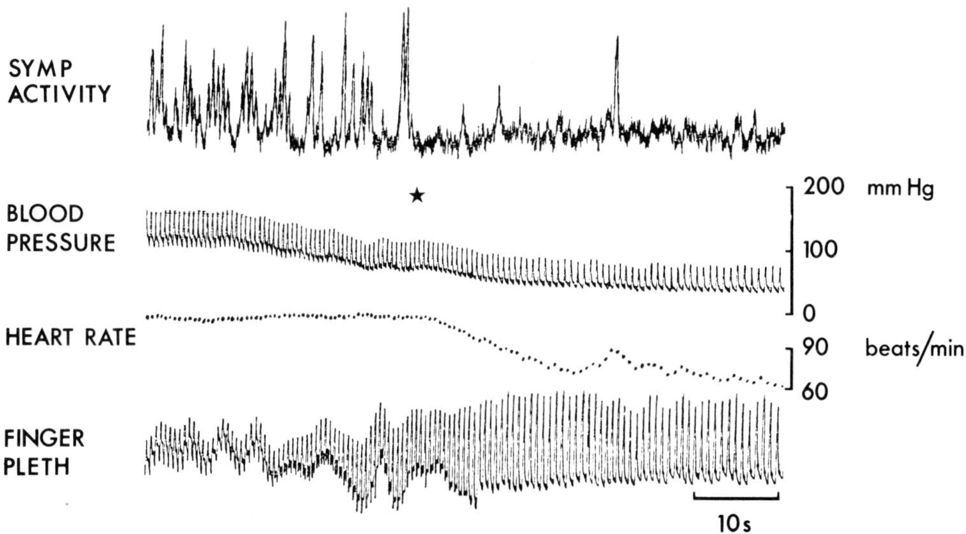

Fig. 7.4. Changes in muscle nerve sympathetic activity, blood pressure, heart rate and finger pulse plethysmogram during syncope (*). From Wallin and Sundlöf,[72] with permission.

condition it has been suggested that pain impulses from the throat are misdirected to brainstem vasomotor centres, where they cause profound sympathoinhibition.

Overflow of neurotransmitters in humans

With microneurographic methods only the sympathetic nerves directed to skeletal muscle and skin can be studied. An important limitation in cardiovascular research is the inaccessibility to testing of the sympathetic nerves to internal organs. Biochemical measurements are more helpful in this regard. Techniques measuring organ-specific noradrenaline release are available for studying regional patterns of sympathetic nervous activation in humans. The close relation between spontaneous sympathetic nerve firing rate, electrical stimulation in the physiological range and the rate of spillover of noradrenaline into the venous effluent from the organ being studied provides the experimental justification for using measures of regional noradrenaline release as a clinical index of sympathetic nervous drive to individual organs. During infusion of radiolabelled noradrenaline (NA) at a constant rate the following formula holds true:[51,53,54]

$$\text{Organ NA spillover} = [(C_v - C_a) + (C_a)(NA_e)]\,[PF]$$

where C_v and C_a are the plasma concentration of noradrenaline in venous and arterial plasma, NA_e is the fractional extraction of tritiated noradrenaline and PF is the organ plasma flow. Similar methodology can also be applied to the measurement of rates of release of presumed sympathetic cotransmitters such as neuropeptide Y and adrenaline.[51,74]

Noradrenaline spillover measurements are instructive in the analysis of reflex, sympathetically mediated, circulatory adjustments in humans. They illustrate the severe methodological limitations of making point measurements of plasma noradrenaline concentration. The rise in plasma noradrenaline concentration when the upright posture is assumed has been used extensively, and often uncritically, as a clinical index of reflex sympathetic nervous responsiveness. But plasma clearance of noradrenaline falls when the upright posture is assumed due to the associated reduction in cardiac output and organ blood flow (Fig. 7.5),[54] so contributing to the rise in plasma noradrenaline concentration. In fact, the rise in plasma noradrenaline concentration seems to be due at least as much to the fall in plasma clearance as to any increase in noradrenaline release.[54]

The importance of sympathetic nervous inhibition in the simple faint is illustrated by measuring changes in noradrenaline spillover. The fainting reaction is a hypotensive circulatory response, often abrupt in onset, that may occur with prolonged standing (particularly in young people) or in re-

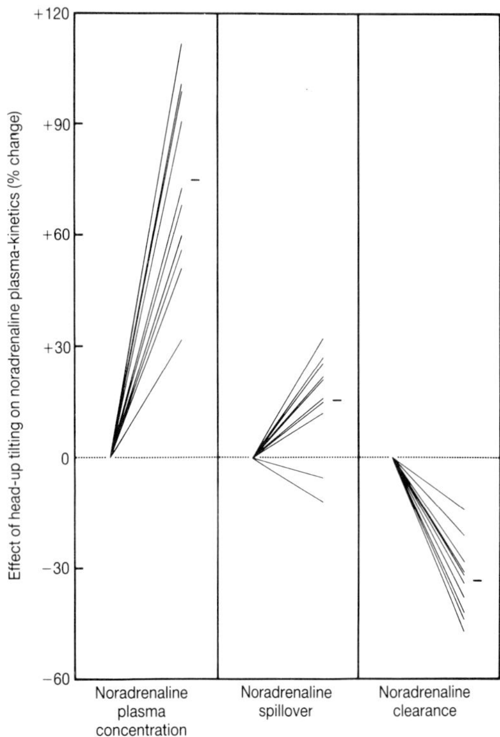

Fig. 7.5. Rise in plasma noradrenaline concentration during 60 min of 40° head-up tilting in 10 subjects with untreated essential hypertension. Note that the rise is attributable to both increased spillover of noradrenaline to plasma and reduced plasma clearance. From Esler *et al.*,[54] with permission.

sponse to unpleasant emotional experiences such as venepuncture. The hypotension is a consequence of the vagal bradycardia and especially the falling vascular resistance: hence the terms 'vasovagal reaction' and 'vasovagal syncope'. The fall in vascular resistance almost certainly results from withdrawal of sympathetic nervous vasoconstrictor drive, as can be demonstrated by sympathetic microneurography (Fig. 7.4), and not to a sympathetic vasodilator mechanism. The reduction in heart rate is also due in part to reduced activity in the cardiac sympathetic nerves, and not solely to increased cardiac vagal drive. Thus, cardiac sympathetic nerve firing, as estimated by measurement of noradrenaline spillover from the heart, falls to near zero during syncope (Fig. 7.6).

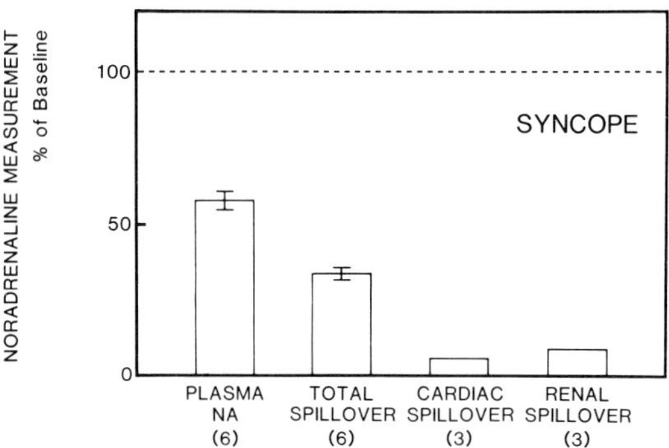

Fig. 7.6. Noradrenaline (NA) measurements, expressed as a percentage of baseline levels, for six subjects who experienced a syncopal reaction during the course of cardiac or renal vein catheterization. Note that cardiac and renal noradrenaline spillover fell to near zero during syncope. From Esler *et al.*,[51] with permission.

Acknowledgements

We are grateful to the colleagues who read this chapter in manuscript, and to those who collaborated in our experimental work. ME and JL are each supported in part by the National Health and Medical Research Council of Australia, and the National Heart Foundation of Australia. GW is supported by the Swedish Medical Research Council (Grant no. B92–04X-03546–21B).

References

1. Ludbrook J and McLachlan E: The autonomic nervous system. In Kyle J and Carey LC (eds): *Scientific Foundations of Surgery*, 4th edn. Oxford, Heinemann Medical Books, 1989, 230–44.
2. Löffelholz K and Pappano AJ: The parasympathetic neuroeffector junction of the heart. *Pharmacological Reviews*, 1985; **37,** 1–24.
3. Randall WC and Rohse WG: The augmentor action of the sympathetic cardiac nerves. *Circulation Research* 1956; **4,** 470–75.
4. Geis GS, Kozelka JW and Wurster RD: Organization and reflex control of vagal cardiomotor neurons. *Journal of the Autonomic Nervous System*, 1981; **3,** 437–50.
5. Kalia M: Brain stem localization of vagal preganglionic neurons. *Journal of the Autonomic Nervous System* 1981; **3,** 451–81.
6. Ciriello J and Calaresu FR: Medullary origin of vagal preganglionic axons to the heart of the cat. *Journal of the Autonomic Nervous System*, 1982; **5,** 9–22.
7. Woolley DC, McWilliam PN, Ford TW and Clarke RW: The effect of selective electrical stimulation of non-myelinated vagal fibres on heart rate in the rabbit. *Journal of the Autonomic Nervous System*, 1987; **21,** 215–21.

8. Ciriello J, Caverson MM and Polosa C: Function of the ventrolateral medulla in the control of the circulation. *Brain Research Reviews*, 1986; **11,** 359–61.
9. Millhorn DE and Eldridge FL: Role of ventrolateral medulla in regulation of respiratory and cardiovascular systems. *Journal of Applied Physiology*, 1986; **61,** 1249–63.
10. Calaresu FR and Yardley CP: Medullary basal sympathetic tone. *Annual Review of Physiology*, 1988; **50,** 511–24.
11. Ruggiero DA, Cravo SL, Arango V and Reis DJ: Central control of the circulation by the rostral ventrolateral reticular nucleus: anatomical substrates. *Progress in Brain Research*, 1989; **81,** 49–79.
12. Dampney RAL: The subretrofacial nucleus: its pivotal role in cardiovascular regulation. *News in Physiological Sciences*, 1990; **5,** 63–7.
13. Dampney RAL: Central mechanisms of cardiovascular control. *Physiological Reviews*; in press.
14. Chalmers J and Pilowsky P: Brainstem and bulbospinal neurotransmitter systems in the control of blood pressure. *Journal of Hypertension*, 1991; **9,** 675–94.
15. McAllen RM and Dampney RAL: The selectivity of descending vasomotor control by subretrofacial neurons. *Progress in Brain Research*, 1989; **81,** 233–42.
16. Agarwal SK and Calaresu FR: Monosynaptic connection from caudal to rostral ventrolateral medulla in the baroreceptor reflex pathway. *Brain Research*, 1991; **555,** 70–74.
17. Blessing WW: Inhibitory vasomotor neurons in the caudal ventrolateral medulla oblongata. *News in Physiological Sciences*, 1991; **6,** 139–41.
18. Li Y-W, Gieroba ZJ, McAllen RM and Blessing WW: Neurons in rabbit caudal ventrolateral medulla inhibit bulbospinal barosensitive neurons in rostral medulla. *American Journal of Physiology*, 1991; **261,** R44–51.
19. Masuda N, Terui N, Koshiya N and Kumada M: Neurons in the caudal ventrolateral medulla mediate the arterial baroreceptor reflex by inhibiting barosensitive reticulospinal neurons in the rostral ventrolateral medulla in rabbits. *Journal of the Autonomic Nervous System*, 1991; **34,** 103–18.
20. Jänig W and McLachlan E: Organization of lumbar spinal outflow to distal colon and pelvic organs. *Physiological Reviews*, 1987; **67,** 1332–404.
21. Jänig W: Pre- and postganglionic vasoconstrictor neurons. Differentiation, type and discharge properties. *Annual Review of Physiology*, 1988; **50,** 525–39.
22. McCall RB: Effects of putative neurotransmitters on sympathetic preganglionic neurons. *Annual Review of Physiology*, 1988; **50,** 553–64.
23. Strack AM, Sawyer WB, Hughes JH, Platt KB and Loewy AD: A general pattern of CNS innervation of the sympathetic outflow demonstrated by transneuronal pseudorabies viral infections. *Brain Research*, 1989; **491,** 156–62.
24. Howe PRC: Blood pressure control by neurotransmitters in the medulla oblongata and spinal cord. *Journal of the Autonomic Nervous System*, 1985; **12,** 95–115.
25. Gilbey MP and Stein RD: Characteristics of sympathetic preganglionic neurones in the lumbar spinal cord of the cat. *Journal of Physiology*, 1991; **432,** 427–43.
26. Polosa C, Yoshimura M and Nishi S: Electrophysiological properties of sympathetic preganglionic neurons. *Annual Review of Physiology*, 1988; **50,** 541–51.
27. Hirst GDS and Edwards FR: Sympathetic neuroeffector transmission in arteries and arterioles. *Physiological Reviews*, 1989; **69,** 546–604.
28. Hirst GDS, Bramich NJ, Edwards FR and Klemm M: Transmission at autonomic neuroeffector junctions. *Trends in Neurosciences*, 1992; **15,** 40–46.
29. Burnstock C and Griffith SG (eds): *Nonadrenergic Innervation of Blood Vessels.* Boca Raton, CA, CRC Press Inc., 1988.
30. Potter E. Neuropeptide Y as an autonomic transmitter. *Pharmacology and Therapeutics*, 1988; **37,** 251–73.
31. Bell C (ed.): *Novel Peripheral Neurotransmitters.* New York, NY, Pergamon Press, 1991.
32. Bolme P and Fuxe K: Adrenergic and cholinergic nerve terminals in skeletal muscle vessels. *Acta Physiologica Scandinavica*, 1970; **78,** 52–9.
33. Schramm LP, Honig CR and Bignall KE: Active muscle vasodilation in primates homologous with sympathetic vasodilation in carnivores. *American Journal of Physiology*, 1971; **221,** 768–77.
34. Rowell LB: Active neurogenic vasodilatation in man. In Vanhoutte PM and Leusen I (eds): *Vasodilatation.* New York, NY, Raven Press, 1981, 1–17.
35. Murray RH and Shropshire S: Effect of atropine on circulatory responses to lower body negative pressure and vasodepressor syncope. *Aerospace Medicine*, 1970; **41,** 717–22.
36. Sanders JS, Mark AL and Ferguson DW: Evidence for cholinergically mediated vasodilation at the beginning of isometric exercise in humans. *Circulation*, 1989; **79,** 815–24.
37. Bevan JA and Brayden JE: Noradrenergic neural vasodilator mechanisms. *Circulation Research*, 1987; **60,** 309–26.
38. Brengelmann GL, Freund PR, Rowell LB, Olerud JE and Kraning KK: Absence of active cutaneous vasodilation associated with congenital absence of sweat glands in humans. *American Journal of Physiology*, 1981; **240,** H571–5.
39. Lundberg J, Norgren L, Ribbe E, Rosén I, Steen S, Thörne J and Wallin BG: Direct evidence of active sympathetic vasodilatation in the skin of the human

foot. *Journal of Physiology*, 1989; **417,** 437–46.
40. Hurley HJ and Mescon H: Cholinergic innervation of the digital arteriovenous anastomoses of human skin. A histochemical localization of cholinesterase. *Journal of Applied Physiology*, 1956; **9,** 82–4.
41. Rand MJ: Nitrergic transmission: nitric oxide as a mediator of non-adrenergic, non-cholinergic neuroeffector transmission. *Clinical and Experimental Pharmacology and Physiology*, 1992; **19,** 147–69.
42. Gibbins IL and Morris JL: Co-location of transmitters in cardiac nerves. *Proceedings of the Australian Physiological and Pharmacological Society*, 1991; **22,** 64–72.
43. Levy MN: Sympathetic : parasympathetic interaction in the heart. *Proceedings of the Australian Physiological and Pharmacological Society*, 1991; **22,** 54–63.
44. Higgins CB, Vatner SF and Braunwald E: Parasympathetic control of the heart. *Pharmacological Reviews*, 1973; **25,** 119–55.
45. Aylward PE, McRitchie RJ, West MJ and Chalmers JP: Relative roles of vagal and sympathetic effector mechanisms in the baroreflex control of myocardial contractility in conscious rabbits. *Pflügers Archiv. European Journal of Physiology (Berlin)*, 1985; **403,** 21–7.
46. Ungar A and Phillips JH: Regulation of the adrenal medulla. *Physiological Reviews*, 1983; **63,** 787–843.
47. McAllen RM and Blessing WW: Neurons (presumably A_1-cells) projecting from the caudal ventrolateral medulla to the region of the supraoptic nucleus respond to baroreceptor inputs in the rabbit. *Neuroscience Letters*, 1987; **73,** 247–52.
48. Day TA and Sibbald JR: A_1 cell group mediates solitary nucleus excitation of supraoptic vasopressin cells. *American Journal of Physiology*, 1989; **257,** R1020–26.
49. Schadt JC and Ludbrook J: Hemodynamic and neurohumoral responses to acute hypovolemia in conscious mammals. *American Journal of Physiology*, 1991; **260,** H305–18.
50. DiCarlo SE, Stahl LK, Hasser EM and Bishop VS: The role of vasopressin in the pressor response to bilateral carotid occlusion. *Journal of the Autonomic Nervous System*, 1989; **27,** 1 10.
51. Esler M, Jennings G, Lambert G, Meredith I, Horne M and Eisenhofer G: Overflow of catecholamine neurotransmitters to the circulation: source, fate and functions. *Physiological Reviews*, 1990; **70,** 963–85.
52. Vallbo ÅB, Hagbarth K-E, Torebjörk E and Wallin BG: Somatosensory, proprioceptive and sympathetic activity in human peripheral nerves. *Physiological Reviews*, 1979; **59,** 919–57.
53. Esler M, Jackman G, Bobik A, Kelleher D, Jennings G, Leonard P, Skews H and Korner P: Determination of norepinephrine apparent release rate and clearance in humans. *Life Sciences*, 1979; **25,** 1461–70.
54. Esler M, Jennings G, Korner P, Willett I, Dudley F, Hasking G, Anderson W and Lambert G: The assessment of human sympathetic nervous system activity from measurements of norepinephrine turnover. *Hypertension*, 1988; **11,** 3–20.
55. Pagani M, Lombardi F, Guzzetti S, Rimoldi O, Furlan R, Pizzinelli P, Sandrone G, Malfatto G, Dell'Orto S, Piccaluga E, Turiel M, Baselli G, Cerutti S and Malliani A: Power spectral analysis of heart rate and arterial pressure variabilities as a marker of sympatho–vagal interaction in man and conscious dog. *Circulation Research*, 1986; **59,** 178–93.
56. Julius S, Pascual A and London R: Role of parasympathetic inhibition in the hyperkinetic type of borderline hypertension. *Circulation*, 1971; **44,** 413–18.
57. LaRovere MT, Specchia G, Mortaro A and Schwartz PJ: Baroreflex sensitivity, clinical correlates and cardiovascular mortality amongst patients with a first myocardial infarction. *Circulation*, 1988; **78,** 816–24.
58. Eckberg DL and Sleight P: *Human Baroreflexes in Health and Disease*. Oxford, Oxford University Press, 1992, 231–65.
59. Wallin BG and Fagius J: Peripheral sympathetic neural activity in conscious humans. *Annual Review of Physiology*, 1988; **50,** 565–76.
60. Oberle J, Elam M, Karlsson T and Wallin BG: Temperature dependent interaction between vasoconstrictor and vasodilator mechanisms in human skin. *Acta Physiologica Scandinavica*, 1988; **132,** 459–69.
61. Hornyak M, Cajner M, Elam M, Matousek M and Wallin BG: Sympathetic muscle nerve activity during sleep in humans. *Brain*, 1991; **114,** 1281–95.
62. Okada H, Iwase S, Mano T, Sugiyama Y and Watanabe T: Changes in muscle sympathetic nerve activity during sleep in humans. *Neurology*, 1991; **41,** 1961–6.
63. Yamada Y, Miyajima E, Tochikubo O, Matsukawa T and Ishii M: Age-related changes in muscle sympathetic nerve activity in essential hypertension. *Hypertension*, 1989; **13,** 870–77.
64. Sanders JS, Mark AL and Ferguson DW: Arterial baroreflex control of sympathetic activity during elevation of blood pressure in normal man: dominance of aortic baroreceptors. *Circulation*, 1988; **77,** 279–88.
65. Saito M, Manbo T, Iwase S, Koga K and Matsukawa T: Sympathetic nervous responses in man to weightlessness simulated by head-out water immersion. In Watanabe S, Miterai G and Mori S (eds): *Biological Sciences in Space*. Tokyo, Myu Research, 1987, 85–92.
66. Saito M, Mano T, Iwase S, Koga K, Abe H and Yamazaki I: Responses in muscle sympathetic nerve

activity to acute hypoxia in humans. *Journal of Applied Physiology*, 1988; **65,** 1548–52.

67. Somers VK, Mark AL, Zavala DC and Abboud FM: Influence of ventilation and hypocapnia on sympathetic nerve responses to hypoxia in normal humans. *Journal of Applied Physiology*, 1989; **67,** 2095–100.
68. Wallin BG, Burke D and Gandevia SC: Coherence between the sympathetic drives to relaxed and contracting muscles of different limbs of human subjects. *Journal of Physiology*, 1992; **455,** 219–33.
69. Fagius J and Berne C: Changes of sympathetic nerve activity induced by 2-deoxy-D-glucose infusions in humans. *American Journal of Physiology*, 1989; **256,** E174–20.
70. Persson B, Andersson OK, Hjemdahl P, Wysocki M, Agewall S and Wallin BG: Adrenaline infusion in man increases muscle sympathetic activity and noradrenaline overflow to plasma. *Journal of Hypertension*, 1989; **7,** 747–56.
71. Wallin BG and Sundlöf G: Sympathetic outflow to muscles during vasovagal syncope. *Journal of the Autonomic Nervous System*, 1982; **2,** 287–91.
72. Scherrer U, Vissing S, Morgan B, Hanson P and Victor RG: Vasovagal syncope after infusion of a vasodilator in a heart-transplant recipient. *New England Journal of Medicine*, 1990; **322,** 602–4.
73. Yatomi A, Iguchi A, Uemura K, Sakamoto N, Iwase S and Mano T: A rare case of recurrent vasodepressive attacks of two hours duration: analysis of the mechanisms by muscle sympathetic nerve activity recording. *Clinical Cardiology*, 1989; **12,** 164–8.
74. Esler M, Eisenhofer G, Chin J, Jennings G, Meredith I, Cox H, Lambert G, Thompson J and Dart A: Is adrenaline released by sympathetic nerves in man? *Clinical Autonomic Research*, 1991; **1,** 103–8.
75. Wallin BG, Kunimoto M and Selgren J: Possible genetic influence on the strength of human muscle nerve activity at rest. *Hypertension*; in press.

Part 3
Regional circulations

8

Cerebral blood flow and hypovolaemic shock

Jes F Schmidt and Olaf B Paulson

Severe blood loss was already associated with cerebral nervous dysfunction as early as 1575 by Ambroise Pare. In severe blood loss a considerable drop in cardiac output occurs.[1] However, this drop is associated with an increase in flow fraction to several regions; namely the brain, the heart and the liver.[1] The blood supply is to a certain degree thereby secured to several vital organs. A contemporary activation of the sympathetic system is a main factor in this redistribution of blood flow.

In the brain activation of the sympathetic nervous system leads to a constriction of the greater resistance vessels (inflow tract), contributing to the maintenance of blood pressure. Despite the favourable redistribution of blood flow to the brain during blood loss cerebral circulation still decreases with the risk of ischaemic damage in severe shock. The present chapter deals with the regulation of cerebral blood flow (CBF) under these conditions.

The mechanisms of regulation of cerebral blood flow

Autoregulation

Autoregulation of cerebral blood flow can be defined in various ways (Fig. 8.1).[2] In clinical settings the concept of a constant flow over a wide range of perfusion pressures seems to be the most appropriate definition (see below), and will be applied in the present chapter. In other circumstances autoregulation can be defined in terms of vascular resistance, by the blood pressure interval in which vascular resistance increases in response to blood pressure increase.[3] Finally, autoregulation can be defined as the blood pressure interval during which there is dilatation of the vessels in response to the drop in perfusion pressure and vasoconstriction in response to an increase in perfusion pressure.[4]

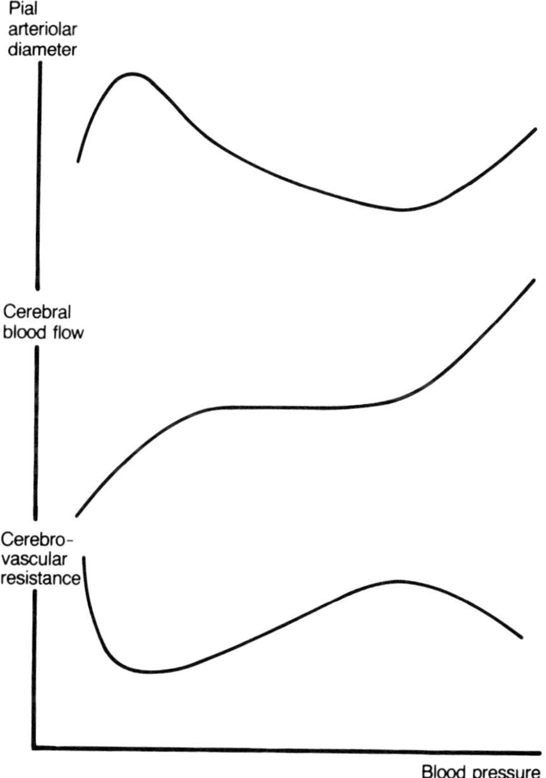

Fig. 8.1. Diagrammatic presentation of pial arteriolar diameter, cerebral blood flow and cerebrovascular resistance with blood pressure. From Paulson *et al.*,[2] with permission.

Neuronal regulation

The cerebral vessels receive sympathetic innervation from the ganglion cervicalis superior. Of this, the greater vessels of the 'inflow tract' receive the major contribution. These nerves have a great effect on cerebral blood volume, intracranial pressure and the formation of cerebrospinal fluid. The resting CBF is left relatively unchanged by stimulation or denervation of the sympathetic nerves. Under activation of CBF by either hypercapnia or intense metabolic stimulation an attenuation of the expected increase is caused by the concomitant increase in sympathetic tone. In addition, a shift of the limits of autoregulation towards higher pressures is induced (see below). The role of parasympathetic nerves, sensory nerves from the trigeminal ganglion and the intrinsic nerves that might sense and quickly change the intracerebral vessel tone needs further investigation.

Chemical regulation

Chemical regulation profoundly influences CBF. Major chemical regulators are the arterial carbon dioxide tension (Pa_{CO_2}) and the oxygen tension (Pa_{O_2}). Hypercapnia and hypoxaemia both induce a global increase in CBF. It has been claimed, based on studies of brainstem lesions, that the response to elevation of Pa_{CO_2} may be mediated in part through brainstem receptors.[5] However, isolated changes of Pa_{CO_2} in the vertebral circulation do not influence flow in the hemispheres.[6]

Oxygen is a major determinant of changes in cerebrovascular resistance. CBF increases when Pa_{O_2} falls below 6.7 kPa.[7,8] In 1948 Kety and Schmidt[9] showed that a decrease of the inspired oxygen fraction to 0.10 (normally 0.21) resulted in an increase in CBF to 35 per cent above resting values. Under these conditions the Pa_{CO_2} must be carefully considered, as hypoxia induces hyperventilation. Dahlgren[10] has investigated the effect on CBF of lowering the Pa_{O_2} thereby inducing hyperventilation. The findings suggest that the response to these two parameters is mediated by different mechanisms: Pa_{O_2} plays no role in CBF regulation in patients at sea level unless they are suffering from a pulmonary and/or a major cardiac disease.

The influence of changes in Pa_{CO_2} on CBF, the cerebral vascular reactivity to CO_2, has been studied in several species. The relation of CBF to Pa_{CO_2} may be described as either an exponential or a linear function in different physiological ranges of Pa_{CO_2}.[11–13] During resting conditions the slope of the linear part of the curve (indicated as change in CBF from baseline value per mmHg change in Pa_{CO_2} has been reported as varying from between 1 and 6 per cent, depending on the method used to measure CBF.[14–16] One report suggested different responses for white and gray matter.[17] When only small changes in Pa_{CO_2} are registered the changes can be calculated by a linear function, while for major changes a logarithmic relation must be considered.[12]

CO_2 regulation at different blood pressures

Harper and Glass[18] found sigma-shaped curves in normotensive anaesthetized dogs with linearity in the Pa_{CO_2} range from 2.7 to 8.1 kPa (20–60 mmHg), the slope being approximately 2.2 per cent. The slope was approximately 1.5 per cent at mild hypotension. At severe hypotension, however, CBF did not react to changes in Pa_{CO_2} (Fig. 8.2). The influence of arterial blood pressure on the CO_2 reactivity of the cerebral vessels has been evaluated in humans by Schmidt *et al.*,[16] who found a diminished CO_2 reactivity when mean pressure was 20 per cent or less of resting values. Henriksen[19] found that the Pa_{CO_2} exerts an important influence on CBF before, during and following cardiac surgery. The relation of CBF to Pa_{CO_2} was unaffected by temperature and haematocrit; and only hypotension significantly reduced the reactivity of the cerebral vessels to changes in Pa_{CO_2}.

A diminished response of cerebral vessel reactivity to CO_2 changes at mean arterial pressure levels more than 20 per cent above the baseline values was shown by Schmidt *et al.*[16]

This indicates that the increase in blood pressure *per se* induced some alterations in the cerebral vessels.

Metabolic regulation

The term metabolic regulation denotes a close coupling between CBF and cerebral metabolism, and this coupling is present in normal individuals[20] and during certain pathophysiological or altered physiological states, i.e. seizures, changes in temperature and during anaesthesia.[21]

In general, increasing cerebral metabolic demand during increased neuronal activity increases CBF. The increase is highly localized. A variety of vasoactive molecules have been proposed as mediators of the coupling between neuronal activity and blood flow: these include CO_2, H^+, O_2, adenosine and adenine nucleotides, K^+ and Ca^{++}.[22] The exact role of these substances in the coupling between flow and metabolism remains to be established.

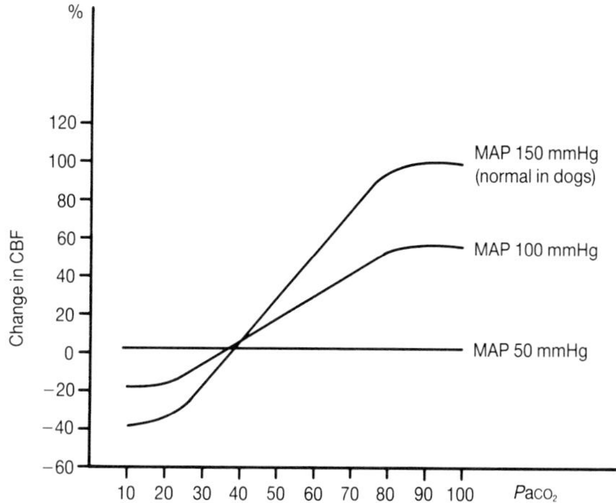

Fig. 8.2. The effect of alterations in arterial carbon dioxide tension ($Pa\text{CO}_2$) on the cortical cerebral blood flow (CBF) in dogs at normotension and two degrees of hypotension. MAP, mean arterial pressure. *Source*: Harper and Glass.[18]

Effects of changes in haematocrit

The level of haematocrit influences CBF substantially, CBF being inversely proportional to the haematocrit.[23] In severe acute and chronic anaemia CBF is increased considerably, and in polycythaemia CBF is reduced.[24,25]

Autoregulation of cerebral blood flow

Autoregulation of CBF as defined above is effective over a wide range of arterial blood pressures, but has a lower as well as an upper pressure limit. Under normal conditions these limits are about mean blood pressures of 60 and 150 mmHg, respectively,[26–28] though the lower limit may be even higher, i.e. 90 per cent of the resting value of mean arterial blood pressure.[29] When blood pressure falls below the lower limit, CBF decreases as vasodilatation becomes inadequate. Autoregulatory vasodilatation reaches a maximum well below the pressure where CBF starts to decrease. Hence, the lower limit of autoregulation is higher than the pressure of maximal dilatation.[30] At the lowest blood pressures the vessels collapse. At levels moderately below the lower limit of autoregulation CBF can be increased by CO_2 inhalation or vasodilatory drugs (Fig. 8.2).[18,31,32] If systemic blood pressure drops moderately below the lower limit of autoregulation (less than around 50 per cent of the resting value, with a CBF decrease of 30 per cent or less), then the oxygen uptake by the brain is maintained at its normal level by an increase of the oxygen extraction from the blood in proportion to the fall in CBF. At this stage clinical symptoms are insignificant. If pressure drops further, symptoms of incipient fainting develop with dizziness, pallor, sweating, yawning, etc. With further pressure reduction consciousness is lost and finally ischaemic brain damage occurs, first reversible and then irreversible.[33] At these stages, with blood pressure markedly below the lower limit of autoregulation, the increase in oxygen extraction from the blood can no longer counterbalance the decrease in CBF and there is a decrease in the cerebral uptake of oxygen, i.e. in the cerebral metabolic rate of oxygen.

CBF autoregulation responds not only to blood pressure changes but also to changes in intracranial pressure.[32,34,35] In the normal situation and in diseases without changes in intracranial pressure the variations in perfusion pressure are nearly identical to those in arterial blood pressure. In brain diseases with increased intracranial pressure the situation may be different (see below) and intracranial pressure changes may be of significance for the autoregulatory limits.

CBF autoregulation and its limits are modulated by the sympathetic nervous system, the vessel wall renin–angiotensin system and any factor that causes cerebral vasodilatation or vasoconstriction (see below). Hence, the limits of autoregulation are not completely fixed, but may vary somewhat as they are under dynamic physiological control.

The mechanisms of autoregulation

The myogenic mechanism

According to the myogenic mechanism theory[36] the smooth muscle of cerebral vessels are responsive to changes in transmural pressure, i.e. the small arteries and arterioles constrict or dilate in response to increases or decreases in the transmural pressure, respectively. The rapidity of the autoregulatory response, which is initiated within a few seconds after a change in transmural pressure of the resistance vessels,[37–39] and largely completed within 15–30 seconds, favours a myogenic response. According to this hypothesis a quick change in intravascular pressure alters the state of the actin and myosin filaments in the smooth muscle cells. This may induce a myogenic response according to the principle outlined by Bayliss in 1902.[40]

The metabolic mechanism
The metabolic theory of cerebral autoregulation states that a reduction in local blood flow results in the release of a chemical factor that elicits dilatation of cerebral vessels. Of the existing metabolic factors only adenosine has received experimental support.[41] Other studies, however, have indicated that adenosine does not play a major role in autoregulation.[42–44] Although the rapidity of the autoregulatory response has been considered to favour the myogenic hypothesis, it should be mentioned that flow changes may occur essentially instantaneously in response to metabolic changes. Thus, CBF increases within seconds in response to seizure activity, and here rapid 'siphoning' of K^+ by the glial cells may be of significance for the rapidity of the response.[45]

Perivascular nerves
Extrinsic nerves Nerve fibres originating from cranial ganglia, such as the superior cervical, trigeminal and sphenopalatine, provide a dense sympathetic, parasympathetic and sensory input to cerebral circulation. The innervation density is greatest in large cerebral vessels at the base of the brain and sparser in more distal and intraparenchymal arteries.[46,47]

Stimulation or denervation of the *sympathetic* nerve supply changes resting CBF only marginally;[48] however, these nerves have a marked effect on cerebral blood volume, i.e. cerebral capacitance,[49] intracranial pressure[50] and cerebrospinal fluid formation.[51] Furthermore, they may attenuate the flow increase caused by hypercapnia[2] and intense metabolic stimulation.[52] Finally, an important effect is to shift the limits of autoregulation (see below).

The *parasympathetic* nerve supply from the VIIth nerve elicits a modest vasodilatation by stimulation,[53] and cutting the facial nerve does not change autoregulation.[54] However, it is difficult to study complete parasympathetic denervated models because of its widespread anatomic localizations.[55]

Intrinsic nerves Over the last 20–30 years there has been discussion over whether the cerebral circulation is regulated by intrinsic nerve fibres that might sense and quickly regulate intraparenchymal vessel tone.[56,57] Ishitsuka *et al.*[58] have reported that the NTS can modify cerebrovascular autoregulation without modifying resting local blood flow. Further details are necessary in order to be able to ascertain the importance of these findings.

The cerebrovascular endothelial cell related factors
NO is an EDRF that has been shown to cause relaxation of vascular smooth muscle.[59,60] The presence of an endothelium-derived contractile factor (EDCF) has been advocated as well.[61] Increments in flow without changes in transmural pressure induce vasodilatation, through isolated vessel sections both *in situ* and *in vitro*, that can be abolished by removal of the endothelium.[62–64] These observations suggest that endothelial cells release a vasodilator mediator (or mediators) in response to increases in flow. Rubanyi *et al.*[65] addressed the role of the endothelium in pressure-induced vasoconstriction in the cerebral vessels. A rapid increase in transmural pressure triggered active contraction which was prevented by removal of the endothelium. However, *in vivo* studies where the production of NO was blocked by nitro-L-arginine did not modify autoregulation of CBF.[66]

Physiological regulation of autoregulation

Sympathetic nervous system
Activity in the perivascular sympathetic fibres around cerebral vessels does not influence resting CBF within the autoregulation range or has a very modest effect.[67–69] Activation of the sympathetic nerves may shift the upper limit of autoregulation towards higher pressures whereas acute denervation may shift the limits of the autoregulation towards lower blood pressure levels.[2] Chronic sympathetic denervation does not shift the limits of autoregulation.[70] The shift of the upper limit of cerebral autoregulation towards higher pressures during sympathetic activation is probably a physiological mechanism, protecting the brain against blood pressure increases during activation.

Reductions in blood pressure within the physiological range, e.g. during sleep or after physical exercise, are often associated with a low sympathetic tone. The consequent tendency to shift towards lower pressures affords some protection to the brain against hypotension-induced ischaemia. In other settings sympathetic tone is not low at low blood pressure but may in some instances be high, for example during haemorrhagic hypotension (see below).

The sympathetic nervous system exerts its vasomotor function predominantly in the larger cerebral resistance vessels (the 'inflow tract'), whereas autoregulation is predominantly a function of the smaller resistance vessels.[2] During sympathetic activation, with constriction of the larger resistance vessels, the smaller resistance vessels further downstream dilate, an autoregulatory response in order to keep CBF constant as long as blood pressure is within the autoregulatory range. The opposite takes place if the sympathetic tone is reduced. Only at the limits of autoregulation may the vasomotor function of the larger resistance vessels affect CBF because the smaller resistance vessels no longer have the full autoregulatory capacity.

Renin–angiotensin system

The renin–angiotensin system has some tone in the cerebral resistance vessels.[71] The ACE inhibitor appears to influence the vessel wall renin system rather than the brain renin system.[72] Probably, the renin–angiotensin system mainly influences the larger cerebral resistance vessels and ACE inhibition causes dilatation of these vessels.[2] The limits for cerebral autoregulation are thereby shifted to lower pressure levels for reasons quite similar to those discussed above for the sympathetic nervous system. An interaction can be shown between the renin–angiotensin system and the sympathetic nervous system. Thus, the downward shift of the upper limit of autoregulation is attenuated by simultaneous stimulation of the superior cervical sympathetic ganglion in the rat.[73] That the renin–-angiotensin system influences CBF autoregulation independent of the sympathetic nervous system has been shown by Waldemar.[74]

In humans the effect of ACE inhibition with captopril is less pronounced than in the rat. In patients with heart failure, captopril caused a marked fall in blood pressure with no changes in CBF, suggestive of a shift in autoregulation towards low pressures.[75] In one study the observations suggested some downward shift of the lower limit of autoregulation, but statistically only at the limits of significance;[76] however, in another study of the same group, a significant reduction was reached.[77] The upper limit of autoregulation was not reached by moderate blood pressure increase in either of the studies.

The level of cerebral blood flow

The level of CBF influences the autoregulation as the autoregulatory plateau is shortened at high CBF and widened at low CBF. $Paco_2$ is one of the strongest physiological modulators of cerebral blood flow: hypocapnia induces vasoconstriction whereas hypercapnia causes vasodilatation. The modification of the autoregulatory curve at high and low CBF is typically found at high and low levels of $Paco_2$ (Fig. 8.3).[32,78,79] At high CBF the resistance vessels are dilated and do not have enough dilatory capacity to keep CBF constant down to the normal lower limit of autoregulation. At the upper limit of autoregulation the dilated resistance vessels will be more vulnerable and resist the increased intravascular pressure less well. Hence the upper limit of autoregulation will be shifted downwards at high flow levels. Both hypercapnia and pharmacological vasodilatation may ultimately altogether abolish autoregulation.

Age

In fetal lamb the cerebral circulation has been shown to be pressure dependent on increases or decreases in perfusion pressure. One might speculate that this is because fetal cerebral vasculature is already maximally dilated. After 3 to 9 days autoregulation of CBF was found to be present.[80]

Pryds *et al.*[81] found heterogeneity of cerebral vasoreactivity in preterm infants supported by mechanical ventilation, i.e. in the first living day

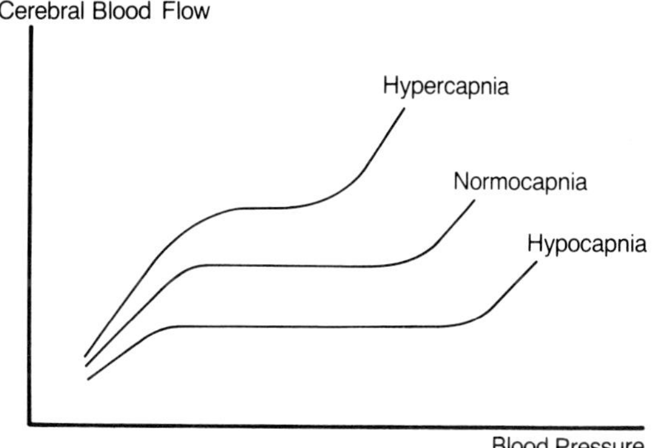

Fig. 8.3. Effect of vasodilatation and vasoconstriction on autoregulation of cerebral blood flow. From Paulson *et al.*,[2] with permission.

a CO_2 reactivity of 12 per cent change in CBF per kPa change in Pa_{CO_2}, which increased to normal values (33 per cent) on day 2. On the other hand, the autoregulation of CBF by changes in mean arterial blood pressure was maintained constantly.

In the early fifties Schieve and Wilson[82] demonstrated that CBF and $CMRO_2$ (the cerebral metabolic rate of oxygen) did not change with age and that even CO_2 reactivity was unchanged in normal elderly people.

Pathophysiology

Acute haemorrhage

The influence of blood loss and shock has been widely studied, using different methods for different species to obtain the blood loss. The changes in CBF mostly have been evaluated globally, especially in humans. In shock blood pressure drops below the lower limit of autoregulation. The autoregulatory protection of the brain is thus impaired and may even be abolished.

Bleeding

In 1944 Shenkin *et al.*[83] published a paper on volunteers that bled large amounts, i.e. up to 15 cc/k. No CBF measurements were made in these subjects, however they all showed signs of impaired CBF: nausea, dizziness, faintness, and some lost consciousness. Forsyth *et al.*[84] drew 10, 30 and 50 per cent of blood from monkeys and showed, using the microsphere technique, an increase in the fraction of cardiac output that reached the brain. At 30 per cent bleeding CBF decreased but not significantly; however, at 50 per cent bleeding CBF decreased to about one-third, despite an increase to 228 per cent of the concomitantly reduced cardiac output reaching the brain. Fitch *et al.*,[85] in baboons, have shown that CBF remains constant by controlled bleeding down to about 65 per cent of resting mean arterial blood pressure. Thereafter CBF decreases when arterial blood pressure decreases further. They also showed that an α-blockage or surgical sympathectomy enhanced the maintenance of CBF to blood pressure values of approximately 35 per cent of mean arterial pressure. The clinical application of this work is that the cerebral circulation is better protected against hypotension due to autonomic blocking agents than it is to haemorrhagic shock. In 1979 Hamar *et al.*[86] found the same effect of α-blockage, i.e. that pretreatment prevented the fall in CBF and $CMRO_2$ that occurs in systemic hypotension due to bleeding.

Tilting

Acute hypotension has also been induced by a combination of tilting and drug infusion. Finnerty *et al.*,[87] using the Kety and Schmidt method to determine CBF, found signs and symptoms of cerebral ischaemia when CBF was reduced to approximately 31.5 ml/100 g/min from 51 ml/100 g/min (a reduction of approximately 40 per cent). The decrease in mean arterial pressure that resulted in these symptoms varied from between 29 and 80 mmHg. No sign of change in the overall cerebral oxygen consumption was noted. Strandgaard *et al.*[26] found a lower end of the autoregulation curve at mean pressure values of between 50 and 70 mmHg and a lowest tolerated blood pressure of between 35 and 40 mmHg in normotensive subjects. In these studies a combination of ganglion blockage and tilting was used to induce the hypotension and CBF was estimated by the arteriovenous oxygen difference method. The calculated value of CBF was reduced to about 70 per cent of resting values when the lowest tolerated blood pressure was reached.

Lower body negative pressure

Murray *et al.*[88] induced hypovolaemia in humans by progressive LBNP; this regimen resulted in syncope. The syncope was induced at a reduction in mean arterial pressure from 91 mmHg to 55 mmHg in seven healthy volunteers. Using a combination of ganglion blockage and LBNP Schmidt *et al.*[29] showed that a decrease in CBF of 30 per cent from 62 ml/100 g/min to 45 ml/100 g/min occurred during a decrease in mean pressure from 110 mmHg to 68 mmHg. These changes in CBF were well tolerated by the moderate hypertensive patients. CBF was measured by Xenon-133 inhalation and SPECT (single photon emission tomography).

Pharmacological

Drugs may have different effects on the autoregulation of CBF. The brain will be best protected if autoregulation is maintained, as impaired autoregulation may result in uneven (heterogenous) perfusion at even moderately decreased blood pressure.[2] Most drug-induced hypotension (trimetaphan, halothane, isoflurane, nitroprusside, etc.) will preserve CBF better compared to hypotension induced by haemorrhage. The most likely explanation is that haemorrhage induces sympathetic activation with cerebral vasoconstriction in the greater inflow vessels to the brain (as mentioned above).

Regional cerebral blood flow studies
Graham *et al.*[89] used a combination of trimetaphan, tilting and haemorrhage to achieve an isoelectric electroencephalogram (EEG) in baboons. Mean arterial pressure was reduced from 99 to 19 mmHg in the normotensive group and from 140 to 32 mmHg in the hypertensive group. CBF was reduced from 56 ml/100 g/min to 11 ml/100 g/min (an 80 per cent reduction) and this was sustained for 30 min. This led to a pattern of brain damage located particularly in the arterial boundary zones, between the major cerebral arteries. The particular vulnerability of the arterial boundary zone is due to the anatomy of the vascular supply of cerebrum; the inability to supply sufficient blood to the most distal part of the arterial system during hypotension. Schmidt *et al.*[29] showed that a reduction of CBF by 30 per cent did not provoke any changes in regional CBF distribution, i.e. no areas of focal ischaemia exceeding the global flow reduction were provoked by the hypotension. The regional distribution was measured by Xenon-133 inhalation and SPECT.

Hypertension

In chronic hypertension CBF and $CMRO_2$ are unchanged from normal values.[90] However, hypertension influences the autoregulation by shifting its limits towards higher pressures (Fig. 8.4).[91] In treated younger patients the limits revert towards normal values, probably within weeks or a few months. In severe and long-standing cases the changes in the vessels may be irreversible. Despite these changes the brain is still the organ that has benefited most from antihypertensive treatment.

The CO_2 reactivity has been shown to be unchanged at least in cases with moderate hypertension.[15,16]

The significance for shock is that a blood pressure drop to a certain level is less well tolerated by the brain in hypertensives than in normotensives.

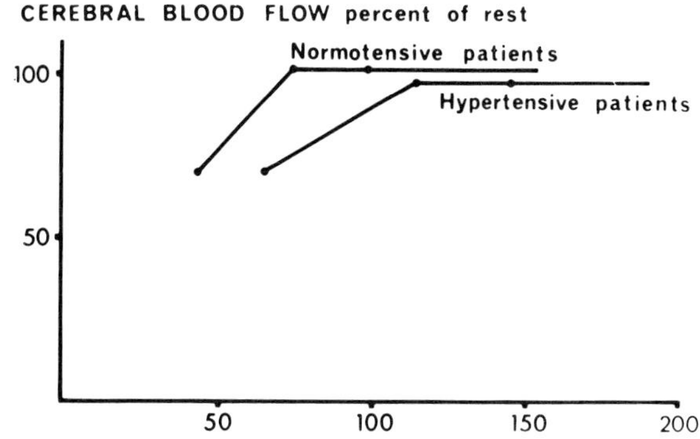

Fig. 8.4. The effect of hypertension on the lower limit in hypertension. From Paulson *et al.*,[2] with permission.

Arteriosclerosis

Vasomotor paralysis with loss of autoregulation is a common and well-known phenomenon in acute ischaemic cerebrovascular diseases.[2] In the ischaemic areas distal to an arterial occlusion the arteriolar pressure will be much lower than normal and obviously below the lower limit of autoregulation. Hence, apparent loss of autoregulation could simply reflect the pressure–flow relation (proportional changes) below the lower limit of autoregulation. However, the ischaemia provokes generalized vasomotor paralysis with true loss of autoregulation, mainly due to tissue acidosis.[92] Loss of autoregulation is also present in the first phase after a spontaneous recanalization of a thromboembolic arterial occlusion where increased flow prevails.[93–95]

Chronic threatening ischaemia is a condition that may be present if an occlusion or stenosis of an artery to the brain results in only a moderate reduction of the local blood pressure distal to the occlusion. In these instances the local blood pressure may be at or slightly below the lower limit of autoregulation[96,97] and CBF may be normal or only slightly reduced in the resting state. However, with a drop in systemic blood pressure the local blood pressure is further reduced resulting in a focal CBF decrease, and symptoms of ischaemia may result from the territory of the artery that no longer is protected by autoregulation (Fig. 8.5).[98]

In an acute cerebral ischaemic lesion there may exist a boundary zone of chronic threatening ischaemia – a penumbra zone.[99,100] It remains a matter of controversy as to how extensive such a zone is and for how long it may survive.[101]

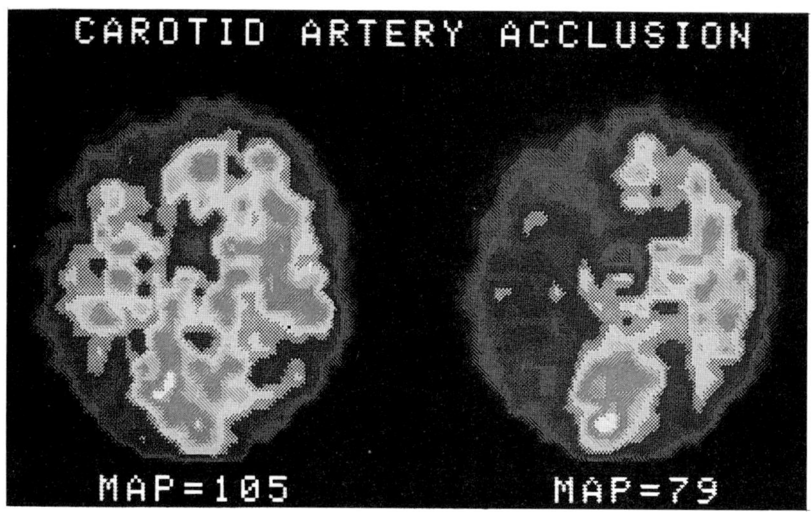

Fig. 8.5. Single photon emission computed tomography (SPECT) before and after moderate hypotension showing focal ischaemia. MAP, mean arterial pressure. From Vorstrup *et al.*,[98] with permission.

As mentioned above CBF autoregulation is a protective mechanism. Reduction of blood pressure below the lower limit of autoregulation can result in patchy (uneven, heterogeneous) blood flow, with ischaemic zones neighbouring on zones with more normal perfusion.[86] The watershed zones between major cerebral arteries seems particularly vulnerable in this regard. Even if CBF is high and above normal baseline values, e.g. due to the application of a cerebral vasodilator, there is risk of patchy ischaemia if blood pressure is below the lower limit of autoregulation.[102]

Diabetes mellitus

Resting CBF is unchanged in patients with diabetes compared with healthy subjects;[103] however, the autoregulation has been shown to be impaired in long-term patients.[103,104] Dandonna *et al.*[105] demonstrated a reduced CO_2 reactivity of the cerebral vessels at least to increases in $Pa\text{CO}_2$.

Infections

Patients with meningitis and/or encephalitis often have impaired CBF autoregulation.[106] In many cases the reactivity of the cerebral vessels to changes in $Pa\text{CO}_2$ has been maintained. This can be used therapeutically, i.e. hyperventilation can restore the autoregulation of CBF.[79]

Trauma

In cerebral trauma autoregulation is impaired.[107] Severe head injury is accompanied by marked disturbances of autoregulation and other regulatory mechanisms of CBF.[2] The lesion in severe head injury is by nature multifocal, with the more and the less diseased tissue adjacent to one other. Corresponding regional flow abnormalities are abundant and the flow patterns often rather complex. Loss of autoregulation and false autoregulation are commonly observed. In some cases of presumed false autoregulation a 'less abnormal' state with only loss of autoregulation could be induced by hypocapnia, decreasing the intracranial pressure.[108] Loss of autoregulation has been found to correlate with changes in intracranial pressure. In patients with intact autoregulation intracranial pressure decreases in response to a blood pressure increase, a consequence of the autoregulatory cerebral vasoconstriction. In contrast, intracranial pressure increases or remains unchanged in response to a blood pressure increase in those patients with widely affected autoregulation.[109] In severe cases the CO_2 reactivity can be lost, and this has been taken as a bad sign.[110] In head trauma, as well as in other acute cerebral diseases, the brain is more vulnerable than usual, and more at risk to complications in cases of shock with blood pressure drop.

Conclusion

Blood loss and shock give rise to an increase in sympathetic tone, constricting the greater arteries of the cerebral circulation. The concomitant autoregulatory response dilates the smaller resistance vessels with the net effect of a higher lower limit of CBF autoregulation. Several studies demonstrate that a 30 per cent reduction in CBF can be well tolerated due to an increase of oxygen extraction in the brain. However, a further decrease in CBF due to haemorrhage will evidently give rise to signs of cerebral ischaemia. Due to the architecture of the cerebral vessels, the so-called boundary zones (watershed areas) are the most vulnerable places in cases of acute haemorrhage. If the blood loss is accompanied with other diseases (chronic hypertension, diabetes, arteriosclerosis, trauma cerebri, etc.) even more complicated conditions may occur.

References

1. Neutze JM, Wyler F and Rudolph AM: Changes in distribution of cardiac output after hemorrhage in rabbits. *American Journal of Physiology*, 1968; **215,** 857–64.
2. Paulson OB, Strandgaard S and Edvinson L: Cerebral autoregulation. *Cerebrovascular and Brain Metabolism Reviews*, 1990; **2,** 161–92.
3. Miller JD, Stanek AE and Langfitt TW: Cerebral blood flow regulation during experimental brain compression. *Journal of Neurosurgery*, 1973; **39,** 186–96.
4. Heistad DD and Kontos HA: Cerebral circulation. In Shepherd JT and Abboud FM (eds): *Handbook of Physiology. Section 2: The Cardiovascular System, Volume 3.* Bethesda, MD, American Physiological Society, 1983, 137–82.
5. Shalit MN, Reinmuth OM, Shinmojyo S and Scheinberg P: Carbon dioxide and cerebral circulatory control. III. The effects of brainstem lesions. *Archives of Neurology*, 1967; **17,** 342–53.
6. Skinhøj E and Paulson OB: Carbon dioxide and cerebral circulatory control. Evidence of nonfocal site of action of carbon dioxide on cerebral circulation. *Archives of Neurology*, 1969; **20,** 249–52.
7. McDowall DG: Interrelationships between blood oxygen tension and cerebral blood flow. In Payne JP and Hill DW (eds): *Oxygen Measurements in Blood and Tissues.* London, Churchill Livingstone, 1966, 205–19.
8. Kogure K, Scheinberg P, Fujishima M, Busto R and Reinmuth OM: Effects of hypoxia on cerebral autoregulation. *American Journal of Physiology*, 1970; **219,** 1393–6.
9. Kety SS and Schmidt CF: The effect of altered arterial tensions of carbon dioxide and oxygen on cerebral blood flow and cerebral oxygen consumption of normal young men. *Journal of Clinical Investigation*, 1948; **27,** 484–92.
10. Dahlgren N: Local cerebral blood flow in spontaneously breathing rats subjected to graded isobaric hypoxia. *Acta Anesthesiologica Scandinavica*, 1990; **34,** 463–7.
11. Alexander SC, Wollman H, Cohen PJ, Chase PE and Behar M: Cerebrovascular response to $Pa\text{CO}_2$ during halothane anesthesia in man. *Journal of Applied Physiology*, 1964; **19,** 561–5.
12. Olesen J, Paulson OB and Lassen NA: Regional cerebral blood flow in man determined by the initial slope of the clearance of intra-arterially injected 133-Xenon. *Stroke*, 1971; **2,** 519–40.
13. Reivich M: Arterial $P\text{CO}_2$ and cerebral hemodynamics. *American Journal of Physiology*, 1964; **206,** 25–35.
14. Waltz AG: Effect of $Pa\text{CO}_2$ on blood flow and microvasculature of ischemic and nonischemic cerebral cortex. *Stroke*, 1970; **1,** 27–37.
15. Tominaga S, Strandgaard S, Uemura K, Ito K, Kutsuzawa T, Lassen NA and Nakamura T: Cerebrovascular CO_2 reactivity in normotensive and hypertensive man. *Stroke*, 1976; **7,** 507–10.
16. Schmidt JF, Waldemar G and Paulson OB: Arterial CO_2 tension and cerebral vascular reactivity during the induction of acute hypertension and hypotension in the awake human. *Journal of Neurosurgical Anesthesiology*, 1990; **2,** 92–6.
17. Willkinson IMS and Browne DRG: The influence of anaesthesia and arterial hypocapnia on regional blood flow in the normal human cerebral hemisphere. *British Journal of Anaesthesiology*, 1970; **42,** 472–82.
18. Harper AM and Glass HI: Effect of alterations in the arterial carbon dioxide tension on the blood flow through the cerebral cortex at normal and low arterial blood pressures. *Journal of Neurology, Neurosurgery and Psychiatry*, 1965; **28,** 449–52.
19. Henriksen L: Brain luxury perfusion during cardiopulmonary bypass in humans. A study of the cerebral blood flow response to changes in CO_2, O_2, and blood pressure. *Journal of Cerebral Blood Flow and Metabolism*, 1986; **6,** 366–78.
20. Raichle ME, Grubb RL Jr, Gado MH, Eichling JO and Ter-Pogossian MM: Correlation between regional cerebral blood flow and oxidative metabolism. *In vivo* studies in man. *Archives of Neurology*, 1976; **33,** 523–6.
21. Nielson B, Rehncrona S and Siesjø BK: Coupling of cerebral metabolism and blood flow in epileptic seizures, hypoxia and hypoglycemia. In Purves M

(ed.): *Cerebral Vascular Smooth Muscle and its Control*, CIBA Foundation Symposium 56 (new series). Amsterdam, Elsevier, 1978, 199–214.
22. Kuschinsky W and Wahl M: Local chemical and neurogenic regulation of cerebral vascular resistance. *Physiological Reviews*, 1978; **58,** 656–89.
23. Paulson OB, Parving HH, Olesen J and Skinhøj E: Influence of carbon monoxide and of hemodilution on cerebral blood flow and blood gases in man. *Journal of Applied Physiology*, 1973; **35,** 111–16.
24. Heyman A, Patterson JL Jr and Duke TW: Cerebral circulation and metabolism in sickle cell and other chronic anemias with observations on the effects of oxygen inhalation. *Journal of Clinical Investigation*, 1952; **31,** 824–8.
25. Humphrey PRD, Marshall JM, Russell RWR, Wetherley-Mein G, Boulay GH, Pearson TC, Symon L and Zilkha E: Cerebral blood flow and viscosity in relative polycythaemia. *Lancet*, 1979; **2,** 873–6.
26. Strandgaard S, Olesen J, Skinhøj E and Lassen NA: Autoregulation of brain circulation in severe arterial hypertension. *British Medical Journal*, 1973; **i,** 507–10.
27. McHenry JLC, West JW, Cooper ES, Goldberg HI and Jaffe ME: Cerebral autoregulation in man. *Stroke*, 1974; **5,** 695–705.
28. Strandgaard S: Autoregulation of cerebral blood flow in hypertensive patients. The modifying influence of prolonged antihypertensive treatment on the tolerance to acute, drug-induced hypotension. *Circulation*, 1976; **53,** 720–27.
29. Schmidt JF, Waldemar G, Vorstrup S, Andersen AR, Gjerris F and Paulson OB: Computerized analysis of cerebral blood flow autoregulation in humans: validation of a method for pharmacologic studies. *Journal of Cardiovascular Pharmacology*, 1990; **15,** 983–8.
30. MacKenzie ET, Farrar JK, Fitch W, Graham DI, Gregory PC and Harper AM: Effects of hemorrhagic hypotension on the cerebral circulation. I: Cerebral blood flow and pial arteriolar caliber. *Stroke*, 1979; **10,** 711–18.
31. Barry DI, Strandgaard S, Graham DI, Svendsen UG, Brændstrup O and Paulson OB: Cerebral blood flow response to intravenous dihydralazine in renal and spontaneously hypertensive rats. *Stroke*, 1984; **15,** 102–7.
32. Häggendal E and Johansson B: Effects of arterial carbon dioxide tension and oxygen saturation on cerebral blood flow autoregulation in dogs. *Acta Physiologica Scandinavica. Supplement*, 1965; **66,** 27–53.
33. Brierly JE, Brown AW, Excell BJ and Meldrum BS: Brain damage in the Rhesus monkey resulting from profounding arterial hypotension. I. Its nature, distribution and general physiological correlates. *Brain Research*, 1969; **13,** 68–100.
34. Sadoshima S, Thames M and Heistad D: Cerebral blood flow during elevation of intracranial pressure: role of sympathetic nerve. *American Journal of Physiology*, 1981; **241,** H78–84.
35. Wagner EM and Traystman RJ: Cerebrovascular transmural pressure and autoregulation. *Annals of Biomedical Engineering*, 1985; **13,** 311–20.
36. Folkow B: Description of the myogenic hypothesis. *Circulation Research*, 1964; **15(suppl. 1),** 279–87.
37. Kontos HA, Wei EP, Navari RM, Levasseur JE, Rosenblum WI and Patterson JL: Responses of cerebral arteries and arterioles to acute hypotension and hypertension. *American Journal of Physiology*, 1978; **234,** H371–83.
38. Symon L, Held K and Dorsch NWC: A study of regional autoregulation in the cerebral circulation to increased perfusion pressure in normocapnia and hypercapnia. *Stroke*, 1973; **4,** 139–47.
39. Johansson BB and Nilsson B: Cerebral vasomotor reactivity in normotensive and spontaneously hypertensive rats. *Stroke*, 1979; **10,** 572–6.
40. Bayliss WM: On the local reaction of the arterial wall to changes of internal pressure. *Journal of Physiology (London)*, 1902; **28,** 220–31.
41. Rubio R, Berne RM and Winn HR: Production, metabolism and possible functions of adenosine in brain tissue *in situ*. In Elliot K and O'Connor M (eds): *Cerebral Vascular Smooth Muscle and its Control*. Amsterdam, Elsevier, 1978, 355–73.
42. Phillis JW: Adenosine in the control of the cerebral circulation. *Cerebrovascular and Brain Metabolism Reviews*, 1989; **1,** 26–54.
43. Phillis JW and de Long RE: The role of adenosine in cerebral vascular regulation during reductions in perfusion pressure. *Journal of Pharmaceutics and Pharmacology*, 1986; **38,** 460–62.
44. Kontos HA and Wei EP: Oxygen-dependent mechanisms in cerebral autoregulation. *Annals of Biomedical Engineering*, 1985; **13,** 329–34.
45. Paulson OB and Newman EA: Does the release of potassium from astrocyte endfeet regulate cerebral blood flow? *Science*, 1987; **237,** 896–8.
46. Edvinsson L: Neurogenic mechanisms in the cerebral circulation. *Acta Physiological Scandinavica. Supplement*, 1975; **427,** 1–35.
47. Uddman R and Edvinsson L: Neuropeptides in the cerebral circulation. *Cerebrovascular and Brain Metabolism Reviews*, 1989; **1,** 230–52.
48. Edvinsson L and MacKenzie ET: Amine mechanisms in the cerebral circulation. *Pharmacological Reviews*, 1977; **28,** 275–348.
49. Edvinsson L, Nielsen KC, Owman C and West KA: Evidence of vasoconstrictor sympathetic nerves in brain vessels of mice. *Neurology*, 1973; **23,** 73–7.
50. Edvinsson L, Owman C and West KA: Changes

in continuously recorded intracranial pressure of conscious rabbits at different time-periods after superior cervical sympathectomy. *Acta Physiologica Scandinavica*, 1971; **83,** 42–50.

51. Lindvall M, Edvinsson L and Owman C: Sympathetic nervous control of cerebrospinal fluid production from the choroid plexus. *Science*, 1978; **201,** 176–8.
52. Mueller SM, Heistad DD and Marcus ML: Effect of sympathetic nerves on cerebral vessels during seizures. *American Journal of Physiology*, 1979; **237,** H178–84.
53. Pinard E, Purves MJ, Seylaz J and Vasquez JV: The cholinergic pathway to cerebral blood vessels. II. Physiological studies. *Pflügers Archiv. European Journal of Physiology (Berlin)*, 1979; **379,**1 65–72.
54. Hoff JT, MacKenzie ET and Harper AM: Responses of the cerebral circulation to hypercapnia and hypoxia after VIIth cranial nerve transection in baboons. *Circulation Research*, 1977; **40,** 258–62.
55. Hara H, Jansen I, Ekman R, Hamel E, MacKenzie ET, Uddman R and Edvinson L: Acetylcholine and vasoactive intestinal peptide in cerebral blood vessels: effect of extirpation of the sphenopalatine ganglion. *Journal of Cerebral Blood Flow and Metabolism*, 1989; **9,** 204–11.
56. Ingvar DH: Cortical state of excitability and cortical circulation. In Jasper HH, Proctor DC, Knighton SR, Noshay CW and Costello TR (eds): *Reticular Formation of the Brain.* Boston, MA, Little, Brown & Co., 1958, 381–408.
57. Molnar L and Szanto J: The effect of electrical stimulation of the bulbar vasomotor centre on the cerebral blood-flow. *Quarterly Journal of Experimental Physiology*, 1964; **49,** 184–93.
58. Ishitsuka T, Underwood MD, Iadecola C and Reis DJ: Bilateral lesions of nucleus tractus solitarii abolishes cerebral vascular autoregulation independently of associated hypertension. *Federation Proceedings*, 1984; **43,** 305.
59. Ignarro LJ, Buga GM, Wood KS, Byrns KS and Chaudhuri G: Endothelium-derived relaxing factor produced and released from artery and vein is nitric oxide. *Proceedings of the National Academy of Sciences (USA)*, 1987; **84,** 9265–9.
60. Palmer RMJ, Ferrige AG and Moncada S: Nitric oxide release accounts for the biological activity of endothelium-derived relaxing factor. *Nature*, 1987; **327,** 524–6.
61. Rubanyi GM: Endothelium-derived vasoconstrictor factors. III. In Ryan US (ed.): *Endothelial Cell.* Boca Ratum, FL, CRC Press, 1988, 61–74.
62. Busse R, Trogisch G and Bassenge E: The role of endothelium in the control of vascular tone. *Basic Research in Cardiology*, 1985; **00,** 475–90.
63. Holtz J, Forstermann U, Pohl U, Giesler M and Bassenge E: Flow-dependent, endothelium-mediated dilatation of epicardial coronary arteries in conscious dogs: effects of cyclooxygenase inhibition. *Journal of Cardiovascular Pharmacology*, 1984; **6,** 1161–9.
64. Smiesko V, Koziak J and Dolezel S: Role of endothelium in the control of arterial diameter by blood flow. *Blood Vessels*, 1985; **22,** 247–51.
65. Rubanyi GM, Romero JC and Vanhoutte PM: Flow-induced release of endothelium-derived relaxing factor. *American Journal of Physiology*, 1986; **250,** H1145–9.
66. Wang Q, Paulson OB and Lassen NA: Is autoregulation of CBF in rats influenced by nitro-L–arginine, a blocker of the synthesis of nitric oxide? *Acta Physiologica Scandinavica*; in press.
67. Harper AM, Deshmukh VD, Rowman JO and Jennett WB: The influence of sympathetic nervous activity on cerebral blood flow. *Archives of Neurology*, 1972; **27,** 1–6.
68. Sercombe R, la Combe P, Aubineau P, Mamo H, Pinard E, Reyneir-Rebuffel AM and Seylaz AJ: Is there any active mechanism limiting the influence of the sympathetic system on the cerebral vascular bed? Evidence for vasomotor escape from sympathetic stimulation in the rabbit. *Brain Research*, 1979; **164,** 81–102.
69. Busija DW, Heistad DD and Marcus ML: Effects of sympathetic nerves on cerebral vessels during acute, moderate increases in arterial pressure in dogs and cats. *Circulation Research*, 1980; **46,** 696–702.
70. Sadoshima S, Fujishima M, Yoshida F, Ibayashi S, Shiokawa O and Omae T: Cerebral autoregulation in young spontaneously hypertensive rats. Effect of sympathetic denervation. *Hypertension*, 1985; **7,** 392–7.
71. Barry DI, Jarden JO, Paulson OB, Graham DI and Strandgaard S: Cerebrovascular effects of converting enzyme inhibition. I: Effects of intravenous captopril in spontaneously hypertensive and normotensive rats. *Journal of Hypertension*, 1984; **2,** 589–97.
72. Jarden JO, Barry DI, Juhler M, Graham DI, Strandgaard S and Paulson OB: Cerebrovascular aspects of converting enzyme inhibition. II. Blood–brain barrier permeability and effect of intracerebroventricular administration of captopril. *Journal of Hypertension*, 1984; **2,** 599–604.
73. Waldemar G, Paulson OB, Barry DI and Knudsen GM: Angiotensin converting enzyme inhibition and the upper limit of cerebral blood flow autoregulation: effect of sympathetic stimulation. *Circulation Research*, 1989; **64,** 1197–1204.
74. Waldemar G: Acute sympathetic denervation does not eliminate the effect of angiotensin converting enzyme inhibition on CBF autoregulation in spontaneously hypertensive rats. *Journal of Cerebral Blood*

Flow and Metabolism, 1990; **10,** 43–7.

75. Paulson OB, Jarden JO, Vorstrup S, Holm S and Godtfredsen J: Effect of captopril on the cerebral circulation in chronic heart failure. *European Journal of Clinical Investigation*, 1986; **16,** 124–32.
76. Waldemar G, Schmidt JF, Andersen AR, Vorstrup S and Paulson OB: Angiotensin converting enzyme inhibition and cerebral blood flow autoregulation in normotensive and hypertensive man. *Journal of Hypertension*, 1989; **7,** 229–35.
77. Schmidt JF, Andersen AR, Paulson OB and Gjerris F: Angiotensin converting enzyme inhibition, CBF autoregulation and ICP in patients with normal-pressure hydrocephalus. *Acta Neurochirurgica*, 1990; **106,** 9–12.
78. Ekstrøm-Jodal B, Hæggendal E, Linder LE and Nielson NJ: Cerebral blood flow autoregulation at high arterial blood pressures and different levels of carbon dioxide tension. *European Neurology*, 1971; **6,** 6–10.
79. Paulson OB, Olesen J and Christensen MS: Restoration of autoregulation of cerebral blood flow by hypocapnia. *Neurology*, 1972; **22,** 286–93.
80. Borel CO, Backofen JE, Koehler RC, Jones MD Jr and Traystman RJ: Cerebral blood flow autoregulation during intracranial hypertension in hypoxic lambs. *American Journal of Physiology*, 1987; **253,** H1342–421.
81. Pryds O, Greisen G, Lou H and Friis-Hansen B: Heterogeneity of cerebral vasoreactivity in preterm infants supported by mechanical ventilation. *Journal of Pediatrics*, 1989; **115,** 638–45.
82. Schieve JF and Wilson WP: The influence of age, anesthesia and cerebral arteriosclerosis on cerebral vascular activity to CO_2. *American Journal of Medicine*, 1953; **142,** 171–4.
83. Shenkin HA, Cheney RH, Govons SR, Hardy JD and Fletcher AG: On the diagnosis of hemorrhage in man: a study of volunteers bled large amounts. *American Journal of Medical Science*, 1944; **208,** 421–36.
84. Forsyth RP, Hoffbrand BI and Melmon KL: Redistribution of cardiac output during hemorrhage in the unanesthetized monkey. *Circulation Research*, 1970; **27,** 311–20.
85. Fitch W, MacKenzie ET and Harper AM: Effects of decreasing arterial blood pressure on cerebral blood flow in the baboon. *Circulation Research*, 1975; **37,** 550–57.
86. Hamar J, Kovach ABG, Reivich M, Nyary I and Durity F: Effect of phenoxybenzamine on cerebral blood flow and metabolism in the baboon during haemorrhagic shock. *Stroke*, 1979; **10,** 401–7.
87. Finnerty FA, Witkin L, Fazekas JF, Langbart M and Young WK: Cerebral hemodynamics during cerebral ischemia induced by acute hypotension. *Journal of Clinical Investigation*, 1954; **33,** 1227–32.
88. Murray RH, Thompson LJ, Bowers JA and Albright CD: Hemodynamic effect of graded hypovolemia and vasopressor syncope induced by lower body negative pressure. *American Heart Journal*, 1968; **76,** 799–811.
89. Graham DI, McGeorge A, Fitch W, Jones JV and MacKenzie ET: Ischaemic brain damage induced by rapid lowering of arterial pressure in hypertension. *Journal of Hypertension*, 1984; **2,** 297–304.
90. Kety SS, Hafkenschiel JH, Jeffers WA, Leopold IH and Shenkin HA: The blood flow, vascular resistance, and oxygen consumption of the brain in essential hypertension. *Journal of Clinical Investigation*, 1948; **27,** 511–14.
91. Jones JV, Fitch W, MacKenzie ET, Strandgaard S, and Harper AM: Lower limit of cerebral blood flow autoregulation in the baboon. *Circulation Research*, 1976; **39,** 555–7.
92. Harris RJ and Symon L: Extracellular pH, potassium, and calcium activities in progressive ischaemia of rat cortex. *Journal of Cerebral Blood Flow and Metabolism*, 1984; **4,** 178–86.
93. Høedt-Rasmussen K, Skinhøj E, Paulson OB, Ewald J, Bjerrum JK, Fahrenkrug A and Lassen NA: Regional cerebral blood flow in acute apoplexy. The 'luxury perfusion syndrome' of brain tissue. *Archives of Neurology*, 1967; **17,** 271–81.
94. Olsen TS, Larsen B, Bech Skriver E, Herning M, Enevoldsen E and Lassen NA: Focal cerebral hyperemia in acute stroke. Incidence, pathophysiology and clinical significance. *Stroke*, 1981; **12,** 598–607.
95. Avery S, Crockard HA and Russell RR: Evolution and resolution of oedema following severe temporary cerebral ischaemia in the gerbil. *Journal of Neurology, Neurosurgery and Psychiatry*, 1984; **47,** 604–10.
96. Shima T, Hossman KA and Date H: Pial arterial pressure in cats following middle cerebral artery occlusion. 1. Relationship to blood flow, regulation of blood flow and electrophysiological function. *Stroke*, 1983; **14,** 713–19.
97. Spetzler RF, Roski RA and Zabramski J: Middle cerebral artery perfusion pressure in cerebrovascular occlusive disease. *Stroke*, 1983; **14,** 512–15.
98. Vorstup S, Waldemar G, Andersen A, Schmidt JF, Haase J and Paulson OB: Selection of patients with occlusive vascular disease for EC–IC bypass. In Crepaldi G, Gotto A, Manzato E and Baggio G (eds): *Atherosclerosis VIII.* Rome, Elsevier Science, 1989, 519–22.
99. Branston NM, Symon L and Crockard HA: Recovery of the cortical evoked response following temporary middle cerebral artery occlusion in baboons: relation to local blood flow and Po_2. *Stroke*, 1976; **7,** 151–7.
100. Astrup J: Energy-requiring cell function in the is-

chemic brain. *Journal of Neurosurgery*, 1982; **56,** 482–97.

101. Olsen TS, Larsen B, Herning M, Bech Skriver E and Lassen NA: Blood flow and vascular reactivity in collaterally prefused brain tissue. Evidence of an ischemic penumbra in patients with acute stroke. *Stroke*, 1983; **14,** 332–41.
102. Harris RJ, Branston NM, Symon L, Bayhan M and Watson A: The effects of a calcium antagonist, nimodipine, upon physiological responses of the cerebral vasculature and its possible influence upon focal cerebral ischaemia. *Stroke*, 1982; **13,** 759–66.
103. Kastrup J, Rørsgaard S, Parving HH and Lassen NA: Impaired autoregulation of cerebral blood flow in long-term type I (insulin-dependent) diabetic patients with nephropathy and retinopathy. *Clinical Physiology*, 1986; **6,** 549–59.
104. Bentsen N, Larsen B and Lassen NA: Chronically impaired autoregulation of cerebral blood flow in long-term diabetics. *Stroke*, 1975; **6,** 497–502.
105. Dandonna P, James IM, Wollard ML, Newsbury P and Beckett AG: Cerebral blood flow in diabetes mellitus: evidence of abnormal cerebrovascular reactivity. *British Medical Journal*, 1978; **2,** 325–6.
106. Paulson OB, Brodersen P, Hansen EL and Kristensen HS: Regional cerebral blood flow, cerebral metabolic rate of oxygen, and cerebrospinal fluid acid-base variables in patients with acute meningitis and with acute encephalitis. *Acta Medica Scandinavica*, 1974; **196,** 191–8.
107. Reivich M, Marshall WJS and Kassell N: Loss of autoregulation produced by cerebral trauma. In Brock M, Fieschi C, Ingvar DH, Lassen NH and Schürmann K (eds): *Cerebral Blood Flow*. New York, NY, Springer-Verlag, 1969, 205–8.
108. Cold GE, Christensen MS and Schmidt K: Effect of two levels of induced hypocapnia on cerebral autoregulation in the acute phase of head injury coma. *Acta Anaesthesiologica Scandinavica*, 1981; **25,** 397–401.
109. Muizelaar JP, Ward JD, Marmarou A, Newlon PG and Wachi A: Cerebral blood flow and metabolism in severely head-injured children. Part 2: Autoregulation. *Journal of Neurosurgery*, 1989; **71,** 72–6.
110. Schalen W, Messeter K and Nordstøm CH: Cerebral vasoreactivity and the prediction of outcome in severe traumatic brain lesions. *Acta Anaesthesiologica Scandinavica*, 1991; **35,** 113–22.

9

Coronary blood flow

Stig Haunsø

Blood loss leading to hypovolaemic shock is important to recognize, particularly in patients with diseases in the coronary arteries or the heart muscle, because of the hazard it poses, and because of the improvement in coronary circulatory dynamics that can be achieved readily and safely by augmentation of vascular volume. The coronary circulation supplies a tissue that is constantly working, has high metabolic requirements, cannot sustain an oxygen debt and by its own contraction (systole) impedes blood flow to the inner layers of the left ventricular free wall, i.e. the subendocardium. Satisfactory blood flow and oxygen supply to the subendocardium of the left ventricle poses problems that in the healthy heart are easily handled. However, with heart diseases and/or blood loss and hypovolaemia these problems are exacerbated, and in order to understand the function of the coronary circulation under such pathophysiological conditions a review of coronary physiology including the smaller parts of the microcirculation is appropriate.

Anatomy and function of the coronary circulation

The weight of the human heart is approximately 300 g, and is dominated by the thick-walled left ventricle. The myocardium of the right and left ventricles is supplied by blood from the coronary system which in simplified terms can be described in humans as consisting of four sections. First, a short left main coronary artery that divides into an anterior descending branch and a circumflex branch. The anterior descending branch courses the intraventricular groove to reach the apex, yielding septal branches in transit while the circumflex branch ends in a posterior descending branch. The right coronary artery passes along the right atrioventricular sulcus towards the back of the heart, where it gives off descending branches to both ventricles. Second, *intramyocardial arteries and arterioles* (10–200 μm), which due to their small diameter and a media packed with smooth muscle cells have the capacity to alter profoundly the resistance to coronary blood flow. Third, a high density network of *capillary vessels* (5 μm) that is uniform throughout the left ventricular wall. The ratio of capillaries to muscle fibres is close to 1 : 1, and the intercapillary distance is approximately 15 μm. Fourth, native thin-walled *collaterals* that link the large conduit vessels to each other. The coronary arteries are well innervated by autonomic nerves and fine unmyelinated nerve fibres running in close association with the coronary vessels, and naked varicose endings are often seen close to the capillaries.[1–6]

The function of the coronary circulation is to supply the myocardium with oxygen and nutrients and to eliminate waste products. This is done by: (1) *convection*, i.e. the movement of blood and its containing substances through the capillaries; and (2) *diffusion*, i.e. the movement of substances across the capillary wall and through the interstitium or vice versa along concentration gradients. The microcirculation of the heart is constructed to deliver a large amount of oxygen and substrates to the myocytes. There are approximately 3500 capillaries/mm^2 and during increased blood flow it seems that previously non-perfused capillaries are perfused. This phenomenon is called *capillary recruitment*, a mechanism probably controlled by the small intramyocardial resistance vessels, leading to a decreased diffusion distance and an increase in the total capillary surface area. Such a mechanism improves the supply of substrates to the myocardium, since this is mainly accomplished by diffusive processes.[7–9]

Aspects of blood loss and hypovolaemia in microcirculation

In patients with blood loss and hypovolaemia, a special problem exists concerning the microcirculation of the heart. In the canine myocardium it has been demonstrated that although hypoxia leads to capillary recruitment the effect is maximal only if the perfusion pressure is normal.[8] If such results can be extrapolated to the human heart, it means that severe hypotension induced by hypovolaemia may lead to less optimal conditions for myocardial oxygen and substrate supply.

Relation between myocardial oxygen metabolism and blood flow

Approximately 5 per cent of cardiac output at rest and during exercise is distributed through the coronary circulation to the myocardium. Left ventricular blood flow in human and canine myocardium is 80–100 ml/min/100 g and can increase to 300–400 ml/min/100 g or even more during pharmacologically induced maximum vasodilatation of the resistance vessels. 'Resting' myocardial oxygen demands are high (8–10 ml/min/100 g) due to a constant workload compared to those of skeletal muscle (approximately 0.15 ml/min/100 g).[9–11]

The relative requirement for oxygen of various types of work carried out by the heart is listed in Table 9.1. Pressure work is much more expensive

Table 9.1 The relative requirement of oxygen during various types of work

Myocardial O_2 consumption
Oxygen needs:
8–10 ml/min/100 g
Basal 20%
Electrical 1%
Volume work 15%
Pressure work 64%
Mycardial O_2 extraction
75% versus 20% systemic

than volume work.[12] With such high oxygen demands, even at 'rest' extraction of oxygen from the coronary vascular bed is very high, resulting in coronary venous oxygen saturation in the range of 20–30 per cent.[12] The close and parallel relation between myocardial metabolism and blood flow is described by the equation:

$$MV_{O_2} = (a-v)_{O_2} \times Q$$

where MV_{O_2} represents the total myocardial oxygen uptake primarily determined by wall stress, contractility and heart rate. The arteriovenous oxygen difference, $(a-v)_{O_2}$, is near maximum at 'rest'. Q equals myocardial blood flow. Thus, coronary circulation meets elevated oxygen demand by increasing myocardial blood flow because oxygen extraction cannot increase much further. The moment-to-moment regulation of local blood flow in response to changing metabolic needs is a function of the intramural resistance vessels.[9–12] The influence of arteriolar resistance and driving pressure on myocardial blood flow (Q) can be defined by the equation:

$$Q = \Delta P / R$$

where δP is the driving perfusion pressure across the coronary vascular bed (usually considered to be the difference between aortic and right atrial pressure) and $1/R$ is the coronary arteriolar conductance.[12]

Distribution of coronary blood flow across the free left ventricular wall

The lower oxygen tension of blood in subendocardial veins and tissue reflects most probably greater work and a marked underperfusion during systole. Due to compressive forces from myocardial contractility during systole, perfusion of the subendocardial layers decreases or ceases. During diastole an excess blood flow is directed to this layer, making the left ventricular free wall of the myocardium homogeneously perfused during a cardiac circle. Consequently, blood flow to the inner layers of the left ventricle is strongly related to the diastolic perfusion pressure and its duration.[13–15]

Factors regulating coronary blood flow

The regulation of coronary blood flow is multifactorial and the major factors regulating coronary tone in intramyocardial resistance vessels are illustrated in Table 9.2. The main determinant of local blood flow regulation is the metabolic mechanism. Neural control, humoral regulation and the endothelial factors are of intermediate importance. The myogenic mechanism remains unproven. Of the physical factors that influence myocardial blood flow, blood flow viscosity is of minor importance. However, extravascular compression of the capillaries can alter blood flow significantly.[2,9–16]

Table 9.2 Factors regulating coronary blood flow

Determinants of coronary vascular tone
Metabolic factors
Adenosine (−)
Adenosine triphosphate (−)
O_2 (+)
CO_2 (−)
H^+ (−)
K^+ (−)
Neural factors
Sympathetic nervous system
α-receptor stimulation (+)
β-receptor stimulation (−)
Vagus (−)
Central control and reflex control (+/−)
Neuropeptide Y (+)
Calcitonin gene-related peptide (−)
Humoral factors
Catecholamines (+)
Angiotensin (+)
Thyroid hormones (+)
Antidiuretic hormone (+)
Endothelial factors
Prostaglandins (−)
EDRF (−)
Endothelin (+)
Myogenic factor
?
Miscellaneous
Thromboxane (+)
Serotonin (+)

EDRF, endothelium-derived relaxing factor. (+), vasoconstriction; (−), vasodilation.

The metabolic hypothesis

A mechanism is required to match myocardial oxygen supply to oxygen demand during increased work, when coronary blood flow must increase. Several 'metabolic' mediators have been suggested as serving as the link between increased metabolic activity and myocardial blood flow. These include adenosine, ATP, oxygen, carbon dioxide, potassium, calcium, pH and osmolality. Of these, adenosine is considered to play an important role in the metabolic hypothesis[2] as reviewed recently by Opie.[17] Adenosine is formed within myocardial cells when, as a result of vigorous work, hypoxia or ischaemia, high energy phosphates, ATP and adenosine diphosphate (ADP), are broken down. Adenosine can readily cross cell membranes and has a very short life time (half-life at 37°C, 10 seconds). Adenosine, after diffusion out of the myocyte, reaches the extracellular space where it acts on arterioles as a powerful vasodilator by opening up ATP-dependent potassium channels. The adenosine hypothesis provides a sensitive feedback mechanism that can restore oxygen supply.[17]

The influence of neural factors on coronary vascular tone

Autonomic nervous system

The afferent neural system includes vagal and sympathetic afferents connected to sensory endings that are activated by mechanical stretch of the myocardium as well as by chemical substances like veratridine, nicotine, sodium diatrizoate (Hypaque^R), prostacyclin and vasopressin. Activation of the afferent nerves leads to reflex vagal-mediated bradycardia, hypotension, sweating and nausea, or pain-induced sympathetically mediated reflex hypertension.[9,16,18–20]

The efferent nerves are parasympathetic and sympathetic subsystems in opposing balance (Table 9.3). The *primary* effect of *parasympathetic* or vagal stimulation is vasodilatation of the coronary arteries with increased myocardial blood flow, decreased heart rate and lowering of arterial blood pressure. The *secondary* effect is a decrease in myocardial blood flow due to a decrease in metabolic needs associated with the decline in heart rate and blood pressure. The result is a fall in myocardial blood flow because metabolic factors override the direct neural effects of parasympathetic stimulation.[9]

The adrenergic sympathetic system involves α, β_1- and β_2-receptors (Tables 9.3 and 9.4). Sympathetic stimulation induces a relatively short decrease in myocardial blood flow before any change in heart rate and contractility, followed by coronary vasodilatation. This biphasic response occurs because

Table 9.3 Neural control of coronary blood flow

Autonomic nervous system and coronary blood flow (Q)		
	Neural (primary) effect	Metabolism (secondary) effect
Parasympathetic		
Vagal stimulation	Vasodilatation, Q ↑	Heart rate, blood pressure ↓, vasoconstriction, Q ↓
Bezold–Jarish reflex		
Sympathetic		
α-stimulation	Vasoconstriction, Q ↓	Blood pressure ↑, Vasodilatation, Q ↑
β-stimulation	Vasodilatation, Q ↑ (β_2)	Heart rate, contractility ↑, Vasodilatation, Q ↑ (β_1)

metabolic coronary vasodilatation after a few seconds completely overrides the vasoconstrictor effect of α-receptor stimulation.

Thus, the physiological role of the autonomic nervous system in the regulation of myocardial blood flow during normal conditions is modest, but neural mechanisms do modify myocardial blood flow response to metabolic needs.[9,20–23]

The influence on coronary vascular tone of neural reflex mechanisms

The important reflex mechanisms that influence coronary vascular tone are the arterial baroreflex and the cardiac mechano- and chemoreflexes. The arterial baroreflex is mediated to the coronary arteries through the cardiac sympathetic nerve fibres, whereas the mechano- and chemoreflexes communicate with the coronary vessels through both sympathetic and parasympathetic fibres as described. The cardiac chemoreflex is known as the Berzold–Jarisch reflex.[19] Experimental and clinical data suggest that this reflex or components of the reflex operates during coronary occlusion, coronary arteriography and during hypovolaemic shock.[19,20,24–27]

Aspects of blood loss and hypovolaemia in neural reflex mechanisms influencing myocardial blood flow

The opposing direct and indirect effects of neural control on myocardial blood flow have clinical implications for the treatment of hypovolaemic shock.

Neuropeptide Y

Neuropeptide Y is found in central and peripheral sympathetic neurones, often costored with nor-

Table 9.4 Cardiovascular neural systems

Receptor	Site	Action
β_1	Myocardium	↑ Contractility
	SA, AV node	↑ Heart rate and conduction
β_2	Epicardial coronary arteries	Vasodilatation
	Intramyocardial arterioles	Vasodilatation
	Peripheral arterioles	Vasodilatation
	Lungs	Bronchodilatation
α	Epicardial coronary arteries	Vasoconstriction
	Intramyocardial arterioles	Vasoconstriction
	Peripheral arterioles	Vasoconstriction

SA, sino-atrial; AV, atrioventricular

adrenaline. Innervation of the coronary arteries by neuropeptide Y is a lot more concentrated compared with other organs. Neuropeptide Y is a potent vasoconstrictor in several organs including the myocardium, and its effect seems more pronounced on intramyocardial arterioles than epicardial arteries.[28]

The influence of humeral factors on coronary vascular tone

Catecholamines, thyroid hormones, angiotensin and antidiuretic hormone all have vasoconstrictor effects on coronary vessels that modulate coronary vascular tone.[16] Under conditions of blood loss, hypovolaemia and concomitant significant coronary artery disease, the effect of humoral factors on vascular tone may be more pronounced.

Endothelial factors and coronary vascular smooth muscle cells

The endothelial cell, interposed between blood and the interstitial space, is considered to be a 'pluripotent cell', able to synthesize and secrete a number of vasoactive substances[29] that act on the innermost layers of the coronary vessel wall (Fig. 9.1). Vascular endothelium has a dual role in promoting either vascular relaxation via EDRF or vascular contraction by release of endothelin.[30] This peptide, composed of 21 amino acids, is the most potent naturally occurring vasoconstrictor substance and acts by calcium channel stimulation.[31] Its biosynthesis is enhanced by thrombin formed during the coagulation process and by oxygen-derived free radicals, and occurs in response to ischaemia and in particular reperfusion.[17]

The endothelium-mediated vasodilatation depends on intact endothelium to manufacture EDRF with a half-life of only a few seconds. Several forms of EDRF exist, of which one is the simple compound NO. ACh and other substances, shear stress and hypertension can promote release of EDRF (Fig. 9.1). Prostaglandin (prostacyclin), synthesized from arachidonic acid, is another vasodilator with a half-life of plasma of 1–2 min. Prostaglandins are released from endothelium cells both to the luminal (blood) side of the cell and to the abluminal side of neighbouring smooth muscle cells in arterioles. They have an antiaggregatory effect on platelets in addition to this effect on the coronary vessels.[32] EDRF and prostaglandin can interact synergistically to cause pronounced vasodilatation. During myocardial ischaemia the release of prostaglandin may activate the sensory endings with vagal afferents that mediate the inhibitory reflex of bradycardia and hypotension.[20]

Nitrates act as coronary vasodilators by conversion to NO in the sarcolemma. Nitrates, papa-

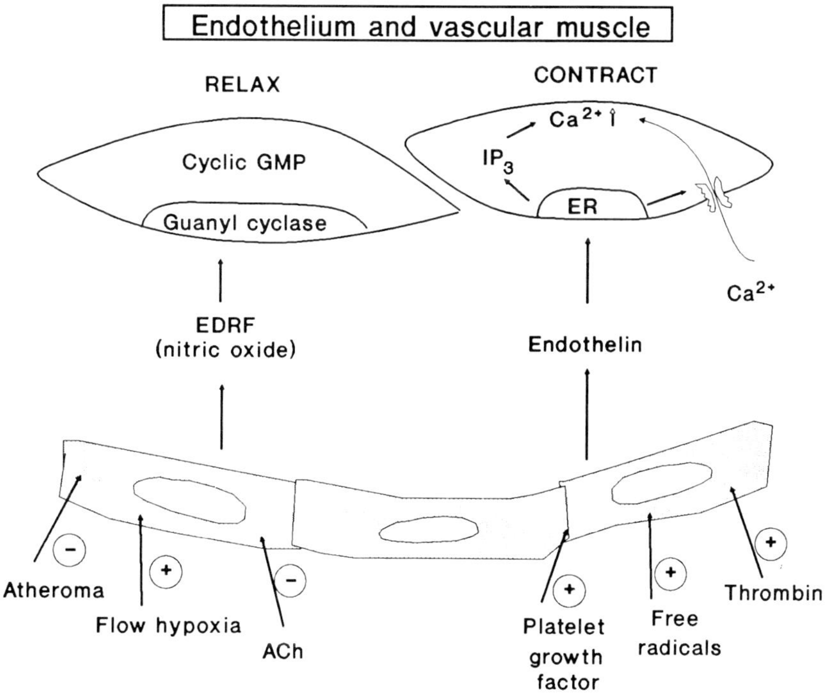

Fig. 9.1. Endothelium and vascular smooth muscle. Vascular endothelium has a dual role in promoting either relaxation via endothelially derived relaxing factor (EDRF; nitric oxide) or vascular contraction by release of endothelin.
GMP, guanosine monophosphate; IP, inositol phosphate; ER, endoplasmic reticulum; ACh, acetycholine. Redrawn from Opie,[17] with permission (originally published in Opie LH, *The Heart, Physiology and Metabolism*, 2nd edn. New York, NY, Raven Press).

verine adenosine and dipyridamole are so-called endothelium-independent vasodilators (Table 9.5). This explains why these compounds can dilate arteries even when the endothelium linings are damaged, whereas the parasympathetic neurotransmitter ACh requires intact endothelium to achieve vasodilatation, as described by Furchgott and Zawadzki in 1980.[33]

Table 9.5 Endothelium-dependent/-independent coronary vasodilators

Endothelium-DEPENDENT (EDRF/NO production)	Endothelium-INDEPENDENT (direct effect on vascular smooth muscle cells)
Acetylcholine	Nitroglycerine
Substance P	Papaverine
Histamine	Adenosine
Serotonin	Dipyridamole
Catecholamines	

EDRF, endothelium-derived relaxing factor; NO, nitric oxide.

Autoregulation of coronary blood flow

If coronary perfusion pressure is decreased with a constant workload and therefore constant oxygen consumption (MVo_2) coronary blood flow will initially fall correspondingly. However, within seconds autoregulatory coronary metabolic vasodilatation of the intramyocardial resistance vessels occurs (see p. 111), with an increase in myocardial blood flow, despite the persisting decrease in perfusion pressure (Fig. 9.2)

In other words, despite changes in coronary perfusion pressure, coronary blood flow remains constant over a wide range of pressures, i.e. *autoregulation* of blood flow. If workload of the heart is increased, the upper curve in Fig. 9.2. illustrates increased blood flow due to metabolic vasodilatation of resistance vessels. However, autoregulation of coronary blood flow is still present but operates on resistance vessels, which are more dilated than at a low workload. In other words the vasodilator reserve is diminished, and the lower limit of autoregulation is shifted upwards. Autoregulation does not determine myocardial blood flow level but ensures constancy of whatever flow

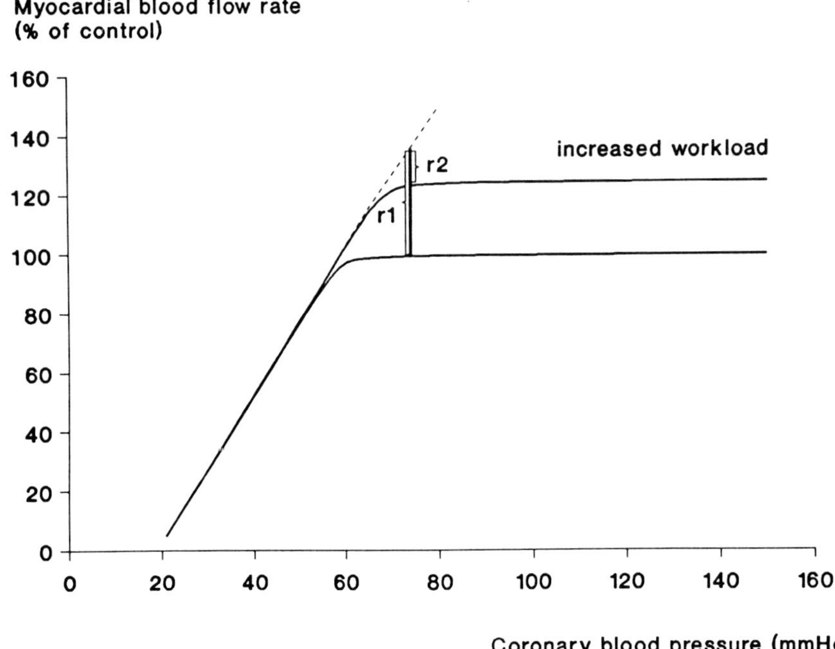

Fig. 9.2. Mean left ventricular myocardial blood flow autoregulatory curves at different workloads of canine hearts. At increased workload (increased oxygen demand) the lower limit of autoregulation of blood flow is shifted towards the right (upper curve). The coronary vasodilator reserve (r2) is diminished compared with the vasodilator reserve (r1) at a lower workload.

level is determined by other factors.[11,13,14,34]

In canine heart autoregulation of myocardial blood flow is much more effective in the outer than in the inner layers of the left ventricular free wall (Fig. 9.3). Myocardial blood flow in the subepicardial and corresponding subendocardial layers of the left ventricle was measured by the local Xenon−133 washout technique.[15] Left ventricular pressure and cardiac work were kept constant and coronary perfusion pressure was varied. When coronary pressure was lowered, blood flow in the corresponding two myocardial layers remained relatively constant until a mean pressure of approximately *75 mmHg*. A reduction in perfusion pressure to *between 60–70 mmHg* induced a reduction in blood flow to the subendocardium of approximately 32 per cent, whereas blood flow remained unchanged in the epicardial layers. When perfusion pressure was lowered further, myocardial blood flow decreased also, indicating that vasodilatation of the resistance vessels could no longer compensate for a decreased perfusion pressure. The reduction in blood flow occurred first in the inner layers of the left ventricle, i.e. the lower end of the autoregulatory range was reached and the resistance vessels maximally dilated, while there still remained some vasodilator reserve in the mid- and subepicardial layers. The vertical distance between the autoregulated and the maximally vasodilated curves at any perfusion pressure is an indicator for vasodilatory ability, i.e. the vasodilator reserve.

Aspects of blood loss and hypovolaemia

Changes in coronary perfusion pressure in *stage II* of a reversible shock are associated with changes in left ventricular pressure.

Because left ventricular pressure has a major influence on myocardial metabolism a steep change in coronary perfusion pressure will activate *metabolic regulation* as well as *autoregulation*.[11,12,16] At the same time there is a parasympathetic increased tone, lowering heart rate and further decreasing the metabolic needs of the myocardium. Consequently, there is a metabolic as well as neurally induced vasorelaxation of the resistance vessels and vasodilator reserve is improved, i.e. the lower limit of autoregulation may be shifted to the left (Figs 9.2

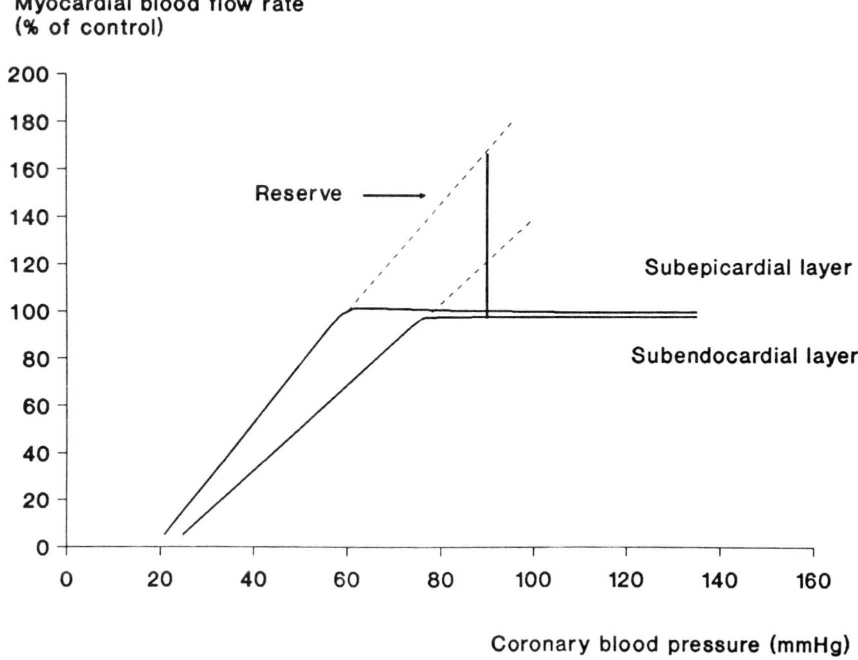

Fig. 9.3. Mean myocardial blood flow autoregulation curves for subepicardium and corresponding subendocardial layers of the left ventricle in canine hearts. During low arterial pressure, when autoregulation is exhausted in both myocardial layers, subendocardial blood flow is lower than in the more superficial layers of the left ventricle. *Source*: Haunsø.[15]

or 9.3). This protects the subendocardium against ischaemia in this stage of hypovolaemia. However, in patients with concomitant coronary artery disease these protective mechanisms against myocardial ischaemia may not be adequate, because the decrease in perfusion pressure behind a severe stenosis is steep, imposing subendocardial myocardial ischaemia, and decreased left ventricular function.

Reactive hyperaemia

Upon release of a temporary coronary artery occlusion, there is an immediate rapid rise in coronary blood flow that is out of proportion to the oxygen debt incurred during the temporary occlusion. In the human and canine myocardium, maximum coronary blood flow during reactive hyperaemia increases with the length of vascular occlusion to approximately 20 seconds. Futher prolongation of ischaemia does not increase maximum blood flow any further indicating that the resistance vessels are maximally dilated. The difference between the preocclusive blood flow and the maximum blood flow following 20 seconds of ischaemia represents the vasodilator reserve of the intramyocardial resistance vessels.

Coronary venous saturation curves demonstrate that adequate oxygen is available to the myocardium, but it is not extracted during the elevated blood flow after release of the occlusion. Thus, some factors other than the lack of oxygen stimulate blood flow. Release of adenosine and other metabolites is strongly suggested. A myogenic response of smooth muscle cells in the coronary resistance vessels may also play a role. A potential explanation for the phenomenon of reactive hyperaemia is that high shear stress associated with sudden restoration of blood flow after occlusion stimulates EDRF release, which causes further vasodilatation and prolongation of higher blood flow than expected on the basis of the oxygen debt caused by brief occlusion.[9–11,16,35]

Reperfusion injury

Early reperfusion is prerequisite for the survival of ischaemic tissue. However, reperfusion is associated with injury known as *reperfusion injury*. The phenomenon is recognized in reperfusion therapy by thrombolysis or percutaneous transluminal angioplasty. The entity of reperfusion injury has grown from laboratory curiosity to clinical recognition and may well be important in patients with reversible haemorrhagic shock.[17]

Reperfusion injury can be defined as events occurring as a consequence of reperfusion that either transiently or permanently subtract from the overall beneficial reperfusion.[36] The events of *reperfusion injury* are: arrhythmias, stunning, induced lethal injury, accelerated necrosis, microvascular injury and no reflow.[37,38]

Reperfusion stunning

Reperfusion stunning is defined as a temporary reversible postischaemic mechanical dysfunction precipitated by reperfusion that is manifest in the absence of any irreversible damage.[39] Stunning is explained by formation of free radicals and/or intracellular cytosolic calcium overload.[37,39] In dogs haemorrhage of approximately 40 per cent of the estimated blood volume causes decreased left ventricular performance. After haemorrhage and augmentation of vascular volume, left ventricular performance remains depressed for at least 30 min despite improved ventricular filling, consistent with stunned myocardium.[40] Clinical evidence of stunned myocardium is related to observations of delayed recovery of left ventricular function following thrombolytic therapy for acute myocardial infarction, reduced compliance following angioplasty and cardiac depression after cardiopulmonary bypass.[37]

Microvascular reperfusion injury

Microvascular reperfusion injury is observed in the canine myocardium and can be defined as a reversible impairment of coronary vasodilatation after reversible ischaemia.[41] Increased capillary permeability to small hydrophilic molecules has been demonstrated.[42,43] The responsible mechanism may well be the free oxygen radicals: superoxide anion (O_2^-), hydrogen peroxide (H_2O_2) and the hydroxyl radical (OH). The three processes for their generation are: (1) mitochondrial generation of free radicals; (2) the activation of neutrophils; and (3) the xanthine oxidase reaction in vascular endothelium (not confirmed in humans).[17,44]

Relation between stage of reversible shock, coronary blood flow and left ventricular performance

Based on the above-mentioned experimental and clinical observations a model for coronary blood flow regulation during hypovolaemic shock in normotensives and patients with coronary artery disease is proposed.

Stage I

In stage I (blood loss of approximately 15 per cent of blood volume) baroreflex sympathetic excitation increases heart rate and restores or even increases arterial blood pressure and cardiac performance by arteriolar vasoconstriction, constriction of splanchnic capacitance vessels and increased cardiac filling pressure. Sympathetic excitation necessary to compensate for haemorrhage leads to increased myocardial oxygen needs (MV_{O_2}). This is met by metabolic adjustments of intramyocardial resistance vessels leading to vasodilatation and increased myocardial blood flow (Q) and thereby increased oxygen delivery ($(a-v)_{O_2} \times Q$). Patients with normal coronary arteries have no cardiac symptoms at this stage except for heart palpitation. However, patients with coronary artery disease may experience angina pectoris, reflecting the reduced coronary blood flow reserve in the area supplied by the coronary artery and leading to subendocardial myocardial ischaemia.

Stage II

In the initial period of stage II (blood loss of between 15 and 40 per cent) a further excessive neurohormonal stimulation of the cardiovascular system increases heart rate and the force of contraction in such a way that myocardial oxygen needs dangerously exceed the capacity of the coronary blood flow reserve even in patients with normal coronary arteries. In addition, increased heart rate (declining diastole) and vigorous ventricular contraction impede blood flow to the subendocardium. Subendocardial myocardial ischaemia is likely. However, as ventricular volume decreases, the powerful ventricular contraction activates sensory endings in the posterior wall of the left ventricle with vagal afferents that mediate an inhibitory reflex bradycardia and hypotension.[45] Consequently, the withdrawal of sympathetic drive, resulting in a rapid decline in arterial pressure and heart rate, leads to a rapid reduction in myocardial oxygen demand and improvement in oxygen supply, especially to the inner layers of the left ventricle. The adjustment of myocardial blood flow in response to changes in myocardial oxygen demand is controlled by metabolic mechanisms and by autoregulation. The inhibitor cardiac reflex is an appropriate adjustment to this stage of haemorrhage, improving blood flow regulation in such a way that autoregulation of transmural blood flow is still in function, protecting the myocardium against subendocardial ischaemia and infarction, especially in patients with coronary artery disease.

Stage III

In stage III (blood loss more than about 40 per cent) severe hypotension is associated with tachycardia.

Although autoregulation of blood flow to declining coronary blood pressure works in resistance vessels that are metabolically less dilated than in stage II, because of decreased cardiac performance (severe hypotension), autoregulation of blood flow becomes exhausted. Consequently, left ventricular blood flow decreases as well as endocardial/epicardial flow ratios, leading to subendocardial ischaemia. If resuscitation from this stage of shock is not immediate, circumferential subendocardial necrosis develops, resulting in the cessation of mechanical contraction. Despite augmentation of vascular volume and left ventricular volume, left ventricular performance and coronary blood flow may remain temporarily depressed because of reperfusion injury of the ischaemic myocardium.

References

1. Gregg DE and Fischer LC: Blood supply of the heart. In Geiger SR (ed.): *Handbook of Physiology*. Bethseda, MD, American Physiological Society, 1963, 1517–84.
2. Berne RM and Rubio R: Coronary circulation. In Geiger SR, Sperelakis N and Berne RM (eds): *Handbook of Physiology*. Bethseda, MD, American Physiological Society, 1979, 873–952.
3. Henquell L and Honig CR: Intercapillary distance and capillary reserve in right and left ventricles. *Microvascular Research*, 1976; **12,** 35–41.
4. Honig CR: *Modern Cardiovascular Physiology*. Boston, MA, Little, Brown & Co., 1981.

5. Schaper W: *The Collateral Circulation of the Heart.* Amsterdam, North Holland Publishing Company, 1971.
6. Abraham A: *Microscopic Innervation of the Heart and Blood Vessels in Vertebrae Including Man.* New York, NY, Pergamon, 1969.
7. Rose PC, Goresky CA, Bélanger P and Chen M-J: Effect of vasodilation and flow rate on capillary permeability surface product and interstitial space size in the coronary circulation. *Circulation Research*, 1980; **47,** 312–28.
8. Haunsø S: Effects of regional hypoxia and blood flow on capillary permeability in canine myocardium. *Acta Physiologica Scandinavica*, 1982; **114,** 59–65.
9. Gould KL: *Coronary Artery Stenosis.* New York, NY, Elsevier, 1991.
10. Haunsø S and Amtorp O: Regional blood flow during reactive hyperaemia in canine myocardium as determined by local washout of Xenon-133. *Acta Physiologica Scandinavica*, 1980; **110,** 285–93.
11. Spaan JAE: *Coronary Blood Flow. Mechanics, Distribution, and Control.* Dordrecht, Kluwer Academic Publishers, 1991.
12. Klocke FJ, Mates RE, Copley DP and Orlic AE: Physiology of the coronary circulation in health and disease. In Paul N and Goodwin JF (eds): *Progress in Cardiology.* Philadelphia, PA, Lea & Febiger, 1976, 1–17.
13. Bache RJ and Dymek DJ: Local and regional regulation of coronary vascular tone. *Progress in Cardiovascular Disease*, 1981; **24,** 191–212.
14. Hoffman JIE: A critical view of coronary reserve. *Circulation*, 1987; **75,** 1–6.
15. Haunsø S: Lower limits of blood flow autoregulation in different layers of the left ventricular wall of dogs. *Acta Physiologica Scandinavica*, 1981; **112,** 349–50.
16. Marcus ML: Humoral control of the coronary circulation. In *The Coronary Circulation in Health and Disease.* New York, NY, McGraw-Hill, 1982, 15–190.
17. Opie LH: Cardiac metabolism – emergence, decline, and resurge, Part II. *Cardiovascular Research*, 1992; **26,** 817–30; first published in Opie LH, *The Heart, Physiology and Metabolism*, 2nd edn. New York, NY, Raven Press.
18. Carson RP and Lazzara R: Hemodynamic responses initiated by coronary stretch receptors with special reference to coronary artery. *American Journal of Cardiology*, 1970; **25,** 571–8.
19. Coleridge HM and Coleridge JCG: Cardiovascular afferents involved in regulation of peripheral vessels. *Annual Review of Physiology*, 1980; **42,** 413–27.
20. Abboud FM: Ventricular syncope. Is the heart a sensory organ? *New England Journal of Medicine*, 1989; **320,** 390–92.
21. Feigl EO: Reflex parasympathetic coronary vasodilation elicited from cardiac receptors in dog. *Circulation Research*, 1975; **37,** 175–82.
22. Young MA, Knight DR and Vatner SF: Autonomic control of large coronary arteries and resistance vessels. *Progress in Cardiovascular Disease*, 1987; **30,** 211–34.
23. Feigl EO: Control of myocardial oxygen tension by sympathetic coronary vasoconstriction in dog. *Circulation Research*, 1975; **37,** 88–95.
24. Ebbert PA, Austen WG and Greenfield LZ: Effect of neurogenic reflexes on heart rate during systemic hypotension. *American Journal of Physiology*, 1962; **203,** 457–60.
25. Little RA, Marshall HW and Kirkman E: Attenuation of the acute cardiovascular responses to haemorrhage by tissue injury in the conscious rat. *Quarterly Journal of Experimental Physiology*, 1989; **74,** 825–33.
26. Sander-Jensen K: *Heart and Endocrine Changes During Central Hypovolaemia in Man.* Copenhagen, Danish Medical Bulletin, 1991.
27. Secher NH, Jacobsen J, Friedman DB and Matzen S: Bradycardia during reversible hypovolaemic shock: associated neural reflex mechanisms and clinical implications. *Clinical and Experimental Pharmacology and Physiology*, 1922; **19,** 733–43.
28. Svendsen JH, Sheikh SP, Jørgensen J, Mikkelsen JD, Paaske WP, Sejrsen P, Haunsø S: Neuropeptide Y modulates regional blood flow in canine myocardium during reactive hyperaemia. *American Journal of Physiology*, 1990; **259,** H1709–17.
29. Thilo-Korner DGS and Freshney RJ: *The Endothelial Pluripotent Control Cell of the Vessel Wall.* Basel, Karger, 1983.
30. Vanhoutte PM and Shimokawa H: Endothelium-derived relaxing factor and coronary vasospasm. *Circulation*, 1989; **80,** 1–90.
31. Yanagisawa M, Kurihara H and Kimira S: A novel potent vasoconstrictor peptide produced by vascular endothelial cells. *Nature*, 1988; **332,** 411–15.
32. Moncada S and Vane JR: Arachidonic acid metabolites and the interactions between platelets and blood-vessel walls. *New England Journal of Medicine*, 1979; **300,** 1142–7.
33. Furchgott R and Zawadzki JV: The obligatory role of endothelial cells in relaxation of arterial smooth muscle by acetylcholine. *Nature*, 1980; **288,** 373–6.
34. Dole WP: Autoregulation of the coronary circulation. *Progress in Cardiovascular Disease*, 1987; **29,** 293–323.
35. Olson RA: Myocardial reactive hyperemia. *Circulation Research*, 1975; **33,** 263–70.
36. Haunsø S: Myocardial blood flow regulation. In Thygesen K and Kjekhus J (eds): *Myocardial Ischaemia.* Oxford, Blackwell Scientific Publications, 1990, 17–30.
37. Opie L: Where do we stand with respect to reperfusion in the 1990s? Clinical and experimental perspectives. In Yellow DM and Jennings RB (eds): *The Pathophysiology of Reperfusion and Reperfusion Injury.* New York, NY, Raven Press, 1992, 197–208.

38. Hearse DJ: Reperfusion injury: a possible role of oxidant stress and its manipulation. *Cardiovascular Drugs Therapy*, 1991; **5,** 225–36.
39. Bolli R, Hartley CJ and Rabinowitz RS: Clinical relevance of myocardial 'stunning'. *Cardiovascular Drugs Therapy*, 1991; **5,** 877–90.
40. Horton JW, Longhurst JC, Coln D and Mitchell JH: Cardiovascular effects of haemorrhagic shock in spleen intact and splenectomized dogs. *Clinical Physiology*, 1984; **4,** 533–48.
41. Bolli R, Triana JF and Jeroudi MO: Prolonged impairment of coronary vasodilation after reversible ischemia. Evidence for microvascular 'stunning'. *Circulation Research*, 1990; **67,** 332–43.
42. Svendsen JH, Bjerrum PJ and Haunsø S: Myocardial capillary permeability after regional ischemia and reperfusion in the *in vivo* canine myocardium. Effect of superoxide dismutase. *Circulation Research*, 1991; **68,** 174–84.
43. Hansen PR, Svendsen JH, Høst NB, Hansen SH and Haunsø S: Effect of 5-aminosalicylic acid on myocardial capillary permeability following ischaemia and reperfusion. *Cardiovascular Research*, 1992; **26,** 798–803.
44. Kukreja RC and Hess ML: The oxygen free radical system: from equations through membrane–protein interactions to cardiovascular injury and protection. *Cardiovascular Research*, 1992; **26,** 641–55.
45. Horton JW and Mitchell JH: Left ventricular dimensions during haemorrhagic shock measured by biplane cinefluorography. *American Journal of Physiology*, 1979; **263,** H1554–9.

10

Regional blood flow – renal

Warwick P Anderson and Gabor Szénási

Introduction

Broadly speaking, renal blood flow is little affected by mild haemorrhage and profoundly reduced in severe blood loss. In mild haemorrhage the clinically obvious effects include oliguria and sodium retention, and this has sometimes led to the erroneous conclusion that renal blood flow is reduced. This chapter presents evidence from experiments in unanaesthetized animals that shows conclusively that renal blood flow is well maintained over the initial phases of progressive haemorrhage. Severe haemorrhage and shock on the other hand can cause anuria, acute tubular necrosis and renal failure.

The renal responses to haemorrhage are influenced by prevailing factors. In the clinical situation the response of the kidney is probably affected by the extent of any trauma associated with the blood loss, the rate of blood loss, the age of the patient, and so on. Experimental haemorrhage in humans is of course limited to relatively modest blood loss, although LBNP is sometimes used as an alternative technique.

Experimental models of haemorrhage in animals vary considerably. Some of the experimental factors that are likely to affect the renal responses to haemorrhage include the initial volume and sodium status of the animal,[1–3] temperature,[4] age, gender, the extent of surgical intervention, the rate of blood loss, whether the animals were pregnant,[5] blood gas status,[6,7] whether heparin was administered,[8] whether the haemorrhage was associated with trauma,[9,10] and probably many other variables.

The most important confounding variable in most experimental studies of haemorrhage however is anaesthesia of the animal, which is known to affect renal haemodynamics and function;[11,12] several studies demonstrate clearly that the renal responses to haemorrhage are altered markedly in anaesthetized animals compared with conscious animals.[13–16]

In this chapter, therefore, we have used results from unanaesthetized animals and humans to build up a description of the renal blood flow responses to haemorrhage. A review of earlier results from anaesthetized animals can be found in Chien[17] and Selkurt.[18]

Renal blood flow responses during mild (non-hypotensive) and moderate haemorrhage

In conscious animals blood flow is well maintained when blood loss is not severe enough to lower arterial pressure, i.e. so-called 'non-hypotensive' haemorrhage. Renal vascular resistance is little changed in this phase, even though there is marked vasoconstriction of other peripheral vascular beds. Amongst the most persuasive experiments are those of Vatner,[15] who studied the effects of slow 'non-hypotensive' haemorrhage (14 ml/kg) in conscious dogs and found that renal blood flow actually rose by about 15 per cent. This vasodilatation became even greater upon further bleeding (26 ml/kg), which lowered arterial pressure by about 25 mmHg (Fig. 10.1), with renal blood flow increasing from about 20 to about 30 per cent of cardiac output.[15] This maintenance of renal blood flow was in marked contrast to the responses in the mesenteric and iliac beds, in which there was powerful vasoconstriction and reduction in blood

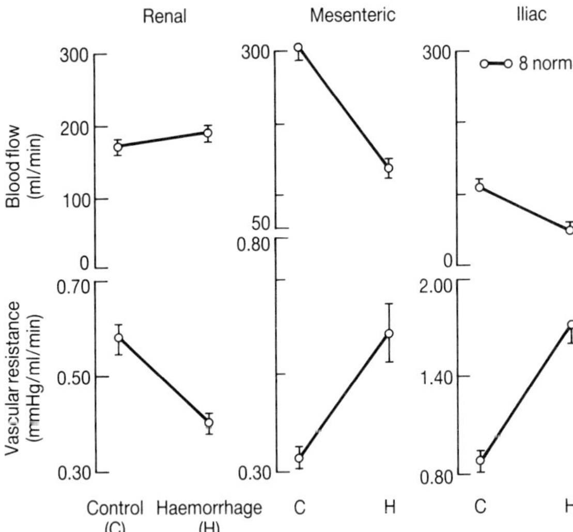

Fig. 10.1. Mean values during control and after moderate hypotensive haemorrhage in dogs (mean arterial pressure reduction of 20–30 mmHg). Values are expressed as means ± SEM. Reproduced from the *Journal of Clinical Investigation* 1974, **54**: 225–35, by copyright permission of the American Society for Clinical Investigation.

flow (Fig. 10.1). Similar rises in total renal blood flow in mild haemorrhage in conscious dogs have also been observed by Gross[19] and several other investigators have reported initial renal vasodilatation in the dog[14,20–23] with good maintenance of blood flow.

In conscious but sedated baboons also, Vatner[15] found that renal blood flow actually increased in non-hypotensive haemorrhage, and further vasodilatation occurred at moderate haemorrhage which reduced arterial pressure by 23 mmHg. In conscious rhesus monkeys Forsyth *et al.*[24] found that renal vascular resistance was not altered in haemorrhage as severe as 30 ml/kg which reduced arterial pressure by 40 mmHg; i.e. renal blood flow fell in proportion to arterial pressure.

There is limited data in humans, but Stone and Stahl[25] reported that there were no significant changes in renal vascular resistance in human volunteers during a haemorrhage which lowered arterial pressure by more than 10 mmHg. However, these subjects were studied after 'preliminary loading' with 10–20 ml/kg 0.45 per cent sodium chloride solution. LBNP is sometimes used as a model of central hypovolaemia and here too there appears to be little or no renal vasoconstriction with mild-to-moderate stimuli,[26] although renal flow is reduced with more severe LBNP.[27]

There have been few studies of the renal effects of haemorrhage in conscious rats. The available results suggest that the response may be different from other animals. In a recent study, for example, Baylis *et al.*[5] found that there was renal vasoconstriction during non-hypotensive haemorrhage in conscious female rats. Similar results have been reported by Seyde and Longnecker[28] and Idvall,[13] although in a subsequent study, Seyde and colleagues[29] reported that renal resistance did not change in a haemorrhage which resulted in a 10 per cent fall in arterial pressure; i.e. similar results to those in other species.

In conscious rabbits both Schadt *et al.*[30] and Banks *et al.*[31] found that renal blood flow was unchanged in mild haemorrhage, while Courneya and Korner[32] reported a mild vasoconstriction (a 10 per cent rise in renal resistance). With more severe haemorrhage (a 26 per cent blood loss), Korner and colleagues[33,34] found an average increase in renal resistance of 25–30 per cent, although this was not apparent in the results of Schadt *et al.*[30] In conscious young pigs renal blood flow was not reduced during mild (7 ml/kg) blood loss.[35]

Thus, results from conscious animals generally indicate good maintenance of renal blood flow during the early stages of progressive blood loss in conscious animals, with a rise measured in some experiments and a small fall in others (particularly in rats). These differences are probably attributable to experimental differences, e.g. in dietary Na^+ intake, or in how well the conscious animal is conditioned to the experimental situation, its level of arousal and activation of the sympathoadrenal system. Good conditioning to the experimental environment may be easier to achieve in larger animals such as dogs than in rats, for example. Other confounding factors sometimes present include minor surgery just prior to the study in the conscious state (e.g. catheter implantation), carotid artery cannulation for blood pressure measurement or microsphere injection in rats (and thus low arterial pressure at the carotid baroreceptors with increased sympathetic nervous tone). Even the posture of the animals may affect the results. Nevertheless, it is certainly apparent that the renal bed is *not* a major target of vasoconstrictor homeostatic mechanisms seeking to maintain arterial pressure initially in haemorrhage.

Severe haemorrhage

Severe haemorrhage causes intense renal vasoconstriction, and combined with the severe hypotension results in very low renal blood flow and tissue ischaemia. For example, Vatner[15] found that, whereas renal blood flow was not reduced following 26 ml/kg haemorrhage, doubling the haemorrhage volume to 50 ml/kg reduced renal blood flow by 70 per cent in conscious dogs (see also Slater *et al.*[36]). He found similar results in the baboon.[15] Chalmers and colleagues[33] reported that severe haemorrhage in conscious rabbits resulted in an increase of renal resistance of about 250 per cent after about 90 min, and Neutze and colleagues[37] found that renal blood flow fell by about 70 per cent in conscious rabbits in response to haemorrhage severe enough to reduce arterial pressure by 35 mmHg and cardiac output by about 60 per cent. Following 50 per cent haemorrhage in rhesus monkey, renal blood flow fell from 16 per cent of cardiac output before haemorrhage to only 10 per cent of the greatly reduced cardiac output; equivalent to an 88 per cent fall in renal perfusion.[24] Profound renal vasoconstriction has also been reported in the pig.[38,39]

Most of these studies measured flow only immediately after haemorrhage. However Korner and colleagues[34] followed the response for up to 5 hours and reported a complex series of changes in renal resistance with time after 32 per cent haemorrhage (Fig. 10.2). After the initial marked vasoconstrictive response to severe haemorrhage, there was a subsequent renal vasodilatation so that renal resistance fell back to only slightly above resting values at 3 hours but rose again by 5 hours (Fig. 10.2). Bartley and Anderson[40] found that renal vascular resistance was increased by only 35 per cent 1–2 hours after less severe 20 per cent haemorrhage. Eventually severe haemorrhage can lead to renal failure (see Brenner and Lazarus,[41] for a description of the mechanisms involved).

Intrarenal distribution of flow

Apart from changes in total renal blood flow, another adaptive response to haemorrhage can be redistribution of blood flow from the outer to the inner cortex. This change in relative blood flow between outer and inner nephrons could affect overall kidney function.[42–44] Most evidence from anaesthetized animals indicates that there is a preferential decrease in outer cortical blood flow in haemorrhage, with inner cortical flow and medullary blood flow relatively better preserved.[45–50] Redistribution of flow from the outer to the inner cortex is also seen when renal perfusion pressure is lowered physically, e.g. by renal artery stenosis in anaesthetized animals.[49,50]

This redistribution may not occur in conscious animals however. Both Lameire *et al.*[22] and Kirkebo and Tyssebotn[51] failed to find redistribution of renal blood flow in haemorrhage in conscious dogs. The study by Lameire and colleagues[22] is of particular interest, since they used microspheres to study redistribution of flow over a wide range of haemorrhage severities (10–30 ml/kg). Kirkebo and Tyssebotn[51] studied severe haemorrhage and used implanted platinum electrodes at different depths of the kidney, but this technique may have caused local tissue reactions to interfere with their measurements. Clearly it is important to resolve whether this redistribution of blood flow is an artefact of anaesthesia.

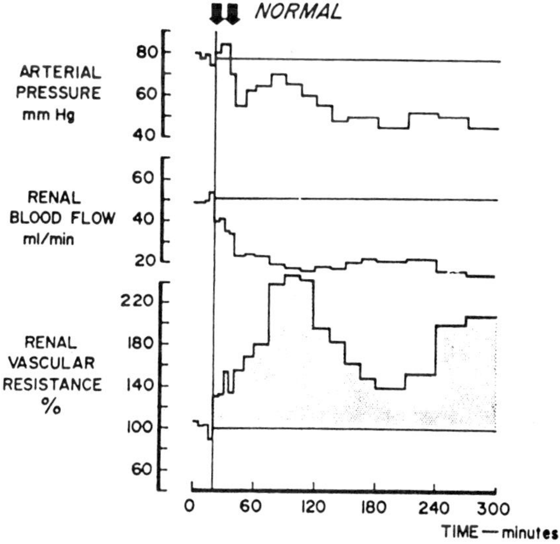

Fig. 10.2. Effects of removal of 32 per cent of the blood volume in a normal rabbit on ear artery pressure, left renal blood flow and vascular resistance (percentage of mean initial control value). The animal was bled between the arrows. From Korner *et al.*,[34] with permission.

Glomerular filtration rate and urine excretion

There is scant data from conscious animals on the effects of haemorrhage on GFR and urinary water and electrolyte excretion. During mild haemorrhage GFR is well maintained.[5,23,35] In moderate haemorrhage in conscious rabbits Korner *et al.*[34] found that GFR was less reduced than renal blood flow; i.e. filtration fraction was increased by about 20 per cent. As haemorrhage becomes progressively more severe GFR changes tend to mirror renal blood flow changes[25,34,35,38,40] until filtration ceases at low arterial pressures.

In LBNP experiments in humans Hirsch *et al.*[26] reported that GFR actually increased (about 15 per cent) during mild LBNP whereas renal blood flow did not change; i.e. filtration fraction rose. GFR still remained elevated at more severe LBNP which reduced renal blood flow by about 10 per cent; i.e. filtration fraction rose further.[26]

There is relatively little data on the glomerular and tubular responses to haemorrhage at the single nephron level. Ichikawa and Brenner[52] found that mild haemorrhage to reduce arterial pressure by less than 10 mmHg markedly reduced the glomerular ultrafiltration coefficient (Kf) in water-loaded, anaesthetized rats, with little apparent change in preglomerular resistance. Heller and Horacek[53] found that efferent arteriolar resistance was elevated in mild haemorrhage in anaesthetized dogs, but that as the haemorrhage became more severe, afferent resistance was also elevated. Both Moore and Mason[54] and Kaufman *et al.*[55] have argued that tubuloglomerular feedback is enhanced in severe haemorrhage. More study is needed on the glomerular and tubular responses to haemorrhage, a situation involving increased activity of the autonomic nervous and renin–angiotensin systems, and on other hormones such as vasopressin which are known to affect mesangial cell contraction *in vitro* and Kf *in vivo*.[56–58]

Mechanisms mediating the renal responses to haemorrhage

Autoregulation

Autoregulatory processes appear to dominate the renal responses to mild haemorrhage. When renal perfusion pressure is reduced by non-haemorrhagic means, such as narrowing of the aorta or the renal artery, renal blood flow is well maintained as arterial pressure is lowered. In conscious animals total renal blood flow may be little changed by pressures as low as 60–70 mmHg.[21,59–61] Kremser and Gewertz[21] have reported that the autoregulatory capacities of the kidney remain unaffected by mild or moderate haemorrhage.

Thus, the powerful renal autoregulatory mechanisms probably explain the good maintenance of renal blood flow in mild-to-moderate haemorrhage in conscious animals. A corollary is that systemic baroreflexes activated by the fall in arterial and cardiopulmonary pressures seem to have little effect on renal haemodynamics while arterial pressure is within the autoregulatory range.

Sympathetic nervous system in the renal responses to haemorrhage

Sympathetic nerves supply the afferent and efferent arterioles of the kidney, the renin secreting cells of the juxtaglomerular apparatus and the renal tubules.[62–64] Thus, activation of these nerves can have a number of physiological effects within the kidney, including vasoconstriction of the arterioles, increased renin secretion and increased tubular water and electrolyte reabsorption.[65,66]

Direct measurement of renal nerve activity during haemorrhage in conscious animals shows that it increases moderately, by about 2–3 fold, during the initial non-hypotensive period of haemorrhage but that it falls again, usually to below prehaemorrhage levels, as arterial pressure begins to fall (Fig. 10.3).[67–71] In very severe haemorrhage there may be a second rise in renal nerve activity,[72,73] but this has been deduced from anaesthetized animal experiments.

The initial increase in renal nerve activity in response to haemorrhage appears to be the result of both arterial and cardiopulmonary baroreflexes. In conscious dogs Morita and Vatner[69] have shown that the initial increase in nerve activity was reduced by 25 per cent in sinoaortic denervated dogs, by 50 per cent in dogs with cardiac denervation (ablation of low pressure baroreceptors), and totally abolished by combined aortic and cardiac denervation.[69] The causes of the paradoxical decrease in renal nerve activity as haemorrhage becomes more severe and arterial pressure begins to fall have attracted considerable interest. There is evidence that the inhibition of nerve activity results

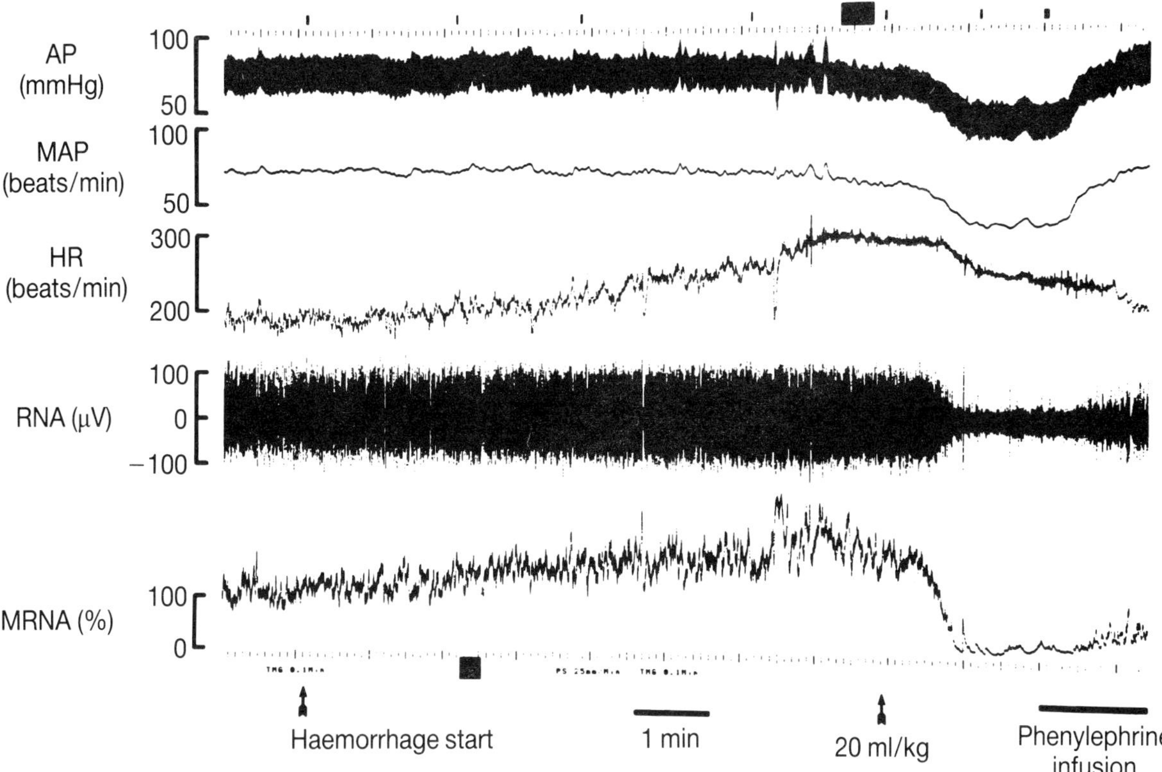

Fig. 10.3. Original record from a rabbit illustrating responses of arterial pressure (AP), mean arterial pressure (MAP), heart rate (HR), renal nerve activity (RNA) and mean renal nerve activity (MRNA) to haemorrhage and subsequent phenylephrine infusion (38 μg/min). MRNA increases initially, until arterial pressure begins to decrease markedly. From Morita *et al.*,[68] with permission.

from reflexes originating from the heart,[67,74] probably from receptors in the left ventricle.[74,75] Thoren *et al.*[74] have suggested that mechanoreceptors sense the high tension which develops in the cardiac wall when cardiac filling is low and the heart is contracting around a near empty ventricular chamber. On the other hand, Morita and Vatner[69] found that neither arterial nor cardiopulmonary reflexes mediate the sympathetic inhibition in conscious dogs. A number of investigators have implicated opioids in this inhibitory phase[67,68,70] but vasopressin and serotonergic mechanisms may also be involved.[71,76] In severe haemorrhage cerebral ischaemia may contribute to the increased RSNA, according to results from anaesthetized animals.[72,73]

The physiological consequences of these changes in RSNA on renal function are not clear at this time. The rise in RSNA in early mild haemorrhage does not seem to affect renal blood flow, since this is mostly reported to be well maintained. Indeed, Morita[77] has confirmed this by measuring renal blood flow and renal nerve activity simultaneously in conscious dogs. It is possible that this increased RSNA may be responsible for the antinatriuresis that occurs at this time, since there is evidence from anaesthetized animals that small increases in RSNA preferentially affect tubular function, and thus electrolyte and water excretion, rather than renal resistance vessels.[65,66,78] Another possible effect of the initial increase in RSNA is stimulation of renin release,[65,66,79] and in this context Thames and DiBona[80] have show that the effects of renal nerve stimulation on renin release are augmented when renal perfusion pressure is lowered.

One way of studying the role of the autonomic nervous system in the renal haemodynamic responses to haemorrhage is to denervate the kidney. However, the results of such experiments are difficult to interpret since these kidneys develop supersensitivity to circulating catecholamines.[81,82] Korner *et al.*[34] showed that the renal vasoconstriction or response to haemorrhage was magnified in denervated kidneys of conscious rabbits, whereas Lifshitz[83] found no effect in dogs.

Plasma levels of adrenal catecholamines also rise in moderate-to-severe haemorrhage[84–87] and contribute to the renal vasoconstriction.[85] In severe hypotensive haemorrhage the strong renal vasoconstriction is mediated largely by the autonomic nervous system,[33,34] as assessed using pharmacological blockade with guanethidine and atropine treatments plus adrenalectomy. Interestingly, the arterial baroreceptors may not be the cause of this activation of the autonomic nervous system to the kidney, in contrast to other organs such as the gut, muscle and skin.[33]

Angiotensin II

Plasma renin and AII levels rise progressively with haemorrhage in conscious animals (Fig. 10.4),[84,87,89–91] though the rise is probably less than in anaesthetized animals.[87–89] There are limited studies in which AII blocking agents have been used in haemorrhage in conscious animals,[31] but such studies are needed, given the powerful systemic and renal physiological actions of AII. Intrarenal actions include vasoconstriction,[92–94] effects on glomerular filtration due to actions on the mesangium[56,57,95,96] and effects on tubular function.[93,94] AII also plays a major role in the maintenance of GFR in other pathophysiological situations when glomerular filtration is under threat, including during renal artery stenosis[59,97–99] and during increased sympathetic nervous system activity.[100,101] It seems likely therefore that this hormone plays a role in the renal responses to haemorrhage; for example, it may be responsible for the increasing filtration fraction seen in the early stages of haemorrhage.[26,34]

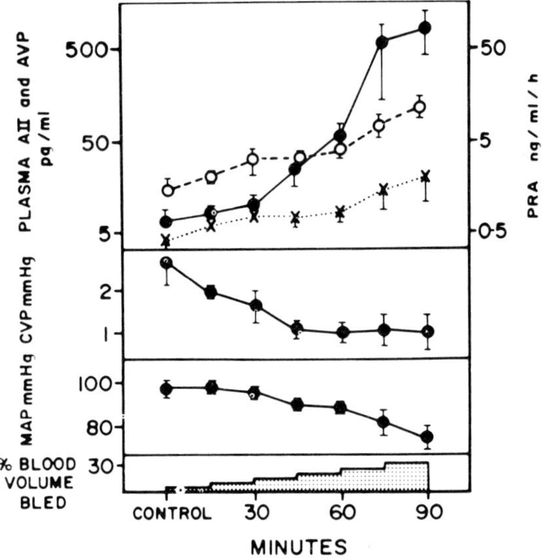

Fig. 10.4. Changes in plasma vasopressin (AVP; ●), plasma angiotensin II (AII; ○) and plasma renin activity (PRA; ×), central venous pressure (CVP) and mean arterial blood pressure (MAP) during stepwise venous haemorrhage in four dogs. Volume of blood removed is indicated as a percentage of total blood volume. From Pullan *et al.*,[91] with permission.

Prostanoids

In anaesthetized dogs blockade of renal prostaglandin production attenuates renal responses to haemorrhage,[102–105] but this may be misleading because renal prostaglandin production is markedly augmented in acute renal preparations in anaesthetized animals.[106] In conscious rabbits Banks *et al.*[31] found that mild haemorrhage had no significant effect on renal blood flow in untreated animals, but that pretreatment with meclofenamate resulted in a marked renal vasoconstriction in response to haemorrhage. Similarly, Vatner[15] found that indomethacin pretreatment changed the initial renal vasodilatatory response in conscious dogs into a vasoconstriction. In contrast, both Lameire *et al.*[22] and Bartley and Anderson[40] have reported that inhibition of prostanoid production did not affect the renal responses to haemorrhage in conscious dogs and rabbits respectively.

Methodological problems in the study of the renal responses to haemorrhage

Most experimental studies of haemorrhage have been performed in anaesthetized animals, but there can be little doubt that anaesthesia and surgery greatly affect the responses to haemorrhage.[13–16,87,89] For example, Vatner[15] demonstrated that both the fall in arterial pressure and the extent of renal vasoconstriction were markedly augmented in pentobarbitone anaesthetized dogs compared with conscious dogs. On the other hand, ethical constraints exist when conscious animals are used, and the quiet haemorrhage used in these animals may not mimic the situation associated with more traumatic haemorrhage in humans and animals. In humans experimental haemorrhage is limited to relatively modest blood loss, and 'sham' haemorrhage procedures such as LBNP do not precisely reproduce the haemodynamic effects of haemorrhage.

Heparin may be another important confounder in studies of haemorrhage. It is frequently given prior to haemorrhage, especially in anaesthetized animals, but Wang *et al.*[8] has shown that preheparinization of conscious rats markedly attenuated the fall in GFR in response to severe haemorrhage.

Areas for future research

Despite several decades of research much still needs to be learnt about the kidney's participation in the responses to haemorrhage. Some of the questions still to be resolved include:

1. How do local autoregulatory mechanisms protect renal blood flow and GFR, and how do they interact with humoral and neural reflexes activated by the haemorrhage?
2. Is there a redistribution of flow within the renal cortex in conscious animals, and if so, what is its significance?
3. What is the role of AII, local and circulating, in the renal response? There are difficulties in planning a convincing experiment to answer this question because AII blockade markedly affects the arterial pressure response to haemorrhage, confounding interpretation of renal responses.
4. How do other factors which might be encountered in the clinical situation affect the renal responses to haemorrhage (e.g. trauma, blood gas derangements, age, pregnancy, obesity)?
5. What role do endothelially derived substances play in the renal responses to haemorrhage? There are already reports suggesting that renal endothelial function may be altered.[107,108]
6. What is the role of hormones and local factors such as mineralocorticoids, vasopressin, opioids, dopamine, 5-HT, kinins, adenosine, etc?

There is also a need to study the responses to haemorrhage over time, since almost all studies have concentrated on the initial responses to haemorrhage only.

Summary

In conscious animals renal blood flow and GFR are little affected by modest, non-hypotensive haemorrhage, despite increased renal nerve activity. As arterial blood pressure begins to fall during progressively more severe haemorrhage, renal blood flow is still quite well maintained initially, and this is probably attributable to the powerful autoregulatory mechanisms of the kidney. Renal nerve activity decreases during this phase of haemorrhage. In severe blood loss renal blood flow is reduced to very low values, and the causes have been little studied. Severe haemorrhage appears to be the only phase in which cardiac output is distributed away from the kidney in conscious animals.

Acknowledgments

The authors' research is supported by grants from the National Health & Medical Research Council and the Alfred Group of Hospitals. Dr Szénási was a Visiting Scientist from MTA-SOTE EKSZ, 2nd Department of Medicine, Semmelweis University School of Medicine, Budapest, Hungary.

References

1. Gothberg G, Lundin S, Aurel M and Folkow B: Response to slow, graded bleeding in salt-depleted rats. *Journal of Hypertension*, 1983; **1(suppl. 2),** 24–6.
2. Kopelman RI, Dzau VJ, Shimabukuro S and Barger AC: Compensatory response to hemorrhage in conscious dogs on normal and low salt intake. *American Journal of Physiology*, 1983; **244,** H351–6.
3. Rocchini AP, Gallagher KP, Botham MJ, Lemmer JH, Szpumar CA and Behrendt D: Prevention of fatal hemorrhagic shock in dog by pretreatment with chronic high-salt diet. *American Journal of Physiology*, 1985; **249,** H577–84.
4. Zager RA, Gmur DJ, Bredl CR and Eng MJ: Temperature effects on ischemic and hypoxic renal proximal tubular injury. *Laboratory Investigation*, 1991; **64,** 766–76.
5. Baylis C, Brango C and Engels K: Renal effects of moderate hemorrhage in the conscious pregnant rat. *American Journal of Physiology*, 1990; **259,** F945–9.
6. Busija DW: Hypercapnia potentiates renal vasoconstriction during hemorrhagic hypotension in awake rabbits. *American Journal of Physiology*, 1984; **246,** H671–4.

7. Busija DW: Interaction between hemorrhagic hypotension and hypoxia in regulation of renal vascular resistance in unanesthetized rabbits. *Circulatory Shock*, 1984; **13,** 353–9.
8. Wang P, Singh G, Rana MW, Ba ZF and Chaudry IH: Preheparinization improves organ function after hemorrhage and resuscitation. *American Journal of Physiology*, 1990; **259,** R645–50.
9. Madias NE, Donohoe JF and Harrington JT: Postischemic acute renal failure. In Brenner BM and Lazarus JM (eds): *Acute Renal Failure*, 2nd edn. New York, NY, Churchill Livingstone, 1988, 251–78.
10. Ratcliffe PJ, Moonen CTW, Ledingham JGG and Radda GK: Timing of the onset of changes in renal energetics in relation to blood pressure and glomerular filtration in haemorrhagic hypotension in the rat. *Nephron*, 1989; **51,** 225–32.
11. Grady HC and Bullivant EMA: Renal blood flow varies during normal activity in conscious unrestrained rats. *American Journal of Physiology*, 1992; **262,** R926–32.
12. Walker LA, Buscemi-Bergin M and Gellai M: Renal hemodynamics in conscious rats: effect of anesthesia, surgery, and recovery. *American Journal of Physiology*, 1983; **245,** F67–74.
13. Idvall J: Influence of ketamine anesthesia on cardiac output and tissue perfusion in rats subjected to hemorrhage. *Anaesthesiology*, 1981; **55,** 297–304.
14. Priano LL: Effect of halothane on renal hemodynamics during normovolemia and acute hemorrhagic hypovolemia. *Anesthesiology*, 1985; **63,** 357–63.
15. Vatner SF: Effects of hemorrhage on regional blood flow distribution in dogs and primates. *Journal of Clinical Investigation*, 1974; **54,** 225–35.
16. Warren DJ and Ledingham JGG: Renal vascular response to haemorrhage in the rabbit after pentobarbitone, chloralose-urethane and ether anaesthesia. *Clinical Science*, 1978; **54,** 489–94.
17. Chien S: Role of the sympathetic nervous system in hemorrhage. *Physiological Reviews*, 1967; **47,** 214–88.
18. Selkurt EE: Current status of renal circulation and related nephron function in hemorrhage and experimental shock I. Vascular mechanisms. *Circulatory Shock*, 1974; **1,** 3–15.
19. Gross R, Ruffmann K and Kirchheim H: The separate and combined influences of common carotid occlusion and nonhypotensive hemorrhage on kidney blood flow. *Pflügers Archiv. European Journal of Physiology (Berlin)*, 1979; **379,** 81–8.
20. Habib BR, Hanet C, van Mechelen H, Keyeux A, Charlier AA and Pouleur H: Effects of atriopentin III on renal function, regional blood flows and left ventricular function in conscious dogs in presence or absence of hypovolemia. *European Journal of Clinical Investigation*, 1986; **16,** 461–7.
21. Kremser PC and Gewertz BL: Effect of pentobarbital and hemorrhage on renal autoregulation. *American Journal of Physiology*, 1985; **249,** F356–60.
22. Lameire NH, Stein JH and Horwitz LD: Hemorrhage and regional renal blood flow in the conscious dog. *Circulatory Shock*, 1980; **7,** 289–98.
23. Levy M and Fechner C: Renal response to hemorrhage in dogs with subacute biliary obstruction. *Canadian Journal of Physiology and Pharmacology*, 1985; **63,** 96–100.
24. Forsyth RP, Hoffbrand BI and Melmon KL: Redistribution of cardiac output during haemorrhage in the unanesthetized monkey. *Circulation Research*, 1970; **27,** 311–20.
25. Stone AM and Stahl WM: Renal effects of hemorrhage in normal man. *Annals of Surgery*, 1970; **170,** 825–36.
26. Hirsch AT, Levenson DJ, Cutler SS, Dzau VJ and Creager MA: Regional vascular responses to prolonged lower body negative pressure in normal subjects. *American Journal of Physiology*, 1989; **257,** H219–25.
27. Gilbert CA, Bricker LA, Springfield WT Jr, Stevens PM and Warren BH: Sodium and water excretion and renal hemodynamics during lower body negative pressure. *Journal of Applied Physiology*, 1966; **21,** 1699–1704.
28. Seyde WC and Longnecker DE: Anesthetic influences on regional hemodynamics in normal and hemorrhaged rats. *Anesthesiology*, 1984; **61,** 686–98.
29. Seyde WC, McGowan L, Lund N, Duling B and Longnecker DE: Effects of anesthetic agents on regional hemodynamics in normovolemic and hemorrhaged rats. *American Journal of Physiology*, 1985; **249,** H164–73.
30. Schadt JS, McKown MD, McKown DP and Franklin D: Hemodynamic effects of hemorrhage and subsequent naloxone treatment in conscious rabbits. *American Journal of Physiology*, 1984; **247,** R497–508.
31. Banks RA, Beilin LJ, Soltys J and Davidson L: Efefct of meclofenamate and captopril on blood flow to the kidney and spleen in conscious rabbits subjected to mild haemorrhage. *Clinical and Experimental Pharmacology and Physiology*, 1981; **8,** 543–8.
32. Courneya CA and Korner PI: Neurohumoral mechanisms and the role of arterial baroreceptors in the reno-vascular response to haemorrhage in rabbits. *Journal of Physiology (London)*, 1991; **437,** 393–407.
33. Chalmers JP, Korner PI and White SW: Effects of haemorrhage on the distribution of the peripheral blood flow in the rabbit. *Journal of Physiology (London)*, 1967; **192,** 561–74.
34. Korner PI, Stokes GS, White SW and Chalmers JP: Role of the autonomic nervous system in the renal vasoconstriction response to hemorrhage in the rabbit. *Circulation Research*, 1967; **20,** 676–85.
35. Sondeen JL, Gonzaludo GA, Loveday JA, Deshon

GE, Clifford CB, Hunt MM, Rodkey WG and Wade CE: Renal responses to graded hemorrhage in conscious pig. *American Journal of Physiology*, 1990; **259,** R119–25.
36. Slater GI, Vladeck BC, Bassin R, Kark AE and Shoemaker WC: Sequential changes in distribution of cardiac output in hemorrhagic shock. *Surgery*, 1973; **73,** 714–22.
37. Neutze JM, Wyler F and Rudolph AM: Changes in distribution of cardiac output after hemorrhage in rabbits. *American Journal of Physiology*, 1968; **215,** 857–64.
38. Sondeen JL, Gonzaludo GA, Loveday JA, Rodkey WG and Wade CE: Hypertonic saline/dextran improves renal function after hemorrhage in conscious swine. *Resuscitation*, 1990; **20,** 231–41.
39. Maningas PA: Resuscitation with 7.5% NaCl in 6% dextran-70 during hemorrhagic shock in swine: Effects on organ blood flow. *Critical Care Medicine*, 1987; **15,** 1121–6.
40. Bartley PJ and Anderson WP: Prostaglandins and the renal responses to haemorrhage, angiotensin II and methoxamine in conscious rabbits. *Clinical and Experimental Pharmacology and Physiology*, 1984; **11,** 71–80.
41. Brenner BM and Lazarus JM: *Acute Renal Failure*, 2nd edn. New York, NY, Churchill Livingstone, 1988.
42. Barger AC and Herd JA: Renal vascular anatomy and distribution of blood flow. In Orloff J and Berliner SR (eds): *Handbook of Physiology. Renal Physiology*. Washington: American Physiological Society, 1973, 249–313.
43. Brenner BM, Zatz R and Ichikawa I: The renal circulation. In Brenner BM and Rector FC (eds): *The Kidney*. Philadelphia, PA, WB Saunders Co., 1986, 93–123.
44. Jacobson HR and Kokko JP: Intrarenal heterogeneity: vascular and tubular. In Seldin DW and Giebisch G (eds): *The Kidney: Physiology and Pathophysiology*. New York, NY, Raven Press, 1985, 531–80.
45. Carriere S, Thornburn GD, O'Morchoe CCC and Barger AC: Intrarenal distribution of blood flow in dogs during hemorrhagic hypotension. *Circulation Research*, 1966; **19,** 167–79.
46. Hardaker WT, Graham TC and Wechsler AS: Renal intracortical blood flow during hemorrhage: role of adrenergic mechanisms. *American Journal of Physiology*, 1975; **229,** 178–84.
47. Jaschke W, Sievers RS, Lipton MJ and Cogan MG: Cine-computed tomographic assessment of regional renal blood flow. *Acta Radiologica*, 1990; **31,** 77–81.
48. Logan A, Jose P. Eisner G, Lilienfield L and Slotkoff L: Intracortical distribution of renal blood flow in hemorrhagic hypotension in dogs. *Circulation Research*, 1971; **29,** 257–66.
49. Montgomery SB, Jose PA, Slotkoff LM, Lilienfield LS and Eisner GM: The regulation of intrarenal blood flow in the dog during ischemia. *Circulatory Shock*, 1980; **7,** 71–82.
50. Stein JH, Boonjaren S, Mauk RC and Ferris TF: Mechanism of redistribution of renal cortical blood flow during hemorrhagic hypotension in the dog. *Journal of Clinical Investigation*, 1973; **52,** 39–47.
51. Kirkebo A and Tyssebotn I: Distribution of renal cortical blood flow during hemorrhagic hypotension in conscious dogs. *Acta Physiologica Scandinavica*, 1974; **91,** 22–31.
52. Ichikawa I and Brenner BM: Evidence for glomerular actions of ADH and dibutyryl cyclic AMP in the rat. *American Journal of Physiology*, 1977; **233,** F102–17.
53. Heller J and Horacek V: Kidney function during deceased perfusion pressure due to aortic clamping and hemorrhagic hypotension: a single nephron study in dog kidney. *Renal Physiology*, 1984; **7,** 90–101.
54. Moore LC and Mason J: Perturbation of tubuloglomerular feedback in hydropenic and hemorrhaged rats. *American Journal of Physiology*, 1983; **245,** F554–63.
55. Kaufman JS, Hamburger RJ and Flamenbaum W: Tubuloglomerular feedback response after hypotensive hemorrhage. *Renal Physiology*, 1982; **5,** 173–81.
56. Anderson WP, Alcorn D, Gilchrist AI and Ryan GB: Antiotensin II-induced contractions of mesangial cells in acute renal artery stenosis in dogs. *Clinical and Experimental Pharmacology and Physiology*, 1987; **14,** 267–71.
57. Anderson WP, Acorn D, Gilchrist AI, Whiting DM and Ryan GB: Glomerular actions of ANG II during reduction of renal artery pressure: a morphometric analysis. *American Journal of Physiology*, 1989; **256,** F1021–6.
58. Kon V and Ichikawa I: Hormonal regulation of glomerular filtration. *Annual Review of Medicine*, 1985; **36,** 515–31.
59. Anderson WP, Denton KM, Woods RL and Alcorn D: Angiotensin II and the maintenance of GFR and renal blood flow during renal artery narrowing. *Kidney International*, 1990; **38(suppl. 30),** S-109–13.
60. Kirchheim H, Ehmke H and Persson P: Role of blood pressure in the control of renin release. *Acta Physiologica Scandinavica Supplement*, 1990; **139,** 40–47.
61. Navar LG: Renal autoregulation: perspectives from whole kidney and single nephron studies. *American Journal of Physiology*, 1978; **234,** F357–70.
62. Barajas L: Innervation of the renal cortex. *Federation Proceedings*, 1978; **37,** 1192–208.
63. Barajas L and Powers K: Monoaminergic inner-

vation of the rat kidney: a quantitative study. *American Journal of Physiology*, 1990; **259,** F503–11.

64. Luff SE, Hengstberger SG, McLachlan EM and Anderson WP: Distribution of sympathetic neuroeffector junctions in the juxtaglomerular region of the rabbit kidney. *Journal of the Autonomic Nervous System*, 1992; **40,** 239–54.
65. DiBona GF: The functions of the renal nerves. *Reviews of Physiology, Biochemistry and Pharmacology*, 1982; **94,** 75–181.
66. Moss NG, Colindres RE and Gottschalk CW: Neural control of renal function. In Windhager EE (ed.): *Handbook of Physiology. Section 8: Renal Physiology, Volume 2.* New York, NY, Oxford University Press and the American Physiological Society, 1992, 1061–128.
67. Burke SL and Dorward PK: Influence of endogenous opiates and cardiac afferents on renal nerve activity during haemorrhage in conscious rabbits. *Journal of Physiology (London)*, 1988; **402,** 9–27.
68. Morita H, Nishida Y, Motochigawa H, Uemura N, Hosomi H and Vatner SF: Opiate receptor-mediated decrease in renal nerve activity during hypotensive hemorrhage in conscious rabbits. *Circulation Research*, 1988; **63,** 165–72.
69. Morita H and Vatner SF: Effects of hemorrhage on renal nerve activity in conscious dogs. *Circulation Research*, 1985; **57,** 788–93.
70. Hasser EM and Schadt JC: Sympathoinhibition and its reversal by naloxon during hemorrhage. *American Journal of Physiology*, 1992; **262,** R444–51.
71. Peuler JD, Schmid PG, Morgan DA and Mark AL: Inhibition of renal sympathetic activity and heart rate by vasopressin in hemorrhaged diabetes insipidus rats. *American Journal of Physiology*, 1990; **258,** H706–12.
72. Koyama S, Aibiki M, Kanai K, Fujita T and Miyakawa K: Role of central nervous system in renal nerve activity during prolonged hemorrhagic shock in dogs. *American Journal of Physiology*, 1988; **254,** R761–9.
73. Skarphedinsson JO, Stage L and Thoren P: Cerebral function during hypotensive hemorrhage in spontaneously hypertensive rats and Wistar Kyoto rats. *Acta Physiologica Scandinavica*, 1986; **128,** 445–52.
74. Thoren P, Skarphedinsson JO and Carlsson: Sympathetic inhibition from vagal afferents during severe haemorrhage in rats. *Acta Physiologica Scandinavica Supplement*, 1988; **571,** 97–105.
75. Oberg B and Thoren P: Increased activity in left ventricular receptors during hemorrhage or occlusion of caval veins in the cat – a possible cause of the vaso-vagal reaction. *Acta Physiologica Scandinavica*, 1972; **85,** 164–73.
76. Morgan DA, Thoren P, Wilczynski EA, Victor RG and Mark AL: Serotonergic mechanisms mediate renal sympathoinhibition during severe hemorrhage in rats. *American Journal of Physiology*, 1988; **255,** H496–502.
77. Morita H: Dissociation between changes in renal nerve activity and renal vascular resistance in conscious dogs. *Japanese Journal of Physiology*, 1986; **36,** 585–93.
78. La Grange RG, Sloop CH and Schmid HE: Selective stimulation of renal nerves in the anaesthetized dog. *Clinical Research*, 1973; **33,** 704–12.
79. Osborn JL and Johns EJ: Renal neurogenic control of renin and prostaglandin release. *Mineral and Electrolyte Metabolism*, 1989; **15,** 51–8.
80. Thames MD and DiBona GF: Renal nerves modulate the secretion of renin mediated by nonneural mechanisms. *Circulation Research*, 1979; **44,** 645–52.
81. Kline RL and Mercer PF: Functional reinnervation and development of supersensitivity to NE after renal denervation in rats. *American Journal of Physiology*, 1980; **238,** R353–8.
82. Szénási G, Bencsáth P and Takacs L: Supersensitivity of the renal tubule to catecholamines in the chronically denervated canine kidney. *Pflügers Archiv. European Journal of Physiology (Berlin)*, 1986; **406,** 57–9.
83. Lifschitz MD: Lack of a role for the renal nerves in renal sodium reabsorption in conscious dogs. *Clinical Science*, 1978; **54,** 567–72.
84. Fejes-Tóth G, Brinck-Johnsen T and Naray-Fejes-Tóth A: Cardiovascular and hormonal response to hemorrhage in conscious rats. *American Journal of Physiology*, 1988; **254,** H947–53.
85. Henrich WL, Pettinger WA and Cronin RE: The influence of circulating catecholamines and prostaglandins on canine renal hemodynamics during hemorrhage. *Circulation Research*, 1981; **48,** 424–9.
86. Togashi H, Yoshioka M, Tochihara M, Matsumoto M and Saito H: Differential effects of hemorrhage on adrenal and renal nerve activity in anesthetized rats. *American Journal of Physiology*, 1990; **259,** H1134–41.
87. Zimpfer M, Manders WT, Barger AC and Vatner SF: Pentobarbital alters compensatory neural and humoral mechanisms in response to hemorrhage. *American Journal of Physiology*, 1982; **243,** H713–21.
88. Schadt JC and Ludbrook J: Hemodynamic and neuronal responses to acute hypovolemia in conscious mammals. *American Journal of Physiology*, 1991; **260,** H305–18.
89. Mzail AH and Noble AR: Haemorrhage-induced secretion of active and inactive renin in conscious and pentobarbitone-anaesthetized sheep. *Clinical and Experimental Pharmacology and Physiology*, 1992; **13,** 131–8.
90. Oliver JR, Korner PI, Woods RL and Zhu JL: Reflex release of vasopressin and renin in hemorrhage is en-

hanced by autonomic blockade. *American Journal of Physiology*, 1990; **258,** H221–8.

91. Pullan PT, Johnston CI, Anderson WP and Korner PI: Plasma vasopressin in blood pressure homeostasis and in experimental renal hypertension. *American Journal of Physiology*, 1980; **239,** H81–7.
92. Denton KM, Fennessy PA, Acorn D and Anderson WP: Morphometric analysis of the actions of angiotensin II on renal arterioles and glomeruli. *American Journal of Physiology*, 1992; **262,** F367–72.
93. Hall JE: Control of sodium excretion by angiotensin II: intrarenal mechanisms and blood pressure regulation. *American Journal of Physiology*, 1986; **250,** R960–72.
94. Navar GL, Saccomani G and Mitchell KD: Synergistic intrarenal actions of angiotensin on tubular reabsorption and renal hemodynamics. *American Journal of Hypertension*, 1991; **4,** 90–96.
95. Baylis C: Glomerular filtration dynamics. In Lote CJ (ed.): *Advances in Renal Physiology*. London, Croom Helm, 1986, 33–83.
96. Blantz RC, Konnen KS and Tucker BJ: Angiotensin II effects upon the glomerular microcirculation and ultrafiltration coefficient of the rat. *Journal of Clinical Investigation*, 1976; **57,** 419–34.
97. Anderson WP and Woods RL: Intrarenal effects of angiotensin II in renal artery stenosis. *Kidney International*, 1987; **31,** 157–67.
98. Dzau VJ, Siwek LG, Rosen S, Fahri ER, Mizoguchi H and Barger AC: Sequential renal hemodynamics in experimental benign and malignant hypertension. *Hypertension*, 1981; **3(suppl. I),** I-63–8.
99. Textor SC, Tarazi RC, Novick AC, Bravo EL and Fouad FM: Regulation of renal hemodynamics and glomerular filtration in patients with renovascular hypertension during converting enzyme inhibition with captopril. *American Journal of Medicine*, 1984; **76,** 29–37.
100. Anderson WP, Korner PI and Selig SE: Mechanisms involved in the renal responses to intravenous and renal artery infusions of noradrenaline in conscious dogs. *Journal of Physiology (London)*, 1981; **321,** 21–30.
101. Johns EJ, Lewis BA and Singer B: The sodium retaining effect of renal nerve activity in the cat: role of angiotensin formation. *Clinical Science*, 1976; **51,** 93–102.
102. Data JL, Chang LCT and Nies AS: Alteration of canine renal vascular response to hemorrhage by inhibitors of prostaglandin synthesis. *American Journal of Physiology*, 1976; **230,** 940–45.
103. Henrich WL, Anderson RJ, Berns AS, McDonald KM, Paulsen PJ, Berl T and Schrier RW: The role of renal nerves and prostaglandins in control of renal hemodynamics and plasma renin activity during hypotensive hemorrhage in the dog. *Journal of Clinical Investigation*, 1978; **61,** 744–50.
104. Henrich WL, Berl T, McDonald KM, Anderson RJ and Schrier RW: Angiotensin II, renal nerves, and prostaglandins in renal hemodynamics during hemorrhage. *American Journal of Physiology*, 1978; **235,** F46–51.
105. Lokhandwala MF and Jandhyala BS: Sympathetic nerve function and renal hemodynamics during hemorrhage: role of pre- and postsynaptic interactions between angiotensin II and prostaglandins. *Journal of Pharmacology and Experimental Therapeutics*, 1979; **211,** 539–45.
106. Terragno NA, Terragno DA and McGiff JC: Contribution of prostaglandins to the renal circulation of conscious, anaesthetized and laparotomized dogs. *Circulation Research*, 1977; **40,** 590–95.
107. Lieberthal W, McGarry AE, Sheils J and Valeri CR: Nitric oxide inhibition in rats improves blood pressure and renal function during hypovolemic shock. *American Journal of Physiology*, 1991; **261,** F868–72.
108. Szabó C, Faragó M, Horváth I, Lohinai Z and Kovách A: Hemorrhagic hypotension impairs endothelium-dependent relaxations in the renal artery of the cat. *Circulatory Shock*, 1992; **36,** 238–41.

11

Skin, muscle and splanchnic circulations

John M Johnson

Sudden marked bradycardia is undoubtedly a primary component of the depressor response in most episodes of vasovagal syncope, including hypovolaemia.[1] Vasomotor responses also contribute to this rapid fall in blood pressure, but the picture is far less clear. The problem relates, in part, to the difficulty in studying an event that is fast to develop and does not follow in a predictable course under laboratory conditions. Of the many studies of the reflex nature of blood pressure control, few were designed to study vasovagal syncope specifically, although it often can accompany such studies. When it does, the onset and degree are not predictable, often relating to other environmental factors such as intravascular catheterization[2] or high thermal loads.[3,4] Moreover, when it occurs the usual response by the investigators is to reverse quickly the falling blood pressure, interrupting the process as it develops. Also, most methods for blood flow measurement in humans are better suited for a more slowly changing haemodynamic pattern. Nevertheless, there is sufficient available information to tender at least tentative conclusions regarding the role of the regional circulations in the bradycardic phase in hypovolaemia.

The design of this chapter is to outline the known vasomotor responses to blood loss at mild, moderate and, finally, severe levels. Incorporated into this is the widely accepted proposal that the sensory elements responsible for initiating the reflex adjustments differ importantly among these levels of blood loss. Focus is placed on responses by humans, but supportive information originating from animal models is included. The focus is also on three major regional circulations: muscle, skin and splanchnic. In humans especially, these regional circulations have been the subject of the greatest amount of study with respect to blood pressure regulation.

Mild blood loss

Methods for studying the cardiovascular adjustments to reduced blood volume include phlebotomy, upright tilting, positive pressure breathing, thigh tourniquets, high footward G-forces and LBNP. With the exception of phlebotomy, these methods reduce the effective blood volume largely by translocating volume from the thorax to the legs, reducing cardiac filling and cardiac output. Over the past 20 years or so, LBNP has proved to be a very useful tool for exploration of cardiovascular reflex control.[2,5–8] Particular advantages include the ability to make measurements without changing the position or posture of the subject and the fact that the level can be tightly controlled, yielding a highly graded perturbation. It is this latter capability of LBNP that has led to some significant advances in our understanding of reflex control of the circulation; specifically, the exploration of the role of cardiopulmonary baroreceptors in responses to hypovolaemia.

Roddie *et al.*[9] noted that stimulation of atrial stretch receptors by raising the legs produced a vasodilatation in the forearm. Because arterial pressure changes were small or inconsistent, the authors reasoned that the sensory elements important in initiating this vasodilatation were in the cardiopulmonary region – the so-called 'low pressure baroreceptors' (an unfortunate term), corresponding to receptors discovered in the cardiopulmonary portion of the circulation.[7,10]

These receptors are involved in the reflex control

of vascular resistance and are well situated to participate in the responses to haemorrhage or its simulation. It was later noted that very mild levels of LBNP could evoke vasoconstrictor responses without measurable changes in arterial pressure parameters such as mean arterial pressure, pulse pressure or the rate of rise of arterial pressure.[11,12] Fig. 11.1 illustrates a variety of the cardiovascular changes and responses over a range of LBNP.[11] Of special interest is the region up to −20 mmHg, in which arterial pressure had no measurable change, but marked forearm vasoconstriction and a milder splanchnic vasoconstriction occurred. Because arterial pressure was well maintained with respect to the parameters felt to be important for sinoaortic baroreceptor activity, the origin of the vasoconstriction in forearm and splanchnic regions is unlikely to be sinoaortic baroreceptors. Instead, it is strongly indicated that cardiopulmonary stretch receptors were being slowly unloaded, leading to a withdrawal of their inhibition of the vasomotor centres and thus to the vasoconstrictor responses.[7,11,12]

Thus, the vasomotor responses to mild blood loss are apparently initiated by cardiopulmonary baroreceptors and lead to vasoconstriction in the limbs and viscera. It is somewhat surprising, but the sinoatrial node does not appear to be an important target for this reflex, as heart rate is not changed (or slightly falls) during this critical period (Fig. 11.1). Although concerns that the sensory signal truly arises from sinoaortic baroreceptors in a simple feedback loop can probably never be fully rebutted, this seems an unlikely scenario because the error signal required for this magnitude of response to originate in the sinoaortic region should be sufficiently large to permit detection.[7,13] Indeed, this points to the value of the feed-forward aspect of the cardiopulmonary receptors. By augmenting vasoconstrictor activity, the necessity for an error signal on the arterial side of the circulation is reduced considerably or even eliminated.

The most frequent and consistent vasomotor re-

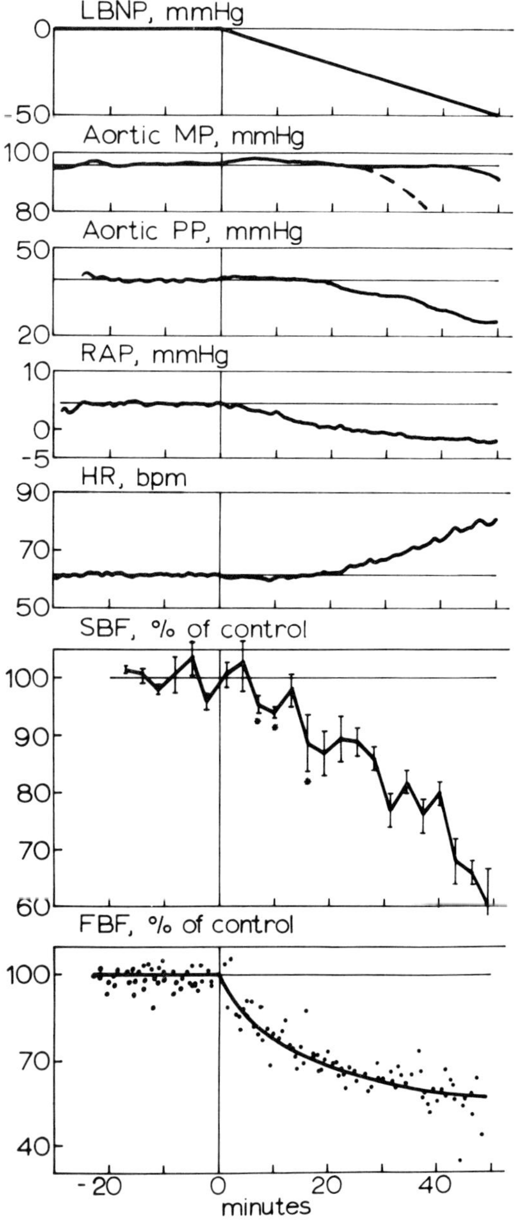

Fig. 11.1. Changes in aortic mean pressure (MP), aortic pulse pressure (PP) and in right atrial pressure (RAP) with lower body negative pressure (LBNP) graded from 0 to −50 mmHg. Reflex responses in heart rate (HR), splanchnic blood flow (SBF) and forearm blood flow (FBF). No changes in aortic pressure are seen prior to reading an LBNP of −20 mmHg, after which aortic PP began to fall. HR showed a similar pattern, beginning to rise at LBNP of −20 mmHg. FBR fell during the earliest stages of LBNP, reaching 67 per cent of control by an LBNP of −20 mmHg. SBF had an intermediate response, falling to 90 per cent of control at an LBNP of −20 mmHg. As LBNP progressed beyond −20 mmHg, FBF and SBF fell further (the latter more markedly) and HR rose. *, Reduction in SBF compared with control ($P < 0.05$); reductions statistically significant ($P < 0.05$) thereafter. FBF was significantly reduced at all times beyond the first minute of LBNP. From Johnson *et al.*,[11] with permission.

sponse is that of a forearm vasoconstriction when cardiopulmonary baroreceptors are selectively unloaded.[7,11–13] At a level of LBNP of −20 mmHg forearm blood flow falls by about one-third.[11] The same level of LBNP only provokes a fall in splanchnic blood flow of about 11 per cent.[11,13] This heterogeneous effect on the regional circulations apparently applies to tissues comprising the forearm circulation as well. It is clear that the skeletal muscle circulation is a primary target.[7] Sympathetic activity specific to skeletal muscle increases markedly, whereas that for the skin is not as obviously affected.[14–18] Low levels of LBNP (−10 mmHg) have no significant effect on forearm skin blood flow[19] at the time of a significant forearm vasoconstriction. However, the cutaneous circulation does become a more obvious target as levels of LBNP are increased further, skin blood flow falling by 20 per cent when LBNP of −20 mmHg is reached[19] and by about one-third at levels of −30 mmHg.[20] At this stage a tentative conclusion is that when cardiopulmonary baroreceptors are selectively withdrawn, the circulation to skeletal muscle is the primary target for vasoconstriction, with the cutaneous circulation second and the splanchnic circulation the least sensitive to this perturbation.

Moderate blood loss

As blood loss (or its redistribution) becomes more severe, the ability of the feed-forward cardiopulmonary baroreceptor system to compensate fully for the decrement in cardiac output becomes limited, ultimately failing and allowing arterial pressure to fall. This fall in arterial pressure represents an error signal to the sinoaortic baroreceptors and initiates feedback control. However, in addition to mean arterial pressure, the sinoaortic baroreceptors are sensitive to other parameters such as pulse pressure and the rate of change of pressure.[21,22] This sensitivity is of more than academic interest because it serves like the feed-forward arrangement of the cardiopulmonary baroreceptors. For example, the sensitivity to a small fall in arterial pulse pressure obviates the requirement for that much error signal in mean blood pressure in engaging reflex adjustments, hence preventing a fall in the latter.

Fig. 11.1 also illustrates the range of LBNP in which arterial baroreceptor unloading becomes engaged, initially through reductions in pulse pressure. Beginning at about −20 mmHg LBNP, arterial pulse pressure begins to fall.[7,11,12] Coincident with this fall in pulse pressure is a rise in heart rate and further increases in forearm and splanchnic vascular resistance (Fig. 11.1).[11–13,20,23] It is during this interval that the splanchnic vasoconstriction becomes more marked, whereas the further increases in forearm vascular resistance are not as steep as earlier.[12,13,20] The usual interpretation of this differential sensitivity among the splanchnic, forearm and sinoatrial node targets is that unloading of the arterial-sided baroreceptors has splanchnic vasoconstriction and tachycardia as the major targets, the limb circulation being less involved.[7,12,13,20] Thus, from a level of −20 to −40 mmHg LBNP approximately 60–70 per cent of the splanchnic vasoconstriction occurs compared with 30–40 per cent of the forearm vasoconstriction. These latter changes may be due largely to unloading of arterial baroreceptors, given the responses to selective cardiopulmonary unloading discussed above. This conclusion is supported by the findings of Abboud *et al.*,[13] who applied increased transmural pressure to the carotid sinus region (neck suction) during rest and LBNP. Neck suction, a reasonably specific stimulus to carotid baroreceptors, had no statistically significant influence on forearm or splanchnic vascular resistance at rest, when little removable vasoconstrictor activity would be expected. Against a background of LBNP of −40 mmHg, when both regional circulations had increased resistances by about 40 per cent, neck suction reversed the splanchnic vasoconstriction but had no measurable influence on that in the forearm. This finding is in keeping with the general conclusion that vasoconstrictor responses to cardiopulmonary baroreceptor unloading primarily target the limb circulation, whereas those from sinoaortic baroreceptor unloading target the splanchnic circulation. Recently, however, Escourrou *et al.*[24] were unable to reverse LBNP-initiated splanchnic vasoconstriction with pulsatile carotid sinus distension. Reasons for differences between these studies[13,24] are not clear, but leave open the question regarding the individual roles of cardiopulmonary and carotid sinus baroreceptors during major blood loss.

With respect to the forearm circulation, at these higher levels of LBNP there is little difference noted in the contributions by skin and muscle to the overall forearm vasoconstriction.[19,23,25] Tripathi and Nadel[19] noted a fall in skin blood flow of about 10 per cent of the control value for each decrement in LBNP of 10 mmHg, which was not strikingly different from that for the entire forearm.

This level of LBNP shares characteristics with other approaches to the simulation of moderate blood loss (or of haemorrhage itself) in that both the cardiopulmonary and sinoaortic baroreceptor inhibition of the vasomotor centre are being withdrawn, yielding an increase in heart rate and vasoconstriction in skeletal muscle, skin and splanchnic regions.[4,8,14,25–38] Collectively, these findings show the combined unloading of cardiopulmonary and sinoaortic receptors to lead to major vasoconstrictor responses in the limbs and viscera. These responses depend on the degree of blood loss and of hypotension, but 30–40 per cent reductions in forearm and splanchnic blood flow can be expected when the challenge to blood pressure regulation approaches its limits of compensation. Based on the available data, this appears to be not a matter of the particular stimulus, as LBNP, high G_z acceleration, upright tilting and venesection give similar results. Furthermore, the responses in the forearm reflect those in the legs.[17,18,34,39] At these levels (e.g. −50 mmHg of LBNP), Rowell *et al.*[20] calculated that the two-thirds of the peripheral vascular compensation to the reduction in cardiac output brought about by this loss of CBV was distributed approximately evenly between the splanchnic and limb circulations, the renal circulation presumably accounting for the remainder.[6,27,35]

Major blood loss

As the translocation of blood from the thorax becomes severe, either through frank blood loss or through pooling in the extremities (LBNP, G_z acceleration, upright tilting, leg tourniquets), the compensatory response by regional vasoconstriction reaches its limit. It is unclear why this limit is reached at this stage, as greater reflex reductions in blood flow to these regions can be seen. For example, intense exercise in the heat can reduce splanchnic blood flow by up to 80 per cent.[40] Similarly, cold stress can reduce skin blood flow by similar amounts or more.[3,41,42] Also, the diving reflex causes there to be almost complete cessation of blood flow to skeletal muscle.[43] Although these circulations are all markedly vasoconstricted at the limits of compensation to blood loss, none appears to be as vasoconstricted as the above maxima might anticipate.

The same is true for heart rate.[1] As blood loss reaches some critical level, the mild tachycardia (80–90 beats/min) accompanying blood loss is suddenly reversed to a marked bradycardia. This is the most frequently observed characteristic of vasovagal syncope with blood loss, and is covered in detail elsewhere in this volume. The receptor groups responsible for this portion of the response to blood loss are thought to be ventricular mechanoreceptors,[44] although other groups may contribute since syncope was induced in a recipient of a cardiac transplant.[45] The focus, here, is how the regional circulations participate in this hypotensive episode. Do they show a further compensatory vasoconstriction as blood pressure falls precipitously; do they have a sustained vascular resistance; or do they show a reversal to a vasodilatation, similar to the response in heart rate but counter to blood pressure regulation? In other words, does peripheral resistance contribute to the hypotensive episode accompanying vasovagal syncope with major blood loss?

Haemodynamic measures strongly support the view that the regional circulations play an important role in precipitating the fall in blood pressure during haemorrhagic syncope. Barcroft *et al.*[46] measured cardiac output and blood pressure before and during syncopal reactions accompanying venesection and/or placement of tourniquets on the thighs. These investigators found cardiac output to fall prior to syncope, but not to change in a consistent pattern during the ensuing faint. Total peripheral resistance showed the usual baroreceptor-mediated increase prior to syncope, but then showed a sharp reversal as syncope developed.

This general observation has been seen in several independent studies[2,39,47,48] and is also the case in patients with various cardiac disorders.[49] Upright tilting,[48] leg tourniquets with venesection[34,46] or a combination of factors[2,49] were used to initiate syncopal reactions. Overall, the results from these various studies are that total peripheral resistance rises during the initial stages of blood loss to perhaps 30–50 per cent above resting values. With syncope, total peripheral resistance falls to control levels or below, often reaching values 20–40 per cent below those of resting conditions.[2,39,46–50] This fall in total peripheral resistance indicates that the vasculature plays a major role in the precipitation of hypovolaemia-induced syncope. Indeed, cardiac output changes inconsistently and, on average, little from its value before blood pressure begins to fall,[2,39,46–50] despite the bradycardia. One would have to conclude from these observations that falling peripheral resistance is the major cause of the fall in blood pressure at that time.

Less clear is which regional circulations are vasodilating to yield the overall reduction in total peripheral resistance, or how those involved might be doing so. Likely places would be those circulations with sufficient capacity for vasodilatation to have pronounced effects on systemic haemodynamics, i.e. the muscle, skin, splanchnic and renal regional circulations.

Answers to the above questions are still speculative to some extent, as there is not a large body of information for this extreme in blood pressure regulation. Nevertheless, there are sufficient solid data to suggest strongly participation in at least some regional circulations. Perhaps the clearest results come from Barcroft *et al.*,[46,51] who extensively studied responses in forearm blood flow accompanying syncope from blood loss. Their findings, illustrated in Fig. 11.2, are surprising in the context of blood pressure regulation. The implication is clear, however. At a time of precipitously falling blood pressure, forearm blood flow was rising as quickly. There is no doubt that the limb was undergoing a significant vasodilatation. Venesection, *per se*, is not required for this forearm vasodilator participation in this hypovolaemic syncope. Bridgen *et al.*[28] found with tilting to the upright posture that a similar increase in forearm blood flow could occur. Epstein *et al.*[52] also noted with upright tilting that there was invariably a reduction in forearm vascular resistance when blood pressure fell markedly. These investigators noted the same pattern of response in subjects who experienced syncope during LBNP. Overall, there was a fall in forearm vascular resistance of about 62 per cent, although a net increase in forearm blood flow was not seen as consistently as in earlier studies.[28,46,51] This response in the forearm is also apparent in the legs, indicating a general response by the limb circulations.[39] It is also important to note that Epstein *et al.*[52] measured reductions in forearm venous compliance during syncope, i.e. venoconstriction, indicating that the site of the vascular contribution to syncope does not include the veins.

Unclear from these data is the extent of participation by the skin and muscle components of limb blood flow. Each has the capacity for a large reflex vasodilatation and, when extrapolated to skin or muscle in general, could have profound effects on total peripheral resistance.[53,54] The available data do not provide support for a vasodilator role for the cutaneous circulation in hypovolaemic syncope. The common observation of a cold, pale skin in shock argues against this role. Hand blood flow tends to follow blood pressure passively.[51] This finding suggests that withdrawal of cutaneous vasoconstrictor activity is not occurring at the time of syncope. Furthermore, the cutaneous active vasodilator system[31,54] does not appear to be engaged. Fig. 11.3 shows data from a single subject who experienced syncope during the application of LBNP while under heat stress sufficient to provide high active cutaneous vasodilator activity.[3] No elevation in forearm blood flow or reduction in forearm vascular resistance was seen, rather a further vasoconstriction. This observation is like that made by Lind *et al.*,[4] who observed forearm vasoconstrictor responses to syncope during upright tilting in the heat. In these cases it is likely that active cutaneous vasodilatation is being withdrawn. Kellogg *et al.*[31] found that LBNP applied to subjects with the active cutaneous vasodilator system engaged reduced cutaneous vascular conductance by withdrawal of active vasodilator activity. Given the further fall of forearm and presumably cutaneous vascular conductance with syncope, further withdrawal of active vasodilatation seems likely. Indeed, it is probable that vasodilatation in forearm muscle is masked by the vasoconstriction in skin in the circumstance of a hot environment, and that is why these studies[3,4] did not observe the net vasodilatation of the forearm seen by Barcroft and Edholm in a neutral environment.[51]

Because skin does not appear to be a source for the limb vasodilatation with syncope, muscle must be the site, in keeping with the original speculation.[46,51] The fact that skeletal muscle is, overall, a major vascular region allows the vasodilatation (as revealed by responses in the forearm) to have a marked effect on total peripheral resistance and blood pressure. Barcroft *et al.*[46] estimated this effect by making various assumptions about the overall response in muscle and applied that to the measured values for cardiac output and total peripheral resistance. These estimates indicate that vasodilatation in skeletal muscle could account for the entire reduction in total peripheral resistance with syncope.

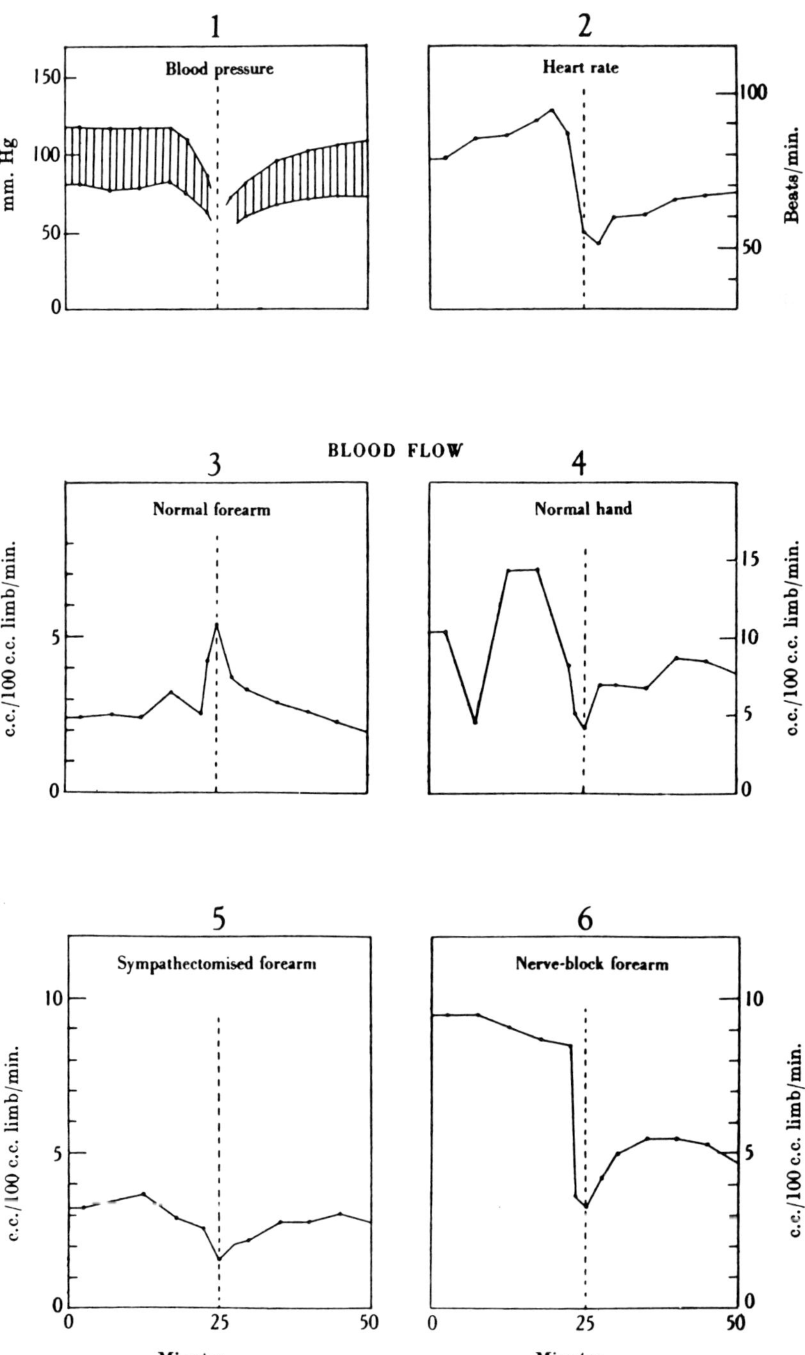

Fig. 11.2. Vasomotor and heart rate changes before, during and after syncope (▥). As arterial pressure fell, forearm blood flow rose by about 100 per cent, heart rate fell by about 45 beats/min and hand blood flow tended to follow blood pressure. Sympathectomy or anaesthetic blockade of forearm nerves prevented the forearm vasodilatation. From Barcroft and Edholm,[46] with permission from The Physiological Society.

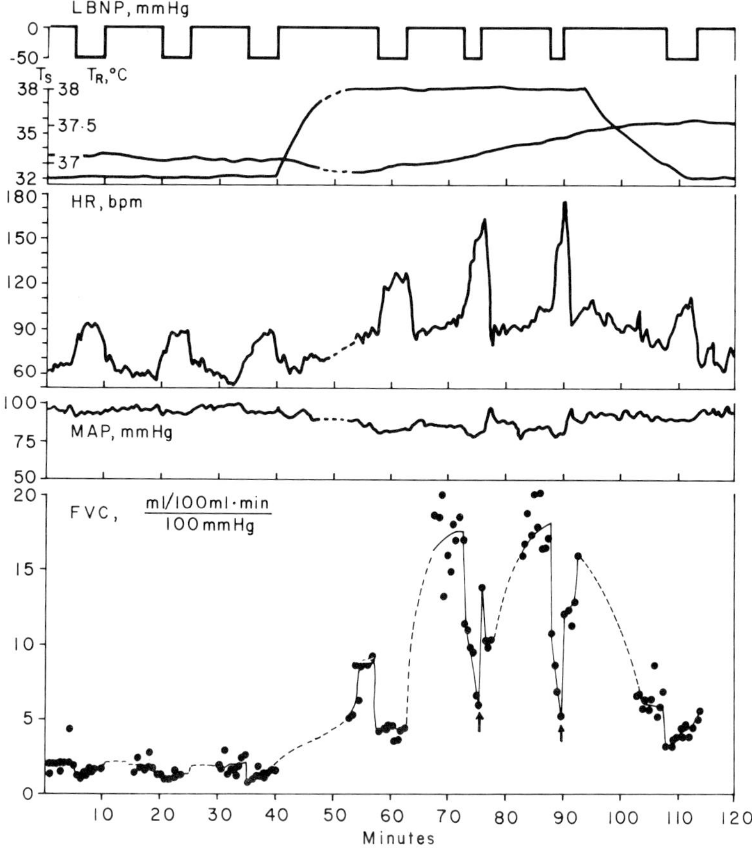

Fig. 11.3. Responses in forearm vascular conductance (FVC), mean arterial pressure (MAP) and heart rate (HR) to lower body negative pressure (LBNP) of −50 mmHg. Responses between 0 and 40 min were from normothermic conditions. At 40 min, skin temperature (T_s) was raised to 38°C by a water-perfused suit, and internal temperature (rectal; T_r) rose progressively. Application of LBNP during whole body heat stress was associated with two bouts of syncope (vertical arrows at 75 and 90 min). Note that FVC rose only when LBNP was terminated, and not during the syncopal episodes. Because skin blood flow is the major component of total forearm blood flow during heat stress, these data indicate skin does not vasodilate during syncope. From Johnson *et al.*,[3] with permission.

It appears that in the case of hypovolaemic syncope, an active vasodilatation in skeletal muscle need not occur to account for the results. The levels of blood flow observed by Barcroft and colleagues[46,51] are in keeping with abolition of vasoconstrictor nerve activity. Indeed, Wallin and Sundlöf[47] found sympathetic activity directed to skeletal muscle to be abolished at the time of syncope. Scherrer *et al.*[45] also noted abolition of sympathetic nerve activity directed to muscle during a syncopal reaction to infused vasodilators. Of special interest is that this subject was a cardiac transplant recipient, suggesting a non-cardiac origin for this response. Active vasodilatation in muscle, as occurs in an emotional faint, has the capacity to vasodilate muscle to three times the levels reported above for haemorrhagic syncope.[53] Furthermore, atropinization does not provide protection against haemorrhagic syncope, indicating that activation of a cholinergic vasodilator system is not responsible for the vasodilatation.[48] However, these arguments do not rule out mechanisms in addition to sympathetic vasoconstrictor withdrawal. For example, increases in circulating adrenaline and CGRP (both vasodilators) have been observed during syncopal reactions.[39] The degree of their participation in the vasodilatation is uncertain, however.

It is less clear whether the splanchnic or renal circulations play a causative role in the sudden fall in total peripheral resistance with hypovolaemic syncope. Bearn *et al.*[50] broached this question for the splanchnic circulation by measuring splanchnic blood flow by the clearance of bromsulphalein. The investigators applied venous congesting cuffs to the thighs and further reduced CBV with venesection of variable volumes. They noted a fall in splanchnic blood flow prior to syncope, which became more pronounced as syncope ensued. These measurements were supported by the observations that hepatic venous oxygen content fell further and there was a sudden marked increase in hepatic venous glucose concentration, a characteristic response to hepatic ischaemia.[50] However, this fall in splanchnic blood flow was less pronounced than the marked fall in blood pressure. Thus, calculated splanchnic vascular resistance fell with the onset of syncope. This result must be considered with some caution, however, because the clearance method for blood flow measurement is not well suited to rapid changes and vascular resistance was estimated from systolic rather than mean arterial pressure.[50] Given this caveat, the measured splanchnic vascular resistance fell from an average of 40 per cent above control to perhaps 17 per cent below values obtained at rest.

The renal vascular participation in syncope is even less clear. Smith[35] observed renal vasoconstriction with tilting to the upright position with no obvious vasodilatation as presyncopal symptoms developed. He also noted renal vasoconstriction to accompany the presyncopal period brought about by emotional alarm (when muscle shows a marked vasodilatation). de Wardener and McSwiney,[55] however, estimated renal vascular resistance from *para*-amino hippurate clearance and auscultatory blood pressure in studies involving venous occlusion at the thighs and venesection or upright tilting. When syncope occurred, there was not a consistent response in renal blood flow, but estimated renal vascular resistance usually fell below the levels prior to syncope. On the other hand, Ladefoged and Munck[56] found renal blood flow, as measured by Xenon-133 washout, to be drastically reduced (to about 5 per cent of control levels) in a single patient during an emotional faint. In rabbits Hasser and Schadt[57] found an increased renal sympathetic activity to accompany the early stages of haemorrhage, but to fall precipitously with blood pressure as haemorrhage became severe. This finding is similar to that by Wallin and Sundlöf[47] for sympathetic activity to skeletal muscle in syncopal humans. Interestingly, the reduction in renal sympathetic activity was blocked by naloxone, suggesting a role for endogenous opioids.[57]

In summary, although bradycardia is the most frequently seen cardiovascular reflex attendant to hypovolaemia-induced syncopal reactions, the vasomotor component is apparently the more important as a causal agent. The sequence of events attending hypovolaemia begin with a vasoconstrictor response in muscle, cutaneous and splanchnic vasculature initiated by the unloading of cardiopulmonary baroreceptors. This reflex response is most prominent in muscle, with smaller reactions in other regions. When compensation from this feed-forward reflex begins to fail, reductions in arterial pulse pressure or mean pressure unload sinoaortic baroreceptors and vasoconstrictor responses become more intense. In this phase of moderate blood loss from the central circulation, splanchnic vasoconstriction, especially, becomes more marked. Additionally, heart rate is increased. The third phase of hypovolaemia is the generation of a syncopal reaction and fainting. Although characterized by a sharp reduction in heart rate, cardiac output is not changed consistently; peripheral vasodilatation is the major source of the fall in arterial pressure. In this case, there is a major vasodilatation in skeletal muscle. Responses in other regions are less clear. The presence of a cold skin in shock underscores the failure to measure any signs of cutaneous vasodilatation. Splanchnic and renal circulation are reported to have reduced vascular resistance, hence contributing to the fall in total peripheral resistance. However, this reduced resistance is less, proportionately, than the fall in blood pressure. Hence, blood flow to these regions falls despite the vasodilatation and signs of hepatic ischaemia, such as an outpouring of glucose, ensue.

The reduced vascular resistance in skeletal muscle and perhaps the kidney appears to be due largely to an abolition of sympathetic activity to these regions. Whether such is the case generally is not known, but does not appear likely, given the intense cutaneous vasoconstriction. Active vasodilatation in skeletal muscle has been postulated, but this role is unclear. Also, the contributions by circulating vasoactive agents and autoregulatory escape remain unknown.

Acknowledgement

The author acknowledges the many contributions by colleagues, the excellent secretarial skills of Rebecca Alexander and the support of his laboratory by Public Health Service Grant HL36080.

References

1. Secher NH and Bie P: Bradycardia during reversible haemorrhagic shock – a forgotten observation? *Clinical Physiology*, 1985; **5,** 315–23.
2. Stevens PM: Cardiovascular dynamics during orthostasis and the influence of intravascular instrumentation. *American Journal of Cardiology*, 1966; **17,** 211–18.
3. Johnson JM, Niederberger M, Rowell LB, Eisman MM and Brengelmann GL: Competition between cutaneous vasodilator and vasoconstrictor reflexes in man. *Journal of Applied Physiology*, 1973; **35,** 798–803.
4. Lind AR, Leithead CS and McNicol GW: Cardiovascular changes during syncope induced by tilting men in the heat. *Journal of Applied Physiology*, 1968; **25,** 268–76.
5. Brown E, Goei JS, Greenfield ADM and Plassaras GC: Circulatory responses to simulated gravitational shifts of blood in man induced by exposure of the body below the iliac crests to sub-atmospheric pressure. *Journal of Physiology (London)*, 1966; **183,** 607–27.
6. Gilbert CA, Bricker LA, Springfield WT Jr, Stevens PM and Warren BH: Sodium and water excretion and renal hemodynamics during lower body negative pressure. *Journal of Applied Physiology*, 1966; **21,** 1699–704.
7. Mark AL and Mancia G: Cardiopulmonary baroreflexes in humans. In Shepherd JT and Abboud FM (eds): *Handbook of Physiology. Section 2: The Cardiovascular System, Volume 3.* Bethesda, MD, American Physiological Society, 1983, 795–813.
8. Samueloff SL, Browse NL and Shepherd JT: Response of capacity vessels in human limbs to head up tilt and suction on lower body. *Journal of Applied Physiology*, 1966; **21,** 47–54.
9. Roddie IC, Shepherd JT and Whelan RF: Reflex changes in vasoconstrictor tone in human skeletal muscle in response to stimulation of receptors in a low pressure area of the intrathoracic vascular bed. *Journal of Physiology (London)*, 1957; **139,** 369–76.
10. Bishop VS, Malliani A and Thorén P: Cardiac mechanoreceptors. In Shepherd JT and Abboud FM (eds): *Handbook of Physiology. Section 2: The Cardiovascular System, Volume 3.* Bethesda, MD, American Physiological Society, 1983, 497–555.
11. Johnson JM, Rowell LB, Niederberger M and Eisman MM: Human splanchnic and forearm vasoconstrictor responses to reductions in right atrial and aortic pressures. *Circulation Research*, 1974; **34,** 515–24.
12. Zoller RP, Mark AL, Abboud FM, Schmid PG and Heistad DD: The role of low pressure baroreceptors in reflex vasoconstrictor responses in man. *Journal of Clinical Investigation*, 1972; **51,** 2967–72.
13. Abboud FM, Eckberg DL, Johannsen UJ and Mark AL: Carotid and cardiopulmonary baroreceptor control of splanchnic and forearm vascular resistance during venous pooling in man. *Journal of Physiology (London)*, 1979; **286,** 173–84.
14. Burke D, Sundlöf G and Wallin BG: Postural effects on muscle sympathetic activity in man. *Journal of Physiology (London)*, 1977; **272,** 399–414.
15. Delius W, Hagbarth K-E, Hongell A and Wallin BG: Manoeuvres affecting sympathetic outflow in human muscle nerves. *Acta Physiologica Scandinavica*, 1966; **84,** 82–94.
16. Delius W, Hagbarth K-E, Hongell A and Wallin BG: Manoeuvres affecting sympathetic outflow in human skin nerves. *Acta Physiologica Scandinavica*, 1972; **84,** 177–86.
17. Victor RG and Leimbach WN Jr: Effects of lower body negative pressure on sympathetic discharge to leg muscles in humans. *Journal of Applied Physiology*, 1987; **63,** 2558–62.
18. Vissing SF, Scherrer U and Victor RG: Relation between sympathetic outflow and vascular resistance in the calf during perturbations in central venous pressure. *Circulation Research*, 1989; **65,** 1710–17.
19. Tripathi A and Nadel ER: Forearm skin and muscle vasoconstriction during lower body negative pressure. *Journal of Applied Physiology*, 1986; **60,** 1535–41.
20. Rowell LB, Detry J-MR, Blackmon J and Wyss C: Importance of the splanchnic vascular bed in human blood pressure regulation. *Journal of Applied Physiology*, 1972; **32,** 213–20.
21. Angel-James JE and Daly M de B: Effects of graded pulsatile pressure on the reflex vasomotor responses elicited by changes of mean pressure in the perfused carotid sinus-aortic arch of the dog. *Journal of Physiology (London)*, 1971; **214,** 51–64.
22. Scher AM and Young AC: Servoanalysis of carotid sinus reflex effects on peripheral resistance. *Circulation Research*, 1963; **12,** 152–62.
23. Rowell LB, Wyss CR and Brengelmann GL: Sustained human skin and muscle vasoconstriction with reduced baroreceptor activity. *Journal of Applied Physiology*, 1973; **34,** 639–43.
24. Escourrou P, Raffestin B, Papelier Y, Pussard E and Rowell LB: Cardiopulmonary and carotid baroreflex control of splanchnic and forearm circulations. *American Journal of Physiology*, 1993; **264,** H777–82.
25. Beiser GD, Zelis R, Epstein SE, Mason DT and Braunwald E: The role of skin and muscle resistance

vessels in reflexes mediated by the baroreceptor system. *Journal of Clinical Investigation*, 1970; **49,** 225–31.

26. Amery A, Bossaert H, Deruyttere M, Vanderlinden L and Verstraete M: Influence of body posture on leg blood flow. *Scandinavian Journal of Clinical and Laboratory Investigation. Supplement*, 1973; **31,** 29–36.
27. Blomqvist CG and Stone HL: Cardiovascular adjustments to gravitational stress. In Shepherd JT and Abboud FM (eds): *Handbook of Physiology. Section 2: The Cardiovascular System, Volume 3.* Bethesda, MD, American Physiological Society, 1983, 1025–63.
28. Bridgen W, Howarth S and Sharpey-Schafer EP: Postural changes in the peripheral blood-flow of normal subjects with observations on vasovagal fainting reactions as a result of tilting, the lordotic posture, pregnancy and spinal anesthesia. *Clinical Science*, 1950; **9,** 79–91.
29. Culbertson JW, Wilkins RW, Ingelfinger FJ and Bradley SE: The effects of upright posture upon hepatic blood flow in normotensive and hypertensive subjects. *Journal of Clinical Investigation*, 1951; **30,** 305–11.
30. Gauer OH and Thron HL: Postural changes in the circulation. In Hamilton WF and Dow P (eds): *Handbook of Physiology. Section 2: Circulation, Volume 3.* Washington, DC, American Physiological Society, 1965, 2409–39.
31. Kellogg DL Jr, Johnson JM and Kosiba WA: Baroreflex control of the cutaneous active vasodilator system in humans. *Circulation Research*, 1990; **66,** 1420–26.
32. McNamara HI, Sikorski JM and Clavin H: The effects of lower body negative pressure on hand blood flow. *Cardiovascular Research*, 1969; **3,** 284–91.
33. Newberry PD and Bryan AC: Effect on venous compliance and peripheral vascular resistance of headward ($+G_z$) acceleration. *Journal of Applied Physiology*, 1967; **23,** 150–56.
34. Skagen K and Bonde-Petersen F: Regulation of subcutaneous blood flow during head-up tilt (45°) in normals. *Acta Physiologica Scandinavica*, 1982; **114,** 31–5.
35. Smith HS: *Principles of Renal Physiology*. New York, NY, Oxford University Press, 1956, 165–8.
36. Stevens PM and Lamb LE: Effect of lower body negative pressure on the cardiovascular system. *American Journal of Cardiology*, 1965; **16,** 506–16.
37. Stone HL and Alexander WC: Abdominal blood flow changes during acceleration stress in anesthetized dogs. *Aerospace Medicine*, 1968; **39,** 115–19.
38. Warren JV, Brannon ES, Stead EA Jr and Merrill AJ: Effect of venesection and the pooling of blood in the extremities on the atrial pressure and cardiac output in normal subjects, with observations on acute circulatory collapse in three instances. *Journal of Clinical Investigation*, 1945; **24,** 337–44.
39. Matzen S, Schifter S, Radvansky J, Knigge U, Warberg J and Secher NH: Calcitonin gene-related peptide (CGRP) and leg vascular resistance during head-up tilt induced hypovolemic shock in man. *Acta Physiologica Scandinavica*, 1991; **142,** 313–18.
40. Rowell LB: Human cardiovascular adjustments to exercise and thermal stress. *Physiological Reviews*, 1974; **54,** 75–159.
41. Greenfield ADM: The circulation through the skin. In Hamilton WF and Dow P (eds): *Handbook of Physiology. Section 2: Circulation, Volume 2.* Washington, DC, American Physiological Society, 1963, 1325–51.
42. Thauer R: Circulatory adjustments to climatic requirements. In Hamilton WF and Dow P (eds): *Handbook of Physiology. Section 2: Circulation, Volume 3.* Washington, DC, American Physiological Society, 1965, 1921–66.
43. Blix AS and Folkow B: Cardiovascular adjustments to diving in mammals and birds. In Shepherd JT and Abboud FM (eds): *Handbook of Physiology. Section 2: The Cardiovascular System, Volume 3.* Bethesda, MD, American Physiological Society, 1983, 917–45.
44. Mark AL: The Bezold–Jarisch reflex revisited: clinical implications of inhibitory reflexes originating in the heart. *Journal of the American College of Cardiology*, 1983; **1,** 90–102.
45. Scherrer U, Vissing S, Morgan BJ, Hanson P and Victor RG: Vasovagal syncope after infusion of a vasodilator in a heart-transplant recipient. *New England Journal of Medicine*, 1990; **322,** 602–4.
46. Barcroft H, Edholm OG, McMichael J and Sharpey-Schafer EP: Post-haemorrhagic fainting. Study by cardiac output and forearm flow. *Lancet*, 1944; **1,** 489–91.
47. Wallin BG and Sundlöf G: Sympathetic outflow to muscles during vasovagal syncope. *Journal of the Autonomic Nervous System*, 1982; **6,** 287–91.
48. Weissler AM, Warren JV, Estes EH, McIntosh HD Jr and Leonard JJ: Vasodepressor syncope. Factors influencing cardiac output. *Circulation*, 1957; **15,** 875–82.
49. Glick G and Yu PN: Hemodynamic changes during spontaneous vasovagal reactions. *American Journal of Medicine*, 1963; **34,** 42–51.
50. Bearn AG, Billing B, Edholm OG and Sherlock S: Hepatic blood flow and carbohydrate changes in man during fainting. *Journal of Physiology (London)*, 1951; **115,** 442–55.
51. Barcroft H and Edholm OG: On the vasodilation of human skeletal muscle during post-haemorrhagic fainting. *Journal of Physiology* (*London*), 1945; **104,** 165–75.
52. Epstein SE, Stampfer M and Beiser GD: Role of the capacitance and resistance vessels in vaso-vagal syncope. *Circulation*, 1968; **37,** 524–33.

53. Blair DA, Glover WE, Greenfield ADM and Roddie IC: Excitation of cholinergic vasodilator nerves to human skeletal muscles during emotional stress. *Journal of Physiology (London)*, 1959; **148,** 633–47.
54. Roddie IC: Circulation to skin and adipose tissue. In Shepherd JT and Abboud FM (eds): *Handbook of Physiology. Section 2: The Cardiovascular System, Volume 3.* Bethesda, MD, American Physiological Society, 1983, 285–317.
55. de Wardener HE and McSwiney RR: Renal haemodynamics in vasovagal fainting due to haemorrhage. *Clinical Science*, 1951; **10,** 209–17.
56. Ladefoged J and Munck O: Renal blood flow during fainting measured with the ^{133}Xenon wash-out technique. *Nephron*,1966; **3,** 59–62.
57. Hasser EM and Schadt JC: Sympathoinhibition and its reversal by naloxone during hemorrhage. *American Journal of Physiology*, 1992; **262,** R444–51.

Part 4
Related clinical aspects

12

Clinical correlates – immunological aspects

Mads Klokker, Else Tønnesen and Bente K Pedersen

A number of stressful conditions induce changes in the immune response. Physical stress includes thermal and traumatic injury,[1] surgery,[2,3] acute myocardial infarction,[4] severe physical exercise,[5] hyperthermia[6] and haemorrhagic shock. Although several studies have examined the aetiology of immunosuppression following mechanical and thermal injury, there have been few systematic investigations addressing haemorrhagic shock in the absence of other forms of significant trauma.

The immune response

The immune system consists of non-specific and specific components, which are closely interrelated.[7] The non-specific immune defences encompass mechanical barriers such as the skin and mucous membranes. Other parts include phagocytotic cells, which are divided into fixed tissue macrophages, circulating polymorphonuclear cells and monocytes. Monocytes produce a number of monokines that can specifically stimulate natural killer (NK) and T-cells. These monokines include interleukin-1α and -1β (IL-1α and IL-1β), interleukin-6 (IL-6) and tumour necrosis factor-α (TNF-α), all of which are involved in the fever response. An important cell subtype is the NK cell. NK cells mediate a non-specific, non-major histocompatibility complex (MHC)-related cytotoxicity of malignant cells and virus infected cells, and are therefore thought to play an important role in the first line of defence against tumours and viral infections.[7]

The specific immune response is composed of mainly two types of lymphoid cells designated the T (thymic-dependent)– and B (bone marrow derived)– cells. According to this classic designation the two cell types are primary mediators of cell-mediated and humoral (antibody-mediated) immunity, respectively. T-cells can be further divided into several subclasses, including helper/inducer cells, expressing a surface molecule called CD4, and suppressor/cytotoxic cells expressing CD8. CD4+ cells coordinate B-cell antibody responses by direct cell to cell interaction and also by production of different cytokines such as IL-2 as well as interferon-γ (IFN-γ). T-suppressor cells play a regulatory role in controlling the T-helper cell. T-cytotoxic cells mediate specific MHC class I associated killing. B-cells are found in the circulation, lymph nodes and spleen. They are characterized by their production of specific antibodies of different immunoglobulin classes (IgG, IgA, IgM, IgD and IgE).[7]

Haemorrhage

Previous study has demonstrated that patients exposed to marked haemorrhagic episodes have an increased risk of infection,[8] and suggests that this enhanced susceptibility to infection is due to depression of non-specific immune functions.[9] Haemorrhagic shock most often accompanies trauma and surgery. Both conditions are known to induce immunosuppression.[1] Furthermore, haemorrhagic shock will always be treated with blood transfusions, which have also been shown to induce immunosuppression (reviewed in Chaudry *et al.*[10]). In order to examine the isolated immunomodulatory effect of haemorrhagic shock it is therefore important to use experimental models. Three experimental models have been developed to examine effects of haemorrhage on the immune system.

Fixed-bleed animal model

Haemorrhage is induced in unanaesthetized rats. After withdrawal of a fixed blood volume, mitogen-induced proliferation of blood lymphocytes and the production of IL-2 are reduced for at least 24 hours after the insult. Infusion of lymphocytes from haemorrhaged rats cannot reverse this depression. It has been suggested that release of a serum factor after haemorrhage is responsible for the inhibition of lymphocyte function. Exposure to serum from haemorrhaged rats induces a marked immunosuppression.[11]

Fixed-pressure animal model of haemorrhage

The fixed blood pressure model of haemorrhagic shock in the mouse was introduced by Stephan *et al.*,[12] who showed marked suppression of IL-2 immediately after haemorrhage, lasting for up to 48 hours. Later it was shown that production of IL-3, IL-6 and IFN-α was depressed after haemorrhage, but that the release of TNF-α and IL-6 was increased.[10]

Passive head-up tilt model in humans with hypotension but no haemorrhage

During passive head-up tilt CBV is reduced.[13] This experiment allows us to obtain information concerning the influence of haemorrhagic shock in humans on both concentration and function of immune competent cells in the blood.

Experiments were performed on a tilt table with a bicycle saddle and no support for the feet. After 1 hour of supine rest, head-up tilt to an angle of 50° was performed over 5 min, and the subject remained in this position until presyncopal symptoms (nausea, dizziness and a flushing sensation) appeared. With the occurrence of such symptoms the subject was immediately returned supine.[14,15] Head-up tilt increased the overall leucocyte concentration. This reflected an increase in lymphocytes and a minor increase in neutrocyte concentration. After recovery the leucocyte concentration was still increased but only because of an increased neutrocyte count. This was analogous to the findings in other forms of stress, e.g. physical exercise.[16] NK cell activity increased during head-up tilt (Fig. 12.1) due to a 3–4-fold increase in CD16+ NK cells in the blood with recovery after 2 hours. Concentrations of the CD3+ and CD4+ T-cell subsets increased at the appearance of presyncopal symptoms, whereas the relative concentration of CD3+ T-cells decreased due to a fall in the CD4+ T-cells. Almost no changes in cell expression of CD19 (B-cells), HLA-DR (a measure of activated cells) or IL-2 receptors (activated lymphocytes) took place. Although changes in blood mononuclear cell composition occurred, the proliferative responses of these cells following stimulation with phytohaemagglutinin (PHA), purified derivative of tuberculin, or with IL-2 did not change.[17]

Increased NK cell activity was also demonstrated during surgery[2,3] and physical exercise,[5] while NK cell activity in these situations was suppressed after the interaction. Other types of physical stress, such as burns and acute myocardial infarction, were also followed by suppressed activity.[1,4]

Possible mechanisms of action

What are the mechanisms behind the immunomodulation induced during head-up tilt? During head-up tilt the plasma concentrations of adrenaline, ACTH and β-endorphin increase.[14,15] These hormones play an important role in the interaction between the endocrine glands and the immune system.

ACTH enhances the B-lymphocyte proliferation but inhibits antibody synthesis. Furthermore, ACTH suppresses the cytokine production of T-cells and monocytes *in vitro*.[18]

The endogenous opiate peptides (i.e. endorphins and enkephalins) are important modulators of the cellular immune response. They bind to monocytes, lymphocytes and granulocytes. *In vitro*, β-endorphin enhances NK cell cytotoxicity over a wide range of concentrations including those concentrations that are believed to be physiologically relevant.[19,20] When Fiatarone *et al.*[21] administered naloxone *in vivo* to persons who underwent a maximal bicycle ergometer test, the rise in NK cell activity was not significant and nor was the rise in cells expressing the CD16 marker (NK cells) compared with the group receiving placebo. However, preliminary results show that when healthy young humans are given epidural analgesia to block afferent impulses, and thereby inhibit the release of β-endorphins and ACTH during exercise, there is no inhibition of the exercise-induced in-

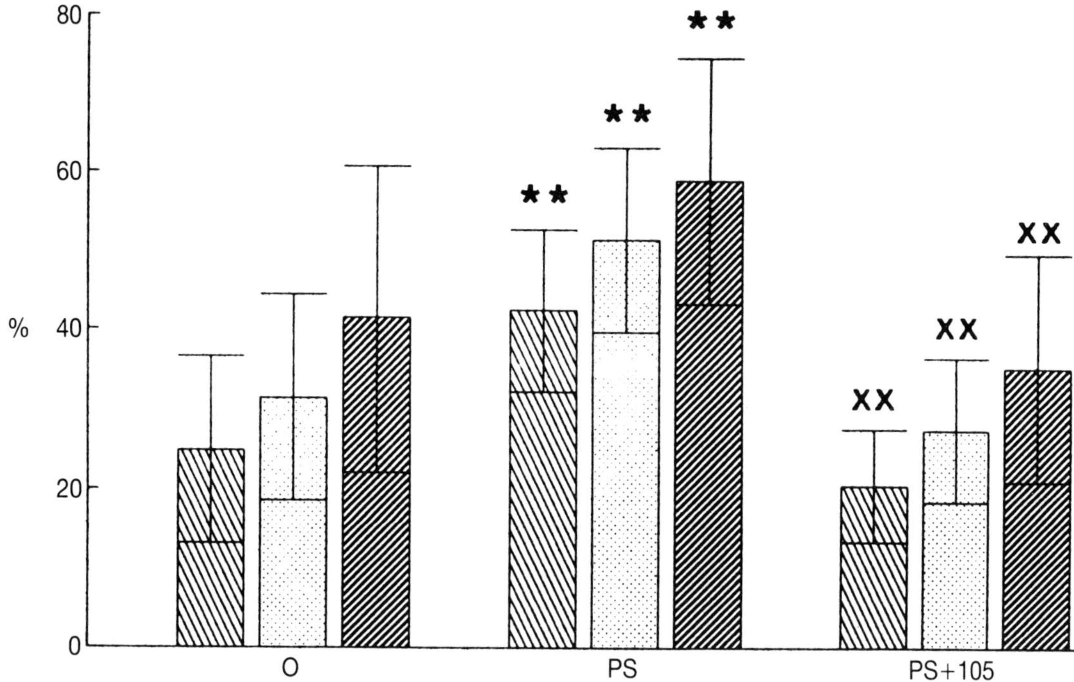

Fig. 12.1. The *in vivo* effect of head-up tilt on natural killer cell activity unstimulated (▧) as well as stimulated with interleukin-2 (▤) and interferon-α (▨) measured as lysis per fixed number of blood mononuclear cells in percentage. The figure shows natural killer cell activities just before head-up tilt (0), at the appearance of presyncopal symptoms but after return of the subject to horizontal position (PS) and 105 min after presyncopal symptoms (PS + 105). Values are expressed as means ± SD of seven observations. Two-way analysis of variance was used. If proven significant, Tukey HSD (honest significant difference) *post hoc* test based on analysis of variance was performed. **, 0 compared with PS and PS + 105 ($P \leqslant 0.01$); ××, PS compared with PS + 105 ($P \leqslant 0.01$).

crease in NK cell activity or numbers in peripheral blood (Klokker *et al.*, 1993, unpublished data). The α-endorphin and enkephalins, but not β-endorphin, are potent suppressors of antibody production,[18] while β-endorphin suppresses PHA-induced T-cell blastogenesis.[22]

Both exogenous and endogenous elevations of adrenaline cause leucocytosis, neutrocytosis and lymphocytosis.[23,24] Adrenaline is a potent stimulator of NK cell activity *in vivo*, as the number of NK cells in peripheral blood is increased instantaneously.[24,25] *In vivo*, adrenaline also decreases the fraction of CD4+ cells and inhibits PHA-induced proliferative responses.[24,26]

It is well established that haemorrhage affects the immune system. The mechanisms behind this immunomodulatory effect have not yet been clarified, but there is increasing evidence that different stress related hormones may be responsible for many of the observed changes in immunity. Adrenaline is one of the stress hormones that is known to increase in response to haemorrhage and may be responsible for most of the effects on the immune system induced during head-up tilt. It also remains to be clarified whether the elevated TNF-α and IL-6 levels are detrimental to the host. In the future, answers to these questions will hopefully allow us to select drugs that can block various mediators and thereby decrease posthaemorrhagic susceptibility to sepsis.

References

1. Blazar BA, Rodrick ML, O'Mahony JB, Wood J, Bessey PQ, Wilmore DW and Mannick JA: Suppression of natural killer-cell function in humans following thermal and traumatic injury. *Journal of Clinical Immunology*, 1986; **6,** 26–36.
2. Lennard TWJ, Shenton BK, Borzotta A, Donnally

PK, White M, Gerriet LM, Proud G and Taylor GMR: The influence of surgical operations on components of the human immune system. *British Journal of Surgery*, 1985; **72,** 771–6.
3. Tønnesen E, Brinkløv MM, Christensen NJ, Olesen AS and Madsen T: Natural killer cell activity and lymphocyte function during and after coronary artery bypass grafting in relation to the endocrine stress response. *Anesthesiology*, 1987; **67,** 526–33.
4. Klarlund K, Pedersen BK, Theander GT and Andersen V: Depressed natural killer cell activity in acute myocardial infarction. *Clinical and Experimental Immunology*, 1987; **70,** 209–16.
5. Pedersen BK: Influence of physical activity on the cellular immune system: mechanisms of action. *International Journal of Sports Medicine Supplement*, 1991; **1,** 23–9.
6. Kappel M, Stadeager C, Tvede N, Galbo H and Pedersen BK: Effects of *in vivo* hyperthermia on natural killer cell activity, *in vitro* proliferative responses and blood mononuclear cell subpopulations. *Clinical and Experimental Immunology*, 1991; **84,** 175–80.
7. Roitt IM, Brostoff J and Male DK: *Immunology*. London, Gower Medical, 1989.
8. Schimpff SC, Miller RM, Polakayetz S and Hornick RB: Infection in the severely traumatized patient. *Annals of Surgery*, 1974; **179,** 352–7.
9. Saba TM: Organ failure with sepsis after trauma and burn: support of the reticuloendothelial host-defence system. In Sibbald WI, Sprung CL (eds): *Perspectives on Sepsis and Septic Shock.* San Francisco, CA, Society of Critical Care Medicine, 1986, 77–95.
10. Chaudry IH, Ayala A, Ertel W and Stephan RN: Hemorrhage and resuscitation: immunological aspects. *American Journal of Physiology*, 1990; **259,** R663–78.
11. Abraham E, Tanaka T and Chang YH: Effects of hemorrhagic serum on interleukin-2 generation and utilization. *Critical Care Medicine*, 1988; **16,** 307–11.
12. Stephan RN, Conrad PJ, Janeway CA, Geha AS, Baue AE and Chaudry IH: Decreased interleukin-2 production following simple hemorrhage. *Surgery Forum*, 1986; **37,** 73–5.
13. Sander Jensen K, Secher NH, Astrup A, Christensen NJ, Giese J, Schwartz TW, Warberg J and Bie P: Hypotension induced by passive head-up tilt: endocrine and circulatory mechanisms. *American Journal of Physiology*, 1986; **251,** R742–8.
14. Matzen S, Knigge U, Schütten HJ, Warberg J and Secher NH: Atrial natriuretic peptide during head-up tilt induced hypovolaemic shock in man. *Acta Physiologica Scandinavica*, 1990; **140,** 161–6.
15. Matzen S, Secher NH, Knigge U, Bach FW and Warberg J: Pituitary–adrenal responses to head-up tilt in humans: Effect of H_1- and H_2-receptor blockade. *American Journal of Physiology*, 1992; **263,** R156–68.
16. Pedersen BK, Tvede N, Klarlund K, Christensen LD, Hansen FR, Galbo H, Kharazmi A and Halkjær-Kristensen J: Indomethacin *in vitro* and *in vivo* abolishes postexercise suppression of natural killer cell activity in peripheral blood. *International Journal of Sports Medicine*, 1990; **11,** 127–31.
17. Klokker M, Secher NH, Matzen S and Pedersen BK: Natural killer cell activity during head-up tilt induced central hypovolemia in humans. *Aviation, Space, and Environmental Medicine*; in press.
18. Scherpereel P: Endocrine problems in anaesthetic practice. *Current Opinion in Anaesthesiology*, 1990; **3,** 437–43.
19. Kay N, Allen J and Morley JE: Endorphins stimulate normal human peripheral blood lymphocyte natural killer cell activity. *Life Sciences*, 1984; **35,** 53–69.
20. Mathews PM, Froelich CJ, Sibbit WL and Bankhurst AD: Enhancement of natural cytotoxicity by β-endorphin. *Journal of Immunology*, 1983; **130,** 1658–62.
21. Fiatarone MA, Morley JE, Bloom ET, Donna M, Maskinodan T and Solomon GF: Endogenous opioids and the exercise-induced augmentation of natural killer cell activity. *Journal of Laboratory Clinic Medicine*, 1988; **112,** 544–52.
22. McCain HW, Lamster IB, Bozzone JM and Grbic JT: β-endorphin modulates human immune activity via non-opiate receptor mechanisms. *Life Sciences*, 1982; **31,** 1619–24.
23. Toft P, Tønnesen E, Svendsen P, Rasmussen JW and Christensen NJ: The redistribution of lymphocytes during adrenaline infusion. *Acta Pathologica Microbiologica et Immunologica Scandinavica*, 1992; **100,** 594–7.
24. Tønnesen E, Christensen NJ and Brinkløv MM: Natural killer cell activity during cortisol and adrenaline infusion in healthy volunteers. *European Journal of Clinical Investigation*, 1987; **10,** 497–503.
25. Tønnesen E, Knudsen F, Nielsen NK and Christensen NJ: Natural killer cell activity during resection of phaeochromocytoma. *British Journal of Anaesthesia*, 1989; **62,** 327–33.
26. Kappel M, Tvede N, Galbo H, Haahr PM, Kjær M, Linstow M, Klarlund K and Pedersen BK: Evidence that the effect of physical exercise on NK cell activity is mediated by epinephrine. *Journal of Applied Physiology*, 1991; **70,** 2530–34.

13

Hypoxaemia and impairment of vasomotor control during orthostasis and simulated haemorrhage

Loring B Rowell

Hypoxaemia is commonly cited as a potential cause of syncope during orthostasis.[1] Hypoxaemia has been observed to impede arterial pressure regulation in normal individuals[2] and in hypoxaemic patients with pulmonary disease.[3] The evidence indicated that sympathetic vasoconstriction was impaired in both groups of individuals. Nevertheless, several of the normal subjects and the patients showed virtually normal vasoconstriction and arterial pressure control during LBNP, a stress that produces central hypovolaemia and thereby simulates haemorrhage and/or orthostasis. In another study the magnitude of vasoconstriction in skeletal muscle during head-up tilt was found to be the same irrespective of whether subjects breathed ambient air (at sea level) or 10 to 11 per cent O_2 in N_2.[4] Henriksen and Rowell[4] proposed that there may be thresholds for central and peripheral effects of hypoxaemia that vary among individuals.

An early report of orthostatic intolerance induced by hypoxaemia showed that 3 of 13 normal individuals experienced sudden bradycardia, hypotension and forearm vasodilatation when they breathed 7–10 per cent oxygen during a 45° head-up tilt.[5] Fig. 13.1 shows one example. Despite the severity of hypoxaemia, which would be expected to reduce Pa_{O_2} to as low as 28 mmHg or below, 10 of the subjects maintained heart rate and arterial pressure despite a progressive rise in forearm blood flow (i.e. rather than the usual vasoconstriction).

The cause of the impairment in arterial pressure control in individuals susceptible to hypoxaemia has not yet been established, but several plausible theories have been put forward. These theories have been directed mainly at the idea that hypoxaemia might impair sympathetic vasoconstriction. Some possible mechanisms by which such impairment might occur are discussed below.

Does local vasodilatation impair vasoconstriction?

A long-held assumption has been that metabolic vasodilatation can severely blunt or even prevent sympathetic vasoconstriction. This phenomenon has been called 'functional sympatholysis'.[6] In contrast to some reports,[7] others concluded that local vasodilator mechanisms do not override sympathetic vasoconstriction.[8–10] When there are marked differences in baseline blood flow, opposite conclusions can be reached about the magnitude of vasoconstriction, depending on whether changes are expressed as resistance or conductance.[11,12] When blood flow is high, vasoconstriction causes large changes in vascular conductance and in blood pressure, but only small changes in resistance. Therefore, a small change in resistance does not necessarily mean that sympathetic vasoconstriction is blunted; it often means simply that blood flow was high.

Severe hypoxaemia does not increase the blood flow to resting muscle, for example, to levels seen even during the mildest exercise. Local vasodilatation in skeletal muscle and also in splanchnic organs is small. For example, when normal subjects inspired 10 per cent oxygen (FI_{O_2} = 10%; Pa_{O_2} = 32–34 mmHg) splanchnic blood flow rose only 15 per cent,[13] and forearm blood flow was observed

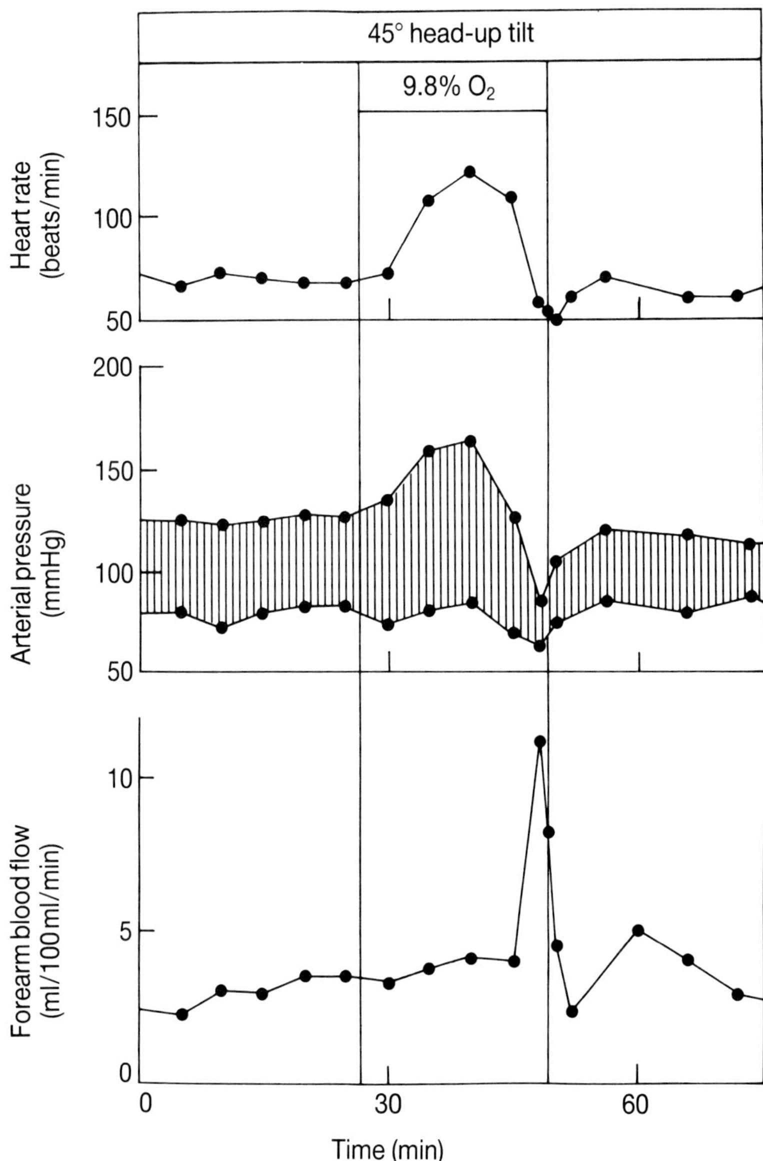

Fig. 13.1. Typical symptoms of a normal young man who was classified as a 'fainter' when exposed to low oxygen during 45° head-up tilt. He represents 3 of 13 individuals who responded similarly to hypoxaemia and orthostatic stress. Shading highlights the difference between systolic and diastolic pressures. *Source*: Anderson *et al.*[5]

either to remain constant[2,14,15] or to increase by a few per cent.[16,17] Such small changes would be unlikely to interfere with effective vasomotor control – and would certainly not alter baseline flow enough to minimize calculated effects on resistance.[16] Renal blood flow does not increase at all during hypoxaemia.[18]

Rowell and Blackmon[13] found no effects of hypoxaemia (FIo_2 = 10 per cent) on either the increase in arterial pressure induced by noradrenaline infusion or on the noradrenaline-induced (transient) splanchnic vasoconstriction. The results indicated that *postjunctional* effects of noradrenaline were not noticeably blunted by hypoxaemia.

However, there have been studies indicating that effects of perfused noradrenaline persist under conditions in which the actions of neurally released noradrenaline are, in contrast, markedly attenuated. For example, intense vasoconstriction in extremely hypoxaemic diving seals (Pa_{O_2} = 20 mmHg) may be maintained by circulating noradrenaline released from the adrenal medulla rather than by noradrenaline released from sympathetic varicosities[19] (see also Burcher and Garlick[20] and below). This suggests that any impairment may reside in the neuronal release of noradrenaline.

Is noradrenaline release inhibited prejunctionally?

Vanhoutte *et al.*[21] listed substances such as potassium and adenosine as those inhibiting noradrenaline release from sympathetic varicosities through their prejunctional effects; however, it is not clear if hypoxaemia can cause these effects in intact animals. Burcher and Garlick[20] found no diminution of vasoconstrictor responses to either neurally released noradrenaline or to circulating noradrenaline in canine skeletal muscle perfused with blood having a P_{O_2} of 17 mmHg. It required an artificial elevation in plasma potassium levels (by infusion) to abolish the neurally mediated vasoconstriction; inasmuch as noradrenaline infusion still caused vasoconstriction, potassium may have blocked neuronal release of noradrenaline.

Vanhoutte *et al.*[21] proposed that any prejunctional inhibition of noradrenaline release would be most pronounced when sympathetic nervous activity is low and when the concentrations of local metabolites are below those that relax vascular smooth muscle. Thus, were hypoxaemia to cause such inhibition, it would be expected at low levels of stress such as supine rest with moderate degrees of hypoxaemia. This could explain the consistent failure of moderate hypoxaemia (e.g. FI_{O_2} = 10–12 per cent, Pa_{O_2} = 32–38 mmHg) to raise plasma noradrenaline concentration in resting individuals, as shown in Fig. 13.2. An alternative hypothesis was that hypoxaemia may not increase sympathetic nerve activity in spontaneously breathing humans (the lung inflation reflex is known to decrease sympathetic nerve activity markedly in dogs[22]).

Rowell and Blackmon[23] found no evidence of prejunctional inhibition of noradrenaline release in human cutaneous veins, as judged by the maintained reflex venoconstrictor responses to local cold or exercise during local or central hypoxaemia, or both. On the other hand, when sympathetic nerve traffic (microneurography) in resting MSNA was increased significantly by moderate to severe hypoxaemia (FI_{O_2} = 12 per cent, 10 per cent and 8 per cent; Fig. 13.3), even the most marked rise (300 per cent at FI_{O_2} = 8 per cent) in MSNA was unaccompanied by increases forearm venous noradrenaline concentration.[24] In contrast, similar per cent increases in MSNA in normoxic subjects exposed to a cold pressor test or to mild exercise raised plasma noradrenaline concentration significantly (see Fig. 7 in Rowell *et al.*[24]).

A recent study suggests that hypoxaemia may not impair neuronal release of noradrenaline, but rather an increase in noradrenaline clearance may prevent or reduce the customary rise in plasma noradrenaline in relation to sympathetic nerve activity.[17] Acute hypoxaemia (FI_{O_2} = 10.5 per cent O_2) increased MSNA, forearm blood flow and [^{3}H] noradrenaline spillover in six normal young people. The rise in both arterial and regional (forearm) noradrenaline spillover was accompanied by increased arterial and regional clearance of noradrenaline. Presumably noradrenaline clearance was increased by increased cardiac output and muscle blood flow.[17]

Does hypoxaemia centrally impair reflexes?

When another stress such as exercise[25] or hyperthermia[26] is superimposed on hypoxaemia, then plasma noradrenaline (and presumably sympathetic nerve activity) increases markedly. The increases far exceed those observed when the same stresses are applied to normoxic subjects. Impairment of vasomotor regulation has not been observed under these conditions. As mentioned earlier, baroreflex-induced vasoconstriction in resting human muscle appeared normal during moderate hypoxaemia (FI_{O_2} = 10–11 per cent).[4] Furthermore, the cutaneous venoconstrictor responses to exercise were unaffected by various combinations of central and local hypoxaemia.[23]

Rowell and Seals[16] applied small (−5 mmHg) increments of LBNP in order to uncover any inhibitory effects of hypoxaemia on autonomic control of the circulation. Levels of LBNP between −5 and −20 mmHg inhibit cardiopulmonary baro-

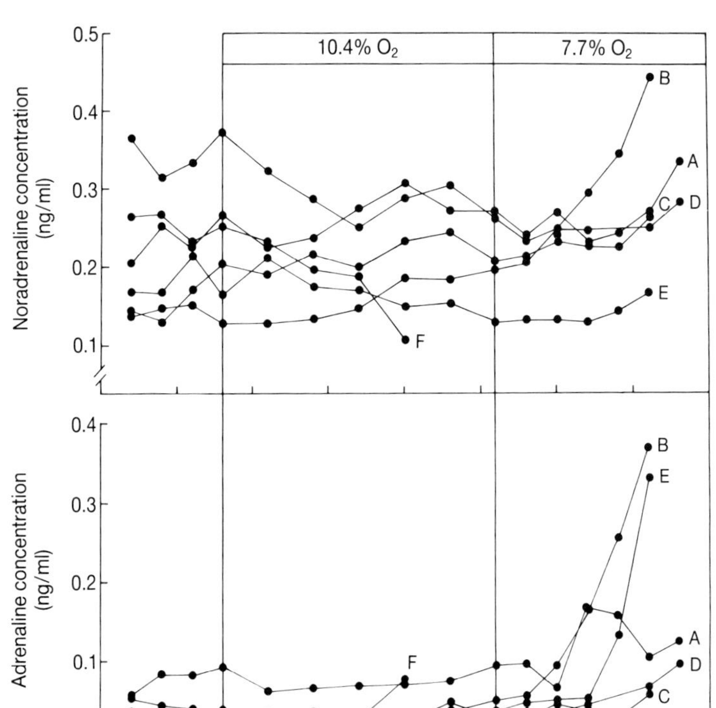

Fig. 13.2. Constancy of forearm venous concentrations of noradrenaline and adrenaline during moderately severe hypoxaemia (FIO_2 = 10.4 per cent, PaO_2 = 32–34 mmHg) in six normal young men. Tolerance to severe hypoxaemia (FIO_2 = 7.7 per cent, PaO_2 = 28 mmHg) was limited to 8 to 12 mins; noradrenaline levels may rise during longer exposures. From Rowell and Blackmon,[13] with permission.

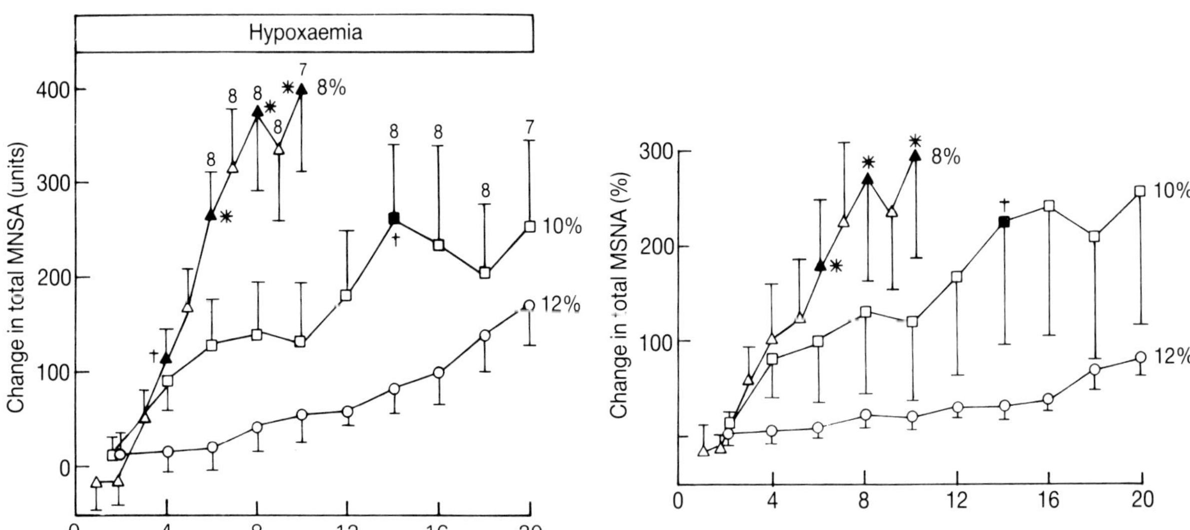

Fig. 13.3. Absolute and relative changes in directly recorded (microneurography) muscle sympathetic nerve activity (MSNA) from nine subjects (or seven to eight subjects shown by numbers) during moderate to severe hypoxaemia (FIO_2 = 12 per cent, 10 per cent and 8 per cent). *, MSNA significantly greater with 8 per cent oxygen than with either 10 per cent or 12 per cent ($P < 0.05$); ▲ and ■, significant differences from next per cent of oxygen used. From Rowell *et al.*,[24] with permission.

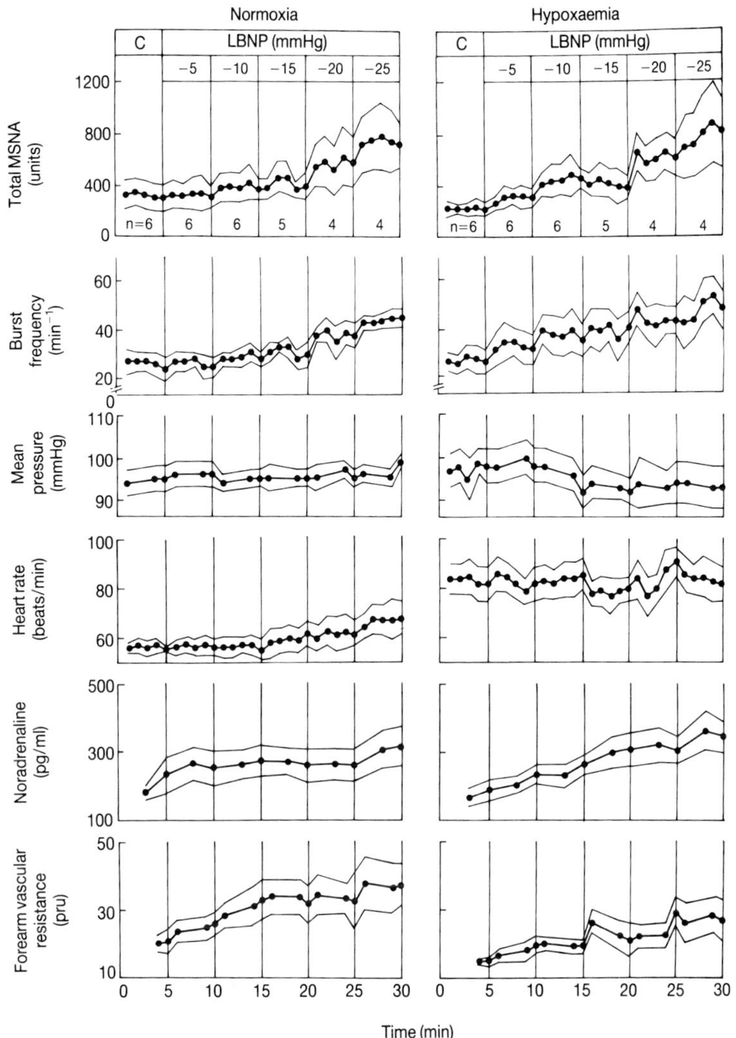

Fig. 13.4. Mean values from six subjects exposed to graded lower body negative pressure (LBNP, −5 to −25 mmHg) during normoxia and hypoxaemia (F_{IO_2}= 10 per cent or 12 per cent in two individuals). Comparisons in each vertical panel for normoxia versus hypoxaemia are between the same subjects. Not all subjects completed the tests as shown by numbers at the bottom of the top panel. MSNA, muscle sympathetic nerve activity. Values are expressed as means ± SEM. From Rowell and Seals,[16] with permission.

receptors and cause significant vasoconstriction without at the same time varying aortic mean pressure, pulse pressure or dp/dt.[27] Beyond −20 mmHg, the initial fall in aortic pulse pressure activates the arterial baroreflex, which initiates the rise in heart rate and a more pronounced splanchnic vasoconstriction.[27]

Fig. 13.4 shows normal time-courses and magnitudes of responses to graded low levels of LBNP during normoxia and hypoxaemia. Hypoxaemia raised heart rate and lowered forearm vascular resistance at rest and at all levels of LBNP. Multiunit recordings of MSNA by microneurography from the right peroneal nerve revealed the expected increases which paralleled the stepwise increments in forearm vascular resistance in both normoxia and hypoxaemia. Fig. 13.5 summarizes the average differences between the responses during hypoxaemia and normoxia over each 5-min period of LBNP. Hypoxaemia significantly increased both

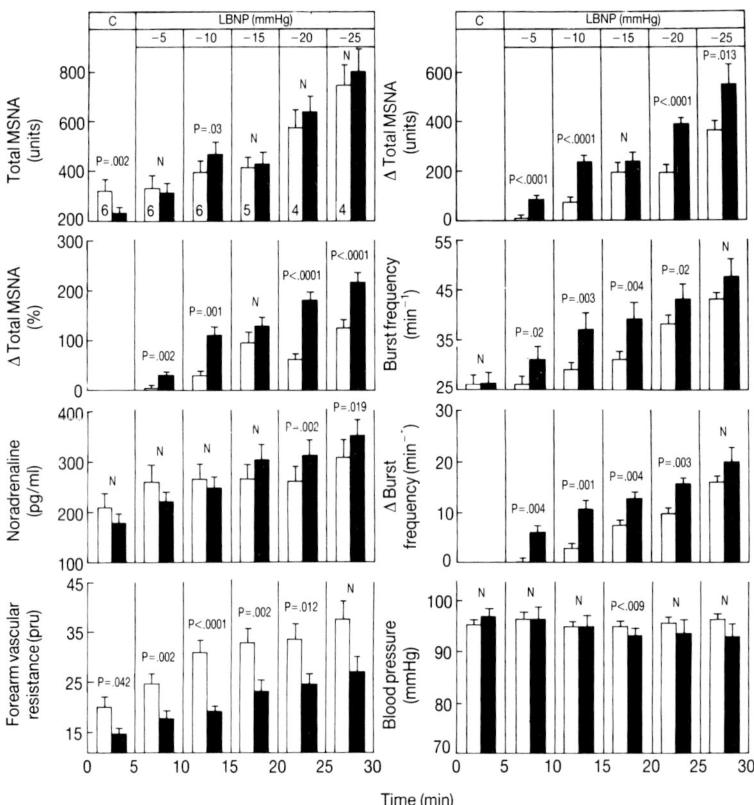

Fig. 13.5. Comparison of responses to lower body negative pressure (LBNP) during normoxia (□) and hypoxaemia (■). Hypoxaemia had minor effects on plasma noradrenaline concentration. The per cent changes in forearm vascular resistance were the same for both conditions, but the lower baseline values in hypoxaemia meant that absolute increases were greater in normoxia. This does not mean that hypoxaemia impaired forearm vasoconstriction. MSNA, muscle sympathetic nerve activity. N, non-significant ($P > 0.05$); P values, normoxia compared with hypoxaemia. Values are expressed as means ± SEM. From Rowell and Seals,[16] with permission.

the absolute and the relative change in total MSNA, and also the sympathetic burst frequency. Plasma noradrenaline concentration rose significantly in both normoxia and hypoxaemia, with no difference between the two states except at the highest levels of LBNP (Fig. 13.5). Arterial mean pressure was maintained equally well throughout LBNP in both conditions.

Although absolute increments in forearm vascular resistance were smaller when subjects were hypoxaemic, the per cent increments were the same in both conditions; that is, baseline forearm vascular resistance was lower and forearm blood flow higher during all periods with hypoxaemia. One could argue that vasoconstriction was diminished by hypoxaemia, or that it was not. The matter is not easily resolved, for even if the per cent changes in vessel diameter were the same in both states, different values for absolute increase in resistance would be obtained owing to the different initial values.[28] The main points revealed in Figs 13.4 and 13.5 are that hypoxaemia did not blunt blood pressure control and release of noradrenaline was not suppressed once a small stress was added to hypoxaemia. The reductions in cardiac output and organ blood flow may contribute to the rise in noradrenaline concentration by reducing noradrenaline clearance.[29] Undoubtedly neuronal release of noradrenaline is also increased along with MSNA. There was, therefore, no apparent central defect in sympathetic control nor in sympathetic effector mechanisms during mild, gradually applied orthostatic stress as long as plasma adrenaline concentration did not increase.

Do hormonal responses to hypoxaemia cause defective regulation?

Before three hypoxaemic subjects of Anderson and colleagues[5] fainted, they experienced precipitous bradycardia and hypotension accompanied by pronounced forearm vasodilatation (Fig. 13.1). The response was much like that observed by Barcroft and Edholm[30] in severe haemorrhage; originally the investigators thought it was caused by neurogenic vasodilatation, but later adrenaline was implicated.[31] Anderson and colleagues assumed this vasodilatation was caused by 'muscle twitching' during hypoxaemia. None of the 'non-fainters' had these symptoms even when they inspired 7 per cent O_2 and gradually became unconscious (not syncopal).

Consistent observations of a close temporal relation between increasing plasma adrenaline levels and presyncopal symptoms first appeared during the last decade.[32–35] The rise in adrenaline often occurred suddenly and its B_2-adrenergic vasodilator effects on skeletal muscle could explain the forearm vasodilatation observed by Anderson *et al.*[5] Perhaps more important are the powerful vasodilator effects on the splanchnic circulation. Failure to vasoconstrict this capacious circuit during orthostasis leads quickly to hypotension and fainting.[36,37]

Hypoxaemia and adrenaline release

In most resting subjects moderate hypoxaemia (FIo_2 = 10–12 per cent) causes no increase in plasma adrenaline concentration (Fig. 13.2). However, when this degree of hypoxaemia was combined with LBNP at −30 mmHg, four of eight normal young subjects developed sudden bradycardia and hypotension, as in Fig. 13.1; at this moment their plasma adrenaline concentrations rose markedly, reaching from 200 up to as high as 1600 pg/ml.[35] Plasma adrenaline did not rise in any subject (when normoxic) during LBNP. In contrast, all subjects showed similar elevations in venous noradrenaline concentration in response to LBNP in both normoxia and hypoxaemia.[35]

Rowell and Seals[16] observed significant increases in plasma adrenaline concentration during LBNP in three of eight hypoxaemic subjects, whereas adrenaline levels were unaffected by LBNP during normoxia (Fig. 13.6). The rise in adrenaline during hypoxaemia altered the cardiovascular adjustments to LBNP. The two cases presented in Fig. 13.7a and 13.7b reveal what is commonly called a vasovagal episode, but neither individual fainted. In both cases the sudden decreases in MSNA, arterial mean pressure and heart rate coincided with the rise in adrenaline concentration. The fall in MSNA was described previously as one of the events in vasovagal syncope.[38] In a third hypoxaemic subject (SS in Fig. 13.6), a progressive rise in adrenaline concentration throughout LBNP was accompanied by a continuous fall in arterial pressure and forearm vascular resistance. These changes occurred despite the fact that this individual's normal rise in MSNA throughout LBNP was unaffected by hypoxaemia. This subject's response may provide a possible cause for the more subtle deficiencies in vasomotor control reported in earlier studies. His adrenaline concentration reached levels that would vasodilate skeletal muscle and splanchnic organs, thereby seriously undermining their major role in reducing peripheral vascular conductance in order to maintain arterial pressure. For example, within the range of 200–500 pg/ml adrenaline will raise peripheral vascular conductance by 40–50 per cent.[39]

Cardiac depressor reflexes

Although the sudden rise in total vascular conductance and the onset of hypotension during LBNP could be explained by β-adrenergic effects of adrenaline on skeletal muscle and splanchnic organs, this would not explain the sudden decreases in MSNA and heart rate (adrenaline normally raises heart rate). These latter events are signs of impending vasovagal syncope. A more sinister possibility is that the powerful inotropic effects of adrenaline, which are imposed on a left ventricle that is low in volume, may trigger a 'cardiac depressor reflex'.

In 1867 von Bezold attributed the sudden vagally mediated decrease in heart rate and arterial pressure in response to an injection of veratrum alkaloids into the heart to direct stimulation of sensory endings in the heart. In 1949 Jarisch suggested

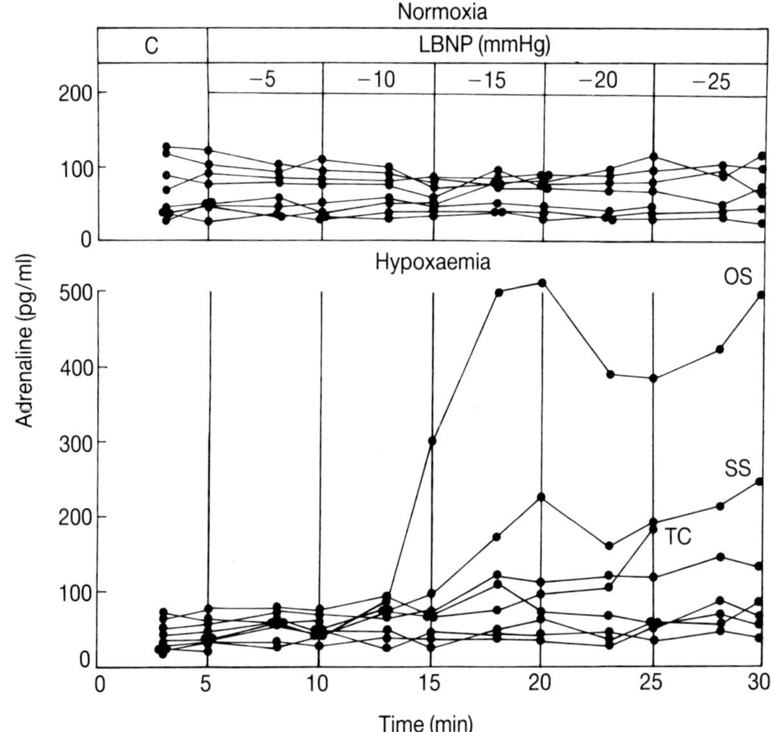

Fig. 13.6. Forearm venous concentration of adrenaline during graded lower body negative pressure (LBNP) in normoxia and in hypoxaemia. Adrenaline concentration did not change during LBNP with normoxia. The sudden increase in subjects OS and TC with hypoxaemia were accompanied by presyncopal symptoms. The gradual rise shown by SS was accompanied by progressive decreases in arterial pressure and forearm vascular resistance. From Rowell and Seals,[16] with permission.

that sensory depressor reflexes from the heart might be the mechanism underlying vasovagal syncope. More recently, Oberg and White[40] have shown in cats that the bradycardia in severe haemorrhage is due to activation of cardiac receptors.

Rowell and Blackmon[35] observed that a marked and sudden reduction in left ventricular end-systolic volume (determined in only one subject by echocardiography) occurred coincidentally with a marked increase in adrenaline concentration to >600 pg/ml, bradycardia and hypotension during combined LBNP and hypoxaemia. These events would be expected to accompany a cardiac depressor reflex.

More recently, Almqvist *et al.*[41] demonstrated that normal subjects experienced bradycardia and hypotension when the β-agonist isoproterenol was infused during a head-up tilt. Syncope could be similarly induced in patients (with normal electrocardiograms) who suffered from recurrent episodes of neurally mediated syncope. Furthermore, their spontaneous neural syncope could be prevented by pharmacological blockade of β_2-adrenergic receptors in the heart. van Lieshout and colleagues[42] studied two patients with hypoadrenergic orthostatic hypotension who had intact vagal cardiac control; vasovagal bradycardiac responses were absent despite a fall in arterial pressure during orthostasis. The investigators suggested that the inability of the patients to release adrenaline protected the heart from too vigorous contractions, thereby preventing initiation of cardiac depressor reflexes.

The evidence that adrenaline by acting gradually on splanchnic and muscle vascular conductance is the factor leading to defective blood pressure control in hypoxaemic individuals is suggestive but not conclusive. The finding that a sudden release of adrenaline during hypoxaemia combined with orthostatic stress is coincident with the onset of vasovagal syncope supports the hypothesis that β-adrenergic stimulation of an empty ventricle triggers a cardiac depressor reflex. This is still unproven and, the cause of the sudden outpouring of adrenaline remains unknown.

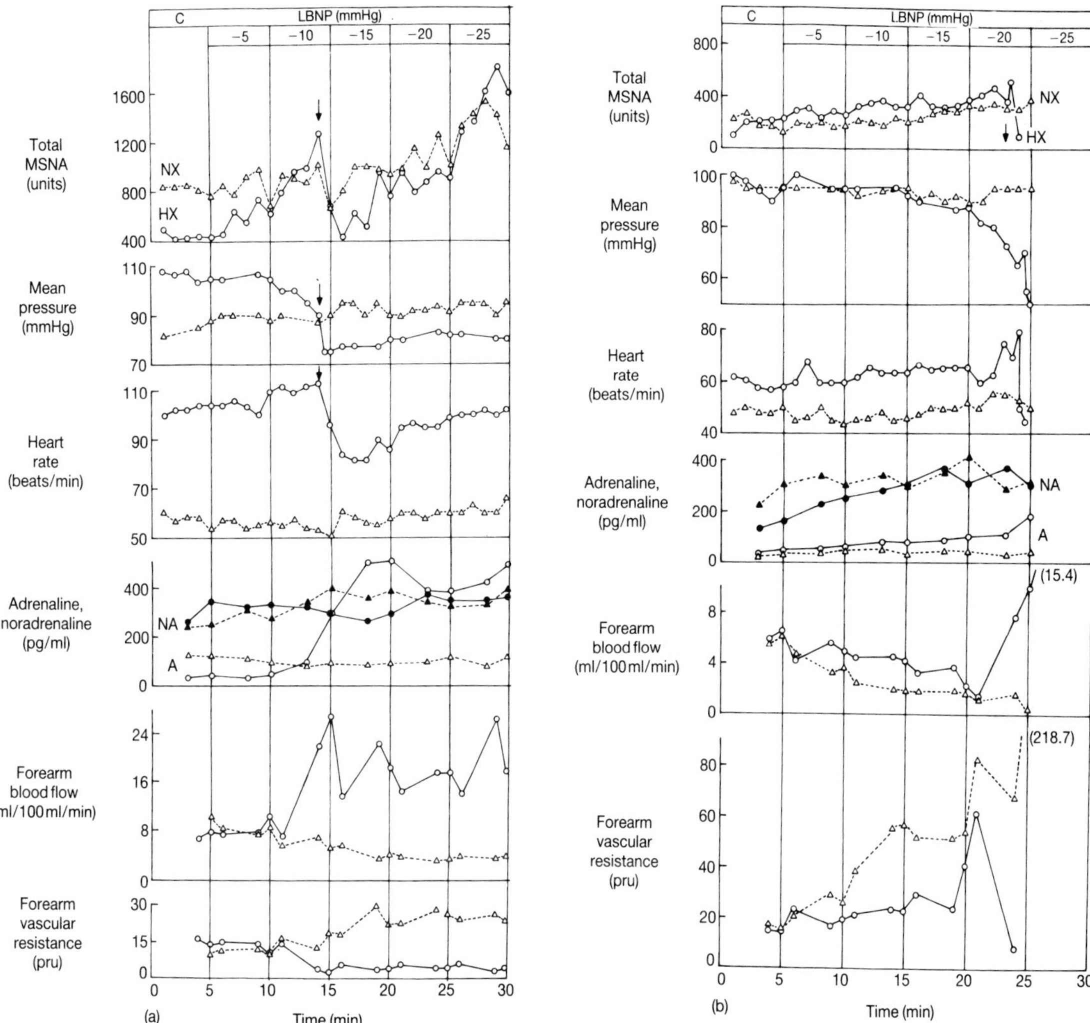

Fig. 13.7. Responses of two subjects (a and b) to sudden increases in plasma adrenaline (A) concentration (see Fig. 13.6) during hypoxaemia (○). Comparison is with responses during normoxia (△). Note the sudden decreases (↓) in muscle sympathetic nerve activity (MSNA), mean pressure, heart rate and forearm vascular resistance (especially for subject b). Plasma noradrenaline (NA) levels are during normoxia (▲) and hypoxaemia (●). From Rowell and Seals,[16] with permission.

References

1. Hurst JW, Schlant RC, Rackley CE, Sonnenblick EH and Wenger NK (eds): *The Heart*, 7th edn. New York, NY, McGraw-Hill, 1990.
2. Heistad DD, Abboud FM, Mark AL and Schmid PG: Impaired reflex vasoconstriction in chronically hypoxemic patients. *Journal of Clinical Investigation*, 1972; **51,** 331–7.
3. Heistad DD and Wheeler RC: Effect of acute hypoxia on vascular responsiveness in man. *Journal of Clinical Investigation*, 1970; **49,** 1252–65.
4. Henriksen O and Rowell LB: Lack of effect of moderate hypoxemia on human postural reflexes to skeletal muscle. *Acta Physiologica Scandinavica*, 1986; **127,** 171–5.
5. Anderson DP, Allen WJ, Barcroft H, Edholm OG and Manning GW: Circulatory changes during

fainting and coma caused by oxygen lack. *Journal of Physiology (London)*, 1946; **104,** 426–33.
6. Remensnyder JP, Mitchell JH and Sarnoff SJ: Functional sympatholysis during muscular activity. *Circulation Research*, 1962; **11,** 370–80.
7. Kjellmer I: On the competition between metabolic vasodilation and neurogenic vasoconstriction in skeletal muscle. *Acta Physiologica Scandinavica*, 1965; **63,** 450–59.
8. Donald DE, Rowlands DJ and Ferguson DA: Similarity of blood flow in the normal and sympathectomized dog hind limb during graded exercise. *Circulation Research*, 1970; **26,** 185–99.
9. Thompson LP and Mohrman DE: Blood flow and oxygen consumption in skeletal muscle curing sympathetic stimulation. *American Journal of Physiology*, 1983; **245,** H66–71.
10. O'Leary DS, Rowell LB and Scher AM: Baroreflex-induced vasoconstriction in active skeletal muscle of conscious dogs. *American Journal of Physiology*, 1991; **260,** H37–41.
11. Lautt WW: Resistance or conductance for expression of arterial vascular tone. *Microvascular Research*, 1989; **37,** 230–36.
12. O'Leary DS: Regional vascular resistance vs. conductance: which index for baroreflex responses? *American Journal of Physiology*, 1991; **260,** H632–7.
13. Rowell LB and Blackmon JR: Lack of sympathetic vasoconstriction in hypoxemic humans at rest. *American Journal of Physiology*, 1986; **251,** H562–70.
14. Richardson DW, Kontos HA, Shapiro W and Patterson JL Jr: Role of hypocapnia in the circulatory responses to acute hypoxia in man. *Journal of Applied Physiology*, 1966; **21,** 22–6.
15. Rowell LB, Freund PR and Brengelmann G: Cutaneous vascular response to exercise and acute hypoxia. *Journal of Applied Physiology*, 1982; **53,** 920–24.
16. Rowell LB and Seals DR: Sympathetic activity during graded central hypovolemia in hypoxemic humans. *American Journal of Physiology*, 1990; **259,** H1197–1206.
17. Leuenberger U, Gleeson K, Wroblewski K, Prophet S, Zelis R, Zwillich C and Sinoway L: Norepinephrine clearance is increased during acute hypoxemia in humans. *American Journal of Physiology*, 1991; **261,** H1659–64.
18. Caldwell FT, Rolf D and White HL: Effects of acute hypoxia in man. *Journal of Applied Physiology*, 1949; **1,** 597–600.
19. Gooden B and Elsner R: What diving animals might tell us about blood flow regulation. *Perspectives in Biology and Medicine*, 1985; **28,** 465–74.
20. Burcher E and Garlick D: Effects of exercise metabolites on adrenergic vasoconstriction in the gracilis muscle of the dog. *Journal of Pharmacology and Experimental Therapeutics*, 1975; **192,** 149–56.
21. Vanhoutte PM, Verbeuren TJ and Webb RC: Local modulation of adrenergic neuroeffector interaction in the blood vessel wall. *Physiological Reviews*, 1981; **61,** 151–247.
22. Angell-James JE and Daly M de B: Cardiovascular responses in apnoeic asphyxia: role of arterial chemoreceptors and the modification of their effects by a pulmonary vagal inflation reflex. *Journal of Physiology (London)*, 1969; **201,** 87–104.
23. Rowell LB and Blackmon JR: Venomotor responses during central and local hypoxia. *American Journal of Physiology*, 1988; **255,** H760–64.
24. Rowell LB, Johnson DG, Chase PB, Comess KA and Seales DR: Hypoxemia raises muscle sympathetic activity but not norepinephrine in resting humans. *Journal of Applied Physiology*, 1989; **66,** 1736–43.
25. Escourrou P, Johnson DG and Rowell LB: Hypoxemia increases plasma catecholamine concentrations in exercising humans. *Journal of Applied Physiology*, 1984; **57,** 1507–11.
26. Rowell LB, Brengelmann GL, Savage MV and Freund PR: Does acute hypoxemia blunt sympathetic activity in hyperthermia? *Journal of Applied Physiology*, 1989; **66,** 28–33.
27. Johnson JM, Rowell LB, Niederberger M and Eisman MM: Human splanchnic and forearm vasoconstrictor responses to reductions of right atrial and aortic pressures. *Circulation Research*, 1974; **34,** 515–24.
28. Rowlands DJ and Donald DE: Sympathetic vasoconstrictive responses during exercise- or drug-induced vasodilation. *Circulation Research*, 1968; **23,** 45–60.
29. Baily RG, Leuenberger U, Leaman G, Silber D and Sinoway L: Norepinephrine kinetics and cardiac output during nonhypotensive lower body negative pressure. *American Journal of Physiology*, 1991; **260,** H1708–12.
30. Barcroft H and Edholm OG: On the vasodilatation in human skeletal muscle during post-haemorrhagic fainting. *Journal of Physiology (London)*, 1945; **104,** 161–75.
31. Barcroft H, Brod J, Hejl Z, Hirsjarvi EA and Kitchin AH: The mechanism of the vasodilatation in the forearm muscle during stress (mental arithmetic). *Clinical Science*, 1960; **19,** 577–86.
32. Sander-Jensen K, Secher NH, Astrup A, Christensen NJ, Giese J, Schwartz TW, Warberg J and Bie P: Hypotension induced by passive head-up tilt: endocrine and circulatory mechanisms. *American Journal of Physiology*, 1986; **251,** R742–8.
33. Tatar P, Bulas J, Kvetnanski R and Strec V: Venous plasma adrenaline response to orthostatic syncope during tilting in healthy men. *Clinical Physiology*, 1986; **6,** 303–9.
34. Robinson BJ and Johnson RH: Why does vasodilatation occur during syncope? *Clinical Science*, 1988; **74,** 347–50.
35. Rowell LB and Blackmon JR: Hypotension induced

by central hypovolaemia and hypoxaemia. *Clinical Physiology*, 1989; **9,** 269–77.
36. van Lieshout JJ: *Cardiovascular Reflexes in Orthostatic Disorders*. Amsterdam, Rodopi, 1989.
37. Wilkins RW, Culbertson JW and Ingelfinger FJ: The effect of splanchnic sympathectomy in hypertensive patients upon estimated hepatic blood flow in the upright as contrasted with the horizontal position. *Journal of Clinical Investigation*, 1951; **31,** 312–17.
38. Wallin BG and Sundlöf G: Sympathetic outflow to muscles during vasovagal syncope. *Journal of the Autonomic Nervous System*, 1982; **6,** 287–91.
39. Stratton JR, Pfeifer MA, Ritchie JL and Halter JB: Hemodynamic effects of epinephrine: concentration –effect study in humans. *Journal of Applied Physiology*, 1985; **58,** 1199–1206.
40. Oberg B and White S: The role of vagal cardiac nerves and arterial baroreceptors in the circulatory adjustments to hemorrhage in the cat. *Acta Physiologica Scandinavica*, 1970; **80,** 395–403.
41. Almqvist A, Goldenberg IF, Milstein S, Chen M-Y, Chen X, Hansen R, Gornick CC and Benditt DG: Provocation of bradycardia and hypotension by isoproterenol and upright posture in patients with unexplained syncope. *New England Journal of Medicine*, 1989; **320,** 346–51.
42. van Lieshout JJ, Wieling W, Karemaker JM and Eckberg DL: The vasovagal response. *Clinical Science*, 1991; **81,** 575–86.

Part 5
Monitoring and treatment

14

Treatment of hypovolaemic shock: monitoring central blood volume

Niels H Secher, Goazina Perko, Per Madsen and Ferdinand Jónsson

Advanced technology allows for monitoring of almost any physiological variable, and ideally such monitoring should be both continuous and non-invasive. Routine monitoring includes assessment of ventilatory and circulatory functions. With the introduction of pulse oxymetry, an integrated, on-line and non-invasive evaluation of ventilation has been made possible. This is in contrast to evaluation of the circulatory system, where no single variable indicates the integrity of the system. Evaluation of the circulatory system needs to indicate the function of the heart, the ability of the system to deliver blood to the heart (preload) and the resultant cardiac output, arterial pressure (afterload) and tissue perfusion. Each of these functions is subject to independent regulation in order to allow for compensation for transient changes, for example in response to redistribution of the blood volume as taking place from the supine to the standing position. Also, the circulatory system can be changed in order to respond to psychological as well as physical stress.

For meaningful evaluation of a given circulatory variable or its derivative, it is often required that the underlying cause is known. For instance, venous oxygen saturation may be low because of a restricted cardiac output in a patient with acute myocardial infarction, or because of low CBV in a bleeding patient. However, venous oxygen saturation is also low during dynamic exercise characterized by an elevated cardiac output because of increased oxygen extraction from the large part of cardiac output serving working muscle. Obviously, the clinical appearance of a patient/subject is very different when the cardiac output is restricted than during dynamic exercise, but the situation is not always so clear. In patients cardiac output and arterial pressure may be elevated due to fear and/or pain while reduced because of haemorrhage. With no explicit measure of pain and little knowledge of the amount of blood lost, it may be difficult to determine what decides a given set of cardiovascular variables. Moreover, many intensive care patients receive potent pharmaceuticals that make an evaluation of patient pathophysiology even more difficult.

Patients with known or suspected bleeding usually have their heart rate and arterial pressure monitored,[1] which evaluates the integrity of the pump including a recording of electrical events in the heart and offers an index of the resultant activity. Most often cardiac filling is monitored by CVP and less often by pulmonary artery and wedge pressures. Pressures are taken as indices of volume, which is true only if venous and pulmonary artery vessels respond passively to changes in volume.

It is suggested that maintaining a normal CBV is the primary goal for monitoring bleeding patients. Determination of CBV by dye dilution determined cardiac output and evaluation of transit time is impractical in a clinical setting. Clinically applicable circulatory variables will be reviewed with respect to their ability to reflect changes in the CBV. At the same time it will be kept in mind to what extent circumstances other than haemorrhage may affect the variable in question. It should also be remembered that many physiological variables show marked interindividual variation not readily explained by gender and body size.[2]

Heart rate

Evaluation of heart rate or rather 'the quality' of the pulse is the classic method of monitoring ill patients. In fact, a low pulse rate in a bleeding patient was recorded as early as 1794. Monitoring of pulse, or more likely the electrocardiogram and derived heart rate, has remained fundamental. Yet, interpretation of heart rate changes is difficult during haemorrhage because the response is complex. This book presents a triphasic heart rate response to haemorrhage with moderate elevation during light bleeding, a decrease in heart rate during moderate to severe bleeding and manifest tachycardia only when haemorrhage is profound in animals[3–5] as well as in patients.[6] Furthermore, the clinical condition of the patient influences the heart rate response to haemorrhage. The pain associated with ileus[5] and injury[7] overrides the reflex inhibition of heart rate during haemorrhage and maintains a value of approximately 120 beats/min.

A low heart rate in an injured patient is often taken to represent 'emotional stress' in parallel with the well known vasovagal syncope.[8,9] However, the vasovagal syncope is usually brief and may be cured instantly by isometric muscle contractions.[10] This means that in a pale, sweating, hypotensive and maybe also bradycardic patient, every effort should be made in order exclude haemorrhage, before emotional factors are considered.

Only with extreme bradycardia are the changes in heart rate during haemorrhage of importance for the clinical condition of the patient. When heart rate decreases in response to haemorrhage the average value is in a 'normal' resting range of approximately 75 beats/min.[6,11] Furthermore, the initial increase in heart rate is so modest that it may not be noticed. However, with knowledge of the different stages of heart rate deviations during haemorrhage heart rate is a reliable monitor. When volume loading results in an increase in heart rate during resuscitation of a bleeding patient, loading should continue until heart rate decreases and end when heart rate is stable (Fig. 14.2 and Chapter 10).

Arterial pressure

With application of Penaz's principle, as with the Finapres® machine, it is possible to monitor arterial pressure both continually and non-invasively, even when it is low due to hypovolaemic shock.[12] Moreover, introduction of disposable transducers with constant flush has made even long lasting monitoring of intraarterial pressure a routine.

During haemorrhage arterial pressure is to be maintained at near normal values because of its importance for organ perfusion. This is especially important for older patients with manifest or potential arteriosclerotic disease, where flow distal to an arterial stenosis is pressure-dependent. It should also be kept in mind that autoregulation is shifted to 'the right' in hypertensive patients, who therefore have reduced tolerance to low blood pressures (see Chapter 3). Furthermore, it is important not to elevate pressure above the normal range. This is pertinent during operations where a vascular stenosis has been corrected, and vascular autoregulation may be lost for hours to weeks.[13] More regularly, overloading will lead to compromised pulmonary diffusion and contribute to (postoperative) hypoxaemia (Table 14.1).

Table 14.1 Fluid balance, indicators of central blood volume and arterial oxygen saturation in 15 patients before and after aortic surgery and on the first postoperative day

	Surgery		First postoperative day
	Before	After	
Body fluid balance (litres)	–	1.8 (−0.1–3.3)	1.4 (0.1–5.4)
Haemoglobin (mmol/l)	6.8 (5.1–8.9)	8.1* (6.5–8.7)	7.4 (5.8–9.4)
Thoracic impedance (ohms)	34 (26–46)	31* (23–39)	28* (21–38)
Central venous pressure (mmHg)	10 (1–17)	5* (−3–14)	6* (−1–12)
Pulmonary arterial mean pressure (mmHg)	24 (12–34)	18* (−1–28)	18 (9–29)
Arterial oxygen saturation	0.98 (0.95–0.99)	0.96* (0.90–0.99)	0.96* (0.90–0.99)

Values are expressed as medians with range. *After compared with before surgery, $P<0.05$.

The importance of maintaining a normal blood pressure is less obvious in a young person. As mentioned in previous chapters, one stage of hypovolaemic shock is characterized by reduced peripheral resistance, perhaps in order to maintain organ perfusion. In fact, Sjöstrand[14] argued that in rats tolerance to haemorrhage is enhanced by maintained ability to induce sympathoinhibition. During general anaesthesia where peripheral vasodilatation is induced, blood pressure may be lowered quite dramatically with no adverse effects. Conversely, blood pressure falls during regional (epidural or spinal) anaesthesia due to the accumulation of blood in veins of the blocked area, with resultant central volume depletion and associated low heart rate.[15,16]

Blood pressure should not be monitored as an index of haemorrhage, but other variables ought to be so sensitive that ongoing haemorrhage is corrected before blood pressure is affected. During central volume depletion blood pressure is maintained at an almost normal value until the reduction amounts to approximately 30 per cent.[17,18] If blood volume is taken to be approximately 5 litres, then monitoring should be able to detect a reduction to the modest precision of 1.5 litres.

The difference between the systolic and diastolic blood pressure, the pulse pressure, is reduced before mean arterial blood pressure falls during haemorrhage.[19] A decrease in pulse pressure may be taken as an early warning and as indicating that immediate intervention is needed in order to prevent blood pressure from falling. Yet the reduction in pulse pressure during haemorrhage is so modest and occurs so late that it is of little clinical importance.

'Central' pressures

Also with the introduction of disposable transducers, monitoring of central venous as well as of pulmonary artery pressures have become relatively routine during major surgery and in the intensive care unit. They are significant only as indicators of CBV, and in turn preload to the heart. Obviously, elevated central pressures may be present in response to increased pulmonary vascular resistance as in patients with chronic pulmonary disease. Also, pertinent to anaesthesia, positive pressure breathing with elevated pulmonary airway pressure will increase CVPs together with a reduction of the CBV. A reduced CBV with positive end-expiratory pressure is demonstrated by a decrease in the plasma level of atrial natriuretic factor (ANF) and reduced diuresis.[20]

During experimental haemorrhage the amount of blood lost is reflected accurately by the reduction in CVP.[21] Also during LBNP CVP decreases in proportion to the reduction in CBV.[17] In contrast, during head-up tilt-induced hypovolaemic shock CVP is a less reliable index of CBV. CVP need not change during tilting, and even when reduced in response to tilting, it remains stable during maintained tilt (Fig. 14.1).[22,23] This contrasts with pulmonary artery mean and wedge pressures, which consistently decline during maintained head-up tilt. Also, in a clinical setting pulmonary artery pressures are more sensitive indices of the CBV than CVP.[24]

Yet, CVP as well as pulmonary artery pressures are unreliable indices of the volume status of a patient both during cardiac[25] and aortic (Table 14.1) operations, where patient volume may be in an excess of more than 3 litres. In these situations central pressures are unchanged, or even reduced (and it may be speculated that patients are overloaded in an attempt to correct the determined variables).

Cardiac output

Monitoring cardiac output in patients has become fairly routine with the introduction of Swan–Ganz catheters.[26] Obviously this method of deriving cardiac output is much easier than that of dye dilution, but it is still both invasive and discontinues procedure. Doppler-derived cardiac output has been introduced; although it is both continuous and non-invasive, the accuracy needed for placement of the probe in the suprasternal notch means that it can be performed only by skilled personnel. Some of these limitations have been overcome by recording of the Doppler signal from the oesophagus,[27] which permits not only a better signal but also a fixed probe position during an operation.

It is puzzling that continuous recording of cardiac output with transthoracic electrical impedance[28] has not generated more interest, when simplicity of apparatus is considered (four electrocardiographic electrodes that are also used for recording). It is often claimed that cardiac output determined by thoracic impedance shows consider-

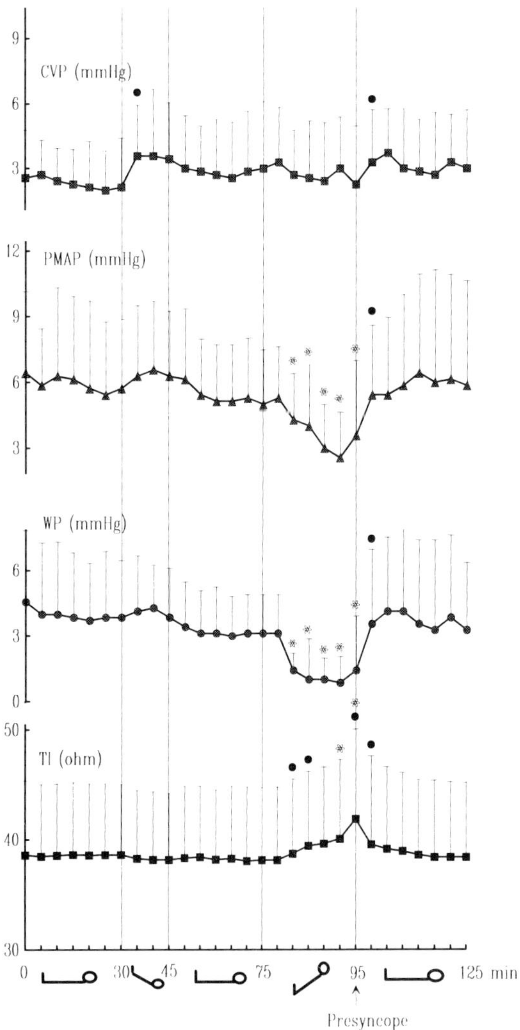

Fig. 14.1. Central venous pressure (CVP), pulmonary mean arterial pressure (PMAP), pulmonary wedge pressure (WP) and thoracic impedance (TI) during head-up tilt-induced hypovolaemic shock. Values are expressed as means ± SD. *, compared with the rest ($P<0.05$); ●, compared with preceding value ($P<0.05$).

ably deviations from values obtained by other means. The measured value for cardiac output is seldom of importance, but it is of interest how the recorded value responds to various interventions. Also of interest, electrical impedance can be used for evaluation of limb vascular control in situations with a reduced CBV.[29]

Calculation of cardiac output from electrical impedance is based on an estimate of stroke volume and should integrate the signal over approximately 1 min before a result is presented as litres per minute. Also, with the use of a Swan–Ganz catheter and thermodilution, the integration period is short relative to that applied during conventional dye dilution, and results ought to represent an average of several determinations in order to give a value in conventional units (l/min).

Cardiac output may be taken as the physiological meaning of the circulation. Yet, in septic shock it may be elevated with compromised organ perfusion. Also, in high output states including hepatic diseases cardiac output may be elevated to 10–15 l/min, and organ perfusion may be affected, if it is reduced to the high normal level of a resting patient. Conversely, in the anhepatic phase of liver transplantation cardiac output is reduced.[30]

With reduced preload cardiac output becomes volume-dependent. The reduction is modest and of interest; when presyncopal symptoms appear with an associated decrease in heart rate, stroke volume may increase more than expected based on the corresponding reduction in heart rate.[31] This reflects the reduction of afterload as blood pressure decreases and emphasizes that circulatory control during haemorrhage is not 'decompensated', but regulated to maintain peripheral flow at the expense of blood pressure.

Venous oxygen saturation

According to Fick's principle pulmonary oxygen uptake is cardiac output times the arteriovenous oxygen difference. Of these variables, pulmonary oxygen uptake will be almost constant in a resting individual. Furthermore, arterial oxygen content corresponds to full saturation. This means that mixed venous oxygen saturation varies directly in relation to changes in cardiac output, and is approximately 0.90 in liver patients with high cardiac output while only 0.75 in a normal individual. In situations with reduced CBV, where cardiac output becomes dependent on preload, venous saturation will reflect the volume status of the patient.

With the introduction of Swan–Ganz catheters, mixed venous saturation can be monitored continually. However, even in patients monitored with a traditional Swan–Ganz catheter, and in patients with a central venous catheter, blood samples can be taken to measure venous saturation. Mixed and central venous oxygen saturation change in parallel with haemorrhage in animals[32] as well as in humans. Central venous oxygen saturation decreases to approximately 0.60 when presyncopal symptoms appear.[31] Using the same approximation as above, a reduction of the blood volume by 100 ml will result in a 1 per cent reduction in saturation.

This type of monitoring can be used to increase blood volume for as long as volume loading results in an increase in venous saturation, and then to stop blood administration when volume results in no further elevation. In other words, blood administration is continued until cardiac output is no longer dependent on preload (of course, ongoing haemorrhage may be balanced by the rate of blood administered).

Of interest, (muscle) venous oxygen saturation can be monitored by near-infrared spectroscopy,[33] which may be both a non-invasive and continuous way of deriving an index of cardiac filling.

Thoracic electrical impedance

Thoracic electrical impedance has been applied to derive cardiac output. The real advantage of impedance monitoring is its dependence on blood volume. Impedance measures the resistance over a given body segment. With placement of electrodes on each side of the thorax, resistance mainly corresponding to CBV blood is assessed.[34] Electrical resistance is elevated with increased content of air in the lungs and has been applied to follow respiration. An elevated CBV will reduce resistance, and conversely, central volume depletion will result in an elevated thoracic impedance. This is reflected during head-up tilt, where thoracic impedance increases in proportion to the tilt angle, while electrical impedance over the legs decreases (Fig. 14.2).[18,35]

With application of different electrical frequencies it is possible to distinguish between the extracellular and cellular (erythrocytes) changes in blood volume. This reflects the fact that a high electrical frequency (100 kHz) penetrates the cells which is not possible for a low frequency signal (e.g. 1–2.5 kHz). Although not fully established experimentally, monitoring of electrical impedance at two frequencies could allow for monitoring of a balanced volume administration. This approach is especially attractive with the introduction of separate administration of erythrocytes, plasma and plasma substitutes. With impedance it is possible to monitor pulmonary oedema[36] and to follow differentiated changes in the distribution of erythrocytes and fluid during head-up tilt.[18,29] A further advantage with the use of thoracic electrical impedance for volume monitoring is that it responds not only to a decrease in CBV, but that it is also an accurate indicator of fluid balance in an overloaded patient (Table 14.1).[35]

Three problems are to be mentioned with the use of thoracic impedance for monitoring CBV. One is that the signal is uncalibrated. Furthermore, during abdominal operations manipulation of the upper abdominal organs may affect the measured value. Finally, it is a conceptual problem that resistance increases with central volume depletion. It would be more logical if the value followed changes in CBV directly. Therefore, conductance ought to be reported rather than resistance.

Assessment of regional flow

If shock can not be defined from blood pressure, maintenance of an adequate organ perfusion may serve the purpose. One such attempt was Ibsen's introduction of toe temperature for evaluation of critically ill patients.[37] Determination of toe temperature is both simple and well functioning. However, its precision in predicting changes in blood volume has not been established. It may be speculated that toe temperature is more reliable for long-term monitoring than for recording acute changes of the circulation.

Clinically, 'regional perfusion' is monitored by the ability to maintain diuresis. Diuresis is reduced during central volume depletion because of an elevated plasma antidiuretic hormone, which reaches vasopressin levels when presyncopal symptoms appear and the skin is pale.[22,38] Of interest, the increase in vasopressin could also explain the associated nausea.[39]

More recently an attempt has been made to monitor splanchnic flow by a calculation of gastric pH.[40] The splanchnic circulation is very sensitive to changes in sympathetic activity but its role during stage II of hypovolaemic shock, including a reduction in sympathetic nerve activity, is not established.[41,42]

Of perhaps more interest is the possibility of monitoring cerebral perfusion by transcranial Doppler.[43] For anaesthesia this possibility allows

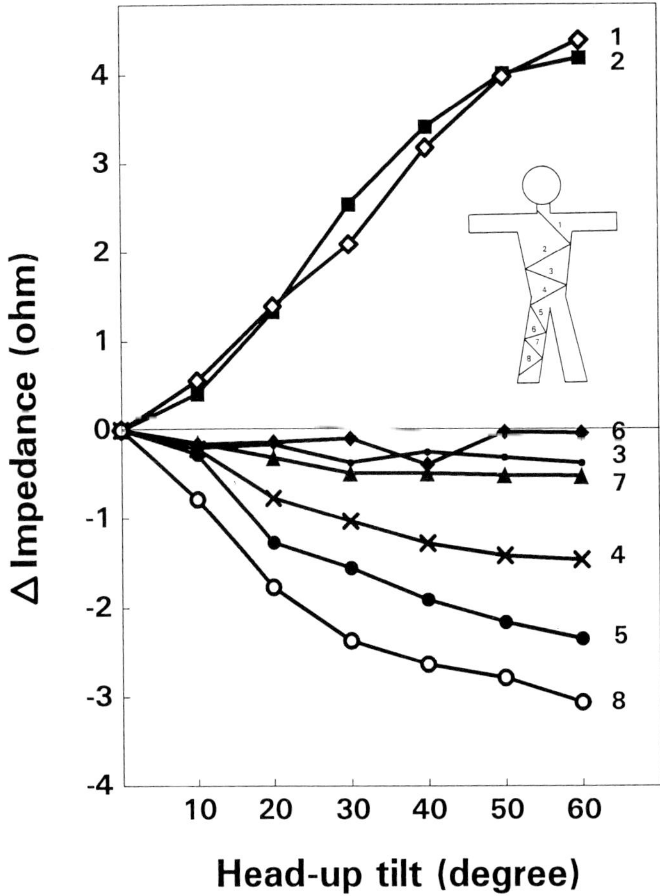

Fig. 14.2. Regional electrical impedance followed over eight body sections during head-up tilting. No significant changes were recorded over the knee. Furthermore, the electrical indifference point was positioned between the umbilicus and trochanter major.

for an evaluation of anaesthetic depth in situations where cerebral metabolism, and in turn CBF, is reduced as with the use of barbiturates.

Conclusion

Maintaining CBV during haemorrhage prevents blood pressure from being affected, and thereby preserves tissue perfusion even in patients with arteriosclerotic disease and hypertension. Traditional monitoring is complicated by a complex heart rate response to haemorrhage. Reliable monitors of a reduced CBV include pulmonary artery and wedge pressures, venous oxygen saturation and thoracic electrical impedance. Of these variables, thoracic impedance shows the highest correlation to changes in volume.

References

1. Cushing H: On routine determination of arterial tension in operation and in clinic. *Boston Medical and Surgical Journal*, 1903; **148,** 250–56.
2. Asmussen E, Secher NH and Andersen EA: Heart rate and ventilatory frequency as dimension dependent variables. *European Journal of Applied Physiology*, 1981; **46,** 379–86.
3. Horton JW, Longhurst JC, Coln D and Mitchell JH: Cardiovascular effects of haemorrhagic shock in spleen intact and in splenectomized dogs. *Clinical Physiology*, 1984; **4,** 533–48.

4. Häggendal J: On the patterns of blood pressure, heart rate and blood levels of noradrenaline and adrenaline during haemorrhage in the rat. *Acta Physiologica Scandinavica*, 1986; **127,** 513–22.
5. Jacobsen J, Hansen OB, Sztuk F, Warberg J and Secher NH: Enhanced heart rate response to haemorrhage by ileus in the pig. *Acta Physiologica Scandinavica*; in press.
6. Jacobsen J and Secher NH: Heart rate during haemorrhagic shock. *Clinical Physiology*, 1992; **12**, 659–66.
7. Little RA, Marchall HW and Kirkman E: Attenuation of the acute cardiovascular responses to haemorrhage by tissue injury in the conscious rat. *Journal of Experimental Physiology*, 1989; **74,** 825–33.
8. Starr I and Collins LH: Physiological studies of faintness and syncope. *Journal of Clinical Investigation*, 1931; **9,** 561–76.
9. Lewis T: Vasovagal syncope and the carotid sinus mechanism. *British Medical Journal*, 1932; **i,** 873–6.
10. Secher NH, Perko G and Olesen HL: Effect of exercise on vasovagal (pre-)syncope. *Scandinavian Journal of Medicine and Science in Sports*, 1992; **2,** 160–61.
11. Sander-Jensen K, Secher NH, Bie P, Warberg J and Schwartz TW: Vagal slowing of the heart during haemorrhage: observations from 20 consecutive hypotensive patients. *British Medical Journal*, 1986; **292,** 364–6.
12. Friedman DB, Jensen FB, Matzen S and Secher NH: Non-invasive blood pressure monitoring during head-up tilt using Penaz principle. *Acta Anaesthesiologica Scandinavica*, 1990; **34,** 519–22.
13. Jørgensen LG and Schroeder T: Defective cerebrovascular autoregulation after carotic endarectomy. *European Journal of Vascular Surgery*; in press.
14. Sjöstrand T: Regulation of blood volume. *Scandinavian Journal of Clinical and Laboratory Investigation*, 1976; **36,** 209–19.
15. Sander-Jensen K, Marving J, Secher NH, Hansen I-KL, Giese J and Bie P: Does the increase in heart rate prevent a detrimental decrease of the end-systolic volume during central hypovolemia in man? *Angiology*, 1990; **41,** 687–95.
16. Jacobsen J, Søfeldt S, Fernades A, Brocks V, Warberg J and Secher NH: Reduced left ventricular size at onset of bradycardia during epidural anaesthesia. *Acta Anaesthesiologica Scandinavica*; in press.
17. Murray RH, Thompson LJ, Bowers JA and Albright CD: Hemodynamic effects of graded hypovolemia and vasodepressor syncope induced by lower body negative pressure. *American Heart Journal*, 1968; **76,** 799–811.
18. Matzen S, Perko G, Groth S, Friedman DB and Secher NH: Blood volume distribution during head-up tilt induced central hypovolaemia in man. *Clinical Physiology*, 1991; **11,** 411–22.
19. Abboud FM, Eckberg DL, Johannesen UJ and Mark AL: Carotid and cardiopulmonary baroreceptor control of splanchnic and forearm vascular resistance during venous pooling in man. *Journal of Physiology*, 1979; **286,** 173–84.
20. Andrivet P, Adnot S, Brun-Buisson C and Chabrier PE: Involvement of ANF in the acute antidiuresis during PEEP ventilation. *Journal of Applied Physiology*, 1988; **65,** 1967–74.
21. Rea RF, Hamdan M, Clary MP, Randels MJ, Dayton PJ and Strauss RG: Comparison of muscle sympathetic responses to hemorrhage and lower body negative pressure in humans. *Journal of Applied Physiology*, 1991; **70,** 1401–5.
22. Sander-Jensen K, Secher NH, Astrup A, Christensen NJ, Giese J, Schwartz TW, Warberg J and Bie P: Hypotension induced by passive head-up tilt: endocrine and circulatory mechanisms. *American Journal of Physiology*, 1986; **251,** R742–8.
23. Matzen S, Secher NH, Knigge U, Bach FW and Warberg J: Pituitary–adrenal responses to head-up tilt in humans: effect of H_1- and H_2-receptor blockade. *American Journal of Physiology*, 1992; **263,** R156–63.
24. Sørenson MB: *Monitoring of the Surgical Patient.* Copenhagen, 1979.
25. Perko G, Perko MJ, Jansen E and Secher NH: Thoracic impedance as an index of body fluid balance during cardiac surgery. *Acta Anaesthesiologica Scandinavica*, 1991; **35,** 568–71.
26. Swan HJC and Ganz W: The Swan–Ganz catheter: past and present. In Blitt CD (ed.): *Monitoring in Anesthesia and Critical Care Medicine.* New York, NY, Churchill Livingstone, 1990, 211–20.
27. Humphrey LS and Weiss JL: Transesophageal echocardiography. In Blitt CD (ed.): *Monitoring in Anesthesia and Critical Care Medicine.* New York, NY, Churchill Livingstone, 1990, 277–336.
28. Kubicek WG, Karnegis JN, Patterson RP, Witsoe DA and Matterson RH: Development and evaluation of an impedance cardiac output system. *Aerospace Medicine*, 1966; **37,** 1208–12.
29. Matzen S, Schifter S, Radvansky I, Knigge U, Warberg J and Secher NH: Calcitonin gene-related peptide (CGRP) and leg vascular resistance during head-up tilt induced hypovolaemic shock in man. *Acta Physiologica Scandinavica* 1991; **142,** 313–18.
30. Spiess BD: Anesthesia. In Williams JW (ed.): *Hepatic Transplantation.* Philadelphia, PA, WB Saunders Co., 1990, 183–206.
31. Madsen P, Iversen H and Secher NH: Central venous oxygen saturation during hypovolaemic shock in man. *Scandinavian Journal of Clinical and Laboratory Investigation*, 1992; **53,** 67–72.
32. Scalea TM, Holman M, Fuortes M, Baron BJ, Phillips TF, Goldstein AS, Sclafani SJA and Shaftan GW: Central venous blood oxygen saturation: an early, accurate measurement of volume during hemorrhage. *Journal of Trauma*, 1988; **28,** 725–30.

33. Wilson JR, Mancini DM, McCully K, Ferraro N, Lanoce V and Chance B: Noninvasive detection of skeletal muscle underperfusion with near-infrared spectroscopy in patients with heart failure. *Circulation*, 1989; **80,** 1668–74.
34. Ebert TJ, Smith JJ, Barney JA, Merril DC and Smith GK: The use of thoracic impedance for determining thoracic blood volume changes in man. *Aviation, Space, and Environmental Medicine*, 1986; **57,** 49–53.
35. Perko G, Payne G and Secher NH: A volume indifference point determined by electrical impedance in humans. *Acta Physiologica Scandinavica*, 1993; **148,** 125–9.
36. Larsen FF, Mogensen L and Tedner B: Transthoracic electrical impedance at 1 and 100 kHz – a means for separating thoracic fluid compartments. *Clinical Physiology*, 1987; **7,** 105–13.
37. Ibsen B: *Intensiv Shockterapi*, in Danish. Copenhagen, Nyt Nordisk Forlag – Arnold Busck, 1969.
38. Bie P, Secher NH, Astrup A and Warberg J: Cardiovascular and endocrine responses to head-up tilt and vasopressin infusion in humans. *American Journal of Physiology*, 1986; **251,** R735–41.
39. Editorial: Nausea and vasopressin. *Lancet*, 1991; **337,** 1133–4.
40. Fiddian-Green RG: The potential for monitoring gastric intramucosal pH to reduce the costs of critical care. In Vincent JL (ed.): *Yearbook of Intensive Care and Emergency Medicine*. Berlin, Springer-Verlag, 1992, 259–70.
41. Bearn AG, Billing B, Edholm OG and Sherlock S: Hepatic blood flow and carbohydrate changes in man during fainting. *Journal of Physiology (London)*, 1951; **115,** 422–55.
42. Price HL, Deutch S, Marchall BE, Stephen GW, Behar MG and Neufeld GR: Hemodynamic and metabolic effects of hemorrhage in man, with particular reference to the splanchnic circulation. *Circulation Research*, 1966; **18,** 469–74.
43. Newell DW and Aaslid R: *Transcranial Doppler*. New York, NY, Raven Press, 1992.

15

Treatment of hypovolaemic shock: pharmacological intervention

Niels H Secher and Daniel B Friedman

It is the intention of this book to make monitoring of CBV so accurate that correction of hypovolaemia is made before adverse effects become manifest. Three stages of the circulatory responses to central volume depletion have been identified (see Chapter 1). In stage I heart rate increases moderately, blood pressure remains stable and the patient has no symptoms. In stage II both heart rate and blood pressure decrease associated with presyncopal symptoms and the patient is pale. With further blood loss heart rate increases again.

In stage I (preshock) there is no need for fluid or other therapy because of the large compensatory capacity in humans for effective control of plasma volume.[1,2] Patients are often thirsty and in blood banks compensatory drinking of fluid is encouraged. In stage II of shock volume loading results in immediate cure (see Chapter 14).[3,4] In fact, the reduced blood pressure maintains administered fluid in the blood stream.

In some patients volume correction is inadvertently not established before stage III of hypovolaemic shock is reached, and transition to an 'irreversible' stage of shock may follow. Irreversible shock after haemorrhage is defined as a state characterized by temporary restoration of blood pressure as blood volume is reestablished, but death of the animal.[5] The experimental irreversible shock is comparable to the clinical setting where a patient for instance with ruptured aortic aneurysm is resuscitated, operated and treated in the post operative intensive care unit to an apparently stable condition. However, at a later stage blood pressure gradually decrease, and the kidneys ('shock kidney', acute tubular necrosis, (ATN)), and lungs are affected. The patient is consequently kept on mechanically controlled ventilation. Finally liver function is affected, and death by 'multiorgan failure' ensues. Thus in animal studies liver function is not compromised until long after resuscitation from severe haemorrhage,[6] although it shows marked hyperaemia.[7]

A spontaneous decrease of blood pressure in the irreversible stage of shock requires that pharmacological intervention is undertaken to restore blood pressure and enhance tissue perfusion. It has also been proposed that stage II of hypovolaemic shock potentially can be prevented or treated by pharmacological intervention or by other means. Thus, intervention other than volume loading will be reviewed with respect to the stage of hypovolaemic shock.

Prior to such considerations, it should be noticed that whole blood or plasma is administered concomitant with citrate. Accordingly, the plasma level of calcium decreases and hence, by way of its vascular effect, hypotension may follow. Following administration of even modest amounts of whole blood or plasma the plasma concentration of calcium should be monitored and calcium administered in order to maintain an ionized concentration of at least 1.1 mmol/l. It may also be that the patient is on a calcium blocking agent that makes the sensitivity to a reduced plasma calcium concentration even more pronounced. On the other hand, entry of calcium ions in injured cells may trigger various deleterious biochemical reactions, rendering the administration of calcium dubious and, in turn, the use of calcium blocking agents an advantage during resuscitation of patients.[8]

Metabolic (lactate) acidosis develops during hypovolaemic shock, and is usually corrected if severe ('base excess' of less than -10 mmol/l) as base excess $\times$ 0.3 body weight = bicarbonate in mmol. Two considerations may be mentioned. Following administration of bicarbonate the titratable acid is neutralized by formation of carbon dioxide, which is eliminated through the lungs, but carbon dioxide also diffuses across the cell membrane causing a temporary enhanced cell acidosis. A low pH may also protect against reperfusion (e.g. liver) injury *in vitro*.[9]

Stage II of shock

Heart rate in stage I of shock regularly reaches approximately 100 beats/min with a modest reduction of the CBV (stage I) and then decreases to approximately 75 beats/min when blood pressure decreases and the patient or subject becomes ill with presyncopal symptoms (stage II) (see Chapter 1 and Sander-Jensen *et al.*[4]). The decrease in heart rate, however, may be more impressive. In a hypotensive patient with a heart rate of 30 beats/min it is tempting to speculate that the hypotension is secondary to the low heart rate.

However, even an extremely low heart rate is not the cause of hypotension during central volume depletion. Heart rate is restored immediately upon volume loading, even if it decreases to very low values as is the case when a patient faints. Conversely, atropine may restore heart rate to approximately 100–120 beats/min with no effect on blood pressure.[10] In other words, hypotension in stage II of hypovolaemic shock is due to sympathoinhibition[4,11,12] and not to activation of the sympathetic cholinergic pathway.

Of more interest is the suggestion that stage II of hypovolaemic shock is provoked by hypoxaemia (see Chapter 13). The cardioinhibitory–vasodepressor reflex to central volume depletion is not caused by arterial hypoxaemia[4,13,14] and during central volume depletion the electrocardiogram shows no signs of ischaemia. Still, hypoxaemia can provoke a similar reflex,[15] making it likely that the combination of central volume depletion and myocardial hypoxaemia may provoke the response. These considerations are especially relevant to anaesthesia, where bleeding is not the sole cause of central volume depletion. Central volume depletion can also be provoked by the vasodilatory effects of general as well as of regional (spinal and epidural) anaesthesia. Therefore it is good clinical practice to elevate the inspiratory oxygen content above 30 per cent during general anaesthesia, even in patients with normal pulmonary oxygenation capacity. Of even more clinical relevance is the administration of nasal oxygen during regional anaesthesia, where sedative drugs such as opioids and benzodiazepines often are administered in order to reduce anxiety. The combined effect of moderate central volume depletion by way of regional anesthesia and hypoxaemia caused by sedatives may thus explain the reported anaesthetic deaths in these patients.[16] In order to prevent accumulation of blood in the legs during epidural and spinal anaesthesia, patients should be placed in moderate (5 per cent) Trendelenburg's position. Furthermore, if the head is to be elevated after the operation, it is equally mandatory that the feet are raised to the same horizontal level as the head.

It has been speculated that the reflex cardioinhibition–vasodepression during haemorrhage is elicited by activation of unmyelinated vagal (C-) fibres in the posterior wall of the left ventricle. Activation of such fibres may include a serotonergic mechanism.[17] Accordingly, the reflex may be prevented by blockade of such receptors. However, in clinically relevant doses neither serotonergic I+II (methysergide), II (ketanserin) or III (ondansetron) receptor anatagonists affect the reflex during head-up tilt induced hypovolaemic shock,[19] This is the case despite the fact that methysergide diminishes the noradrenaline and β-endorphin responses to head-up tilt and abolishes the increase in prolactin and plasma renin activity. Odansetron reduces the decrease in heart rate and further abolishes the increase in plasma catecholamines while ketanserin reduces tolerance to head-up tilt with no effect on hormonal variables.

In rats the reflex is uninfluenced by blockade of prostaglandin synthesis by endomethacin and bradykinins by aprotinin.[19] Furthermore, the reflex is activated during head-up tilt induced hypovolaemic shock in the presence of a commonly used benzodiazepine dose of 10 mg diazepam although it diminishes the cortisol response.[20] The histamine I receptor blocking agent mepyramine provokes the reflex during head-up tilt, perhaps because of associated α-adrenergic blockade as demonstrated by a reduced plasma noradrenaline response.[21] On the other hand, the histamine 2 receptor antagonist cimetidine has no effect on tilt tolerance despite an attenuation of the adrenaline response. This finding argues against the view that the decrease in peripheral resistance elicited in stage II of shock is dependent on the concomitant increase in plasma adrenaline (see Chapter 13). Accordingly, also during epidural anaesthesia, central volume depletion results in hypotension (and reduced heart rate) although plasma adrenaline need not be increased.[22] Yet, β_2-adrenoceptors contribute to the maintainence peripheral flow during hypovolaemic shock and conversely survival is lessened by β_2-adrenoceptor blockade.[23]

During hyopovolaemic shock β-endorphin increases.[21] As expected morphine induces severe orthostatic intolerance even in a dose commonly used for premedication. Naloxone may restore blood pressure during hypovolaemic shock[24] and this observation has sparked a great deal of interest. The effectiveness of this drug in a wide range of experimental conditions has been recognized (see Chapter 2). Naloxone has no cardiovascular effects in the unbled animal. During central volume depletion the pressor effect of naloxone is related to an increase in peripheral vascular resistance and can be prevented by prior α-blockade. Thus, in rabbits the cardioinhibitory–vasodepressor reflex to central volume depletion is prevented by naloxone[25] and the receptor is of the δ-type located in the brain.[26] In animal studies the intravenous dose of naloxone was 4–8 mg/kg. However, with the clinically more reasonable dose of 0.03–0.1 mg/kg, paradoxically, naloxone has no effect on cardiovascular control during the normotensive phase of central volume depletion, but reduces tilt tolerance time (Klokker, 1993, personal communication).[27] Furthermore, naloxone (and morphine) fails even to increase short-term survival in rats subjected to haemorrhage.[28] Thus, the experience with naloxone during hypovolaemic shock is similar to the original observation by Sjöstrand,[29] that survival of rats is reduced after vagal deafferentation of the heart preventing the cardioinhibitory–vasodepressor reflex.

TRH also improves cardiovascular function during haemorrhagic shock[30] probably without increasing peripheral sympathetic activity. Thus, this means of improving blood pressure may preserve tissue perfusion but human experience is lacking.

Another means of affecting the cardioinhibitory – vasodepressor reflex to haemorrhage has been to use a concentrated saline solution.[31] It is worth noting that this means of restoring blood pressure in a hypotensive animal depends on the route of administration. The hypertonic saline solution needs to pass the lungs in order to be effective. Very likely its effect is to inhibit the cardioinhibitory–vasodepressor reflex. It should be kept in mind that this way of restoring blood pressure adds volume, exceeding the small volume administered due to an osmotic effect mobilizing fluid from the interstitial space to the vascular volume. Accordingly these solutions of 3–7.5 per cent NaCl sometimes with dextran have also been shown to reduce the amount of fluid subsequently needed. Yet, hyperosmotic saline may be disadvantageous in shock states characterized by extensive tissue injury.[32]

Paradoxically, an increased inotropic state induced by isoproterenol provokes bradycardia and hypotension on a tilt table.[33] Conversely, tilt time is increased after heart–lung transplantation.[34] Both observations indicate that the cardioinhibitory–vasodepressor reflex to central volume depletion originates in the heart and is related to increased contractility combined with a reduced chamber volume.[22] On the other hand, when central volume depletion is provoked by redistribution of blood volume, e.g. during epidural or spinal anaesthesia, ephedrine may prevent episodes of hypotension.[35]

Anti-G suits have been used as a non-pharmacological way of increasing blood pressure in bleeding patients.[36] With this means, pressure trousers are inflated around the legs. Obviously this will reduce the vascular blood volume of the legs and thereby increase CBV. On the other hand, if this was the only effect of anti-G trousers it may be easier just to raise the leg above the level of the heart, which is an effective way of mobilizing approximately 500 ml blood. However, the blood raising effect of anti-G trousers is maintained even after an arterial tourniqet is inflated high on the thighs preventing any shift in blood from the legs to the CBV. This observation points to the anti-G trousers stimulating blood pressure raising receptors in the legs. Accordingly, during epidural anaesthesia, the blood pressure raising effect of anti-G trousers is lost.[37] It is known that stimulating a peripheral nerve[38] or subjecting a limp to ischaemia[39] prevents the decrease in heart rate and blood pressure in response to haemorrhage. Thus, the specific cardiovascular response to haemorrhage is a complex balance between input from many receptor systems. The cardioinhibitory–vasodepressor response to haemorrhage is also lost during isometric muscle contractions with clinical application during a vasovagal syncope.[40]

Severe haemorrhage

Survival after haemorrhage is also influenced by the physiological condition. Thus in rats subjected to haemorrhage resulting in a blood pressure of 55 mmHg, all animals survived in the postprandial state, while all rats died when they had been subjected to 24 h of food deprivation.[41]

With marked decrease in blood pressure despite volume loading sympathomimetic agents are indicated in order to increase blood pressure through an increase in cardiac output. Unfortunately the vasoconstricting action of these agents also reduces peripheral flow. Yet, in tissue with marked autoregulation such as the brain, pharmacologically induced increase in blood pressure may increase flow. This is especially relevant in hypertensive patients and is associated with a 'right' shift of cerebral autoregulation (see Chapter 4). Conversely, in anasthetized patients this consideration is of less relevance.[42] Before inotropic or vasoconstrictor agents are applied it should be excluded that a low blood pressure is due to volume depletion. This may be difficult especially in patients with ongoing internal bleeding because of the calculated large volume surplus. An easy test of sufficient volume loading is to measure central venous oxygen saturation following volume expansion. Any increases in saturation in response to volume loading indicate that cardiac output is limited by preload, and volume loading should continue until venous saturation becomes stable (see Chapter 14).

Ahlquist[43] proposed that there are two types of adrenergic agonist receptors which he designated as α and β. He recognized that the α-receptors are responsible for vasoconstriction in contrast to the β-receptors which result in vasodilatation when stimulated. Later two classes of each of these receptors were identified. It was subsequently demonstrated that adrenergic receptor stimulation results in generation of a second messenger cyclic adenosine monophosphate[44] and that the receptors are linked to their effector molecules by guanine nucleotide-binding regulatory (G-) proteins.[45]

The commonly used drugs include dobutamine, dopamine, noradrenaline, adrenaline and isoprenaline. In contrast to noradrenaline and adrenaline, dopamine plays no role in the normal response to haemorrhage. All these agents, except for isoprenaline, have α-adrenergic effects with associated reduced peripheral blood flow, an effect which is less relevant for dobutamine. Amrinone, a phosphodiesterase inhibitor, exerts both inotropic and vasodilator effects. It important to recognize that there are no studies which document any advantage in terms of survival for any of these drugs.

Adrenaline has been widely used in situations such as anaphylaxis and cardiac arrest. It is a potent α- and β_1-agonist with lesser β_2-effects. At a low dose the β-effects are most prominent, with resulting increase in heart rate, stroke volume and decreased peripheral vascular resistance.[46] At higher doses it becomes almost entirely an α-receptor stimulating agent. *Noradrenaline* is both a potent α- and β_1-stimulator. Thus inotropy is increased, but the vasoconstriction results in reduced renal and mesenteric blood flow. *Isoproterenol* is rarely used as an inotrope because its β_1 effects result in marked tachycardia and its vasodilatory β_2 response results in hypotension. It may occasionally be useful prior to temporary pacemaker implantation during profound bradycardia when atropine is inadequate. *Dopamine* is the immediate precursor of noradrenaline and stimulates both directly and by releasing noradrenaline from nerve terminals.[47] At low doses (<2 μg/kg/min) it stimulates renal dopaminergic receptors and increases renal perfusion and diuresis. At a dose of 2–5 μg/kg/min dopamine causes mostly a dose-dependent β-agonist effect increasing heart rate and stroke volume. At a dose of 5–10 μg/kg/min the α-adrenergic effects predominate. *Dobutamine* is a synthetic catecholamine with marked β_1-agonist effects and weak β_2- and α-effects. The latter effects neutralize one another so there is little net effect on the vascular bed. The inotropic response predominates, with much less effect on heart rate. *Amrinone* increases cardiac output and lowers pulmonary artery wedge pressure. It has a long half-life of up to 6 h. It has special relevance for congestive heart failure, but may cause nausea and impair hepatic function.

Irreversible haemorrhagic shock has been related to the release of a 'myocardial depressant factor'.[48] More recently, during apparently irreversible shock after haemorrhage, blood pressure has been made stable by the administration of plasma containing endotoxin-specific antibodies.[49] Furthermore, development of irreversible shock may be related to the release of free oxygen radicals as it can be prevented by the early administration of lazaroid inhibiting lipid peroxidation.[50] In contrast, agents which oppose superoxide generation by xanthine oxidase (oxypurinol), inhibit arachidonic acid generation oxidation by cyclooxygenase (ibuprofen) or clear iron (desferal), have no effect. Blood pressure after haemorrhage is also unaffected by methylprednisolone.[51] These observations are encouraging as they represent the first clinically applicable pharmacological intervention that promises a causal prevention for the irreversible stage of shock.

References

1. Länne T and Lundvall J: Very rapid net transcapillary fluid absorption from skeletal muscle and skin in man during pronounced hypovolaemic circulatory stress. *Acta Physiologica Scandinavica*, 1989; **137,** 1–6.
2. Lundvall J and Länne T: Large capacity in man for effective plasma volume control in hypovolaemia fluid transfer from tissue to blood. *Acta Physiologica Scandinavica*, 1989; **137,** 513–20.
3. Secher NH, Sander-Jensen K, Werner C, Warberg J and Bie P: Bradycardia during severe but reversible hypovolemic shock in man. *Circulatory Shock*, 1984; **14,** 267–74.
4. Sander-Jensen K, Secher NH, Bie P, Warberg J and Schwartz TW: Vagal slowing of the heart during haemorrhage: observations from 20 consecutive hypotensive patients. *British Medical Journal*, 1986; **292,** 364–6.
5. Smith JJ and Kampine JP: Hypovolemic shock. In *Circulatory Physiology – The Essentials*. Baltimore, MD, Williams & Wilkins, 1990, 312–18 (mimeograph).
6. Wang P, Ba ZF, Burkhardt J and Chaudry IH: Measurement of hepatic blood flow after severe hemorrhage: lack of restoration despite adequate resuscitation. *American Journal of Physiology*, 1992; **262,** G92–8.
7. Iversen PO, Benestad HB and Nicolaysen G: Marked splenic hyperaemia during post-haemorrhagic hypotension in the rat, rabbit and cat. *Journal of Physiology* (*London*), 1992; **448,** 437–52.
8. Safar P: Cerebral resuscitation after cardiac arrest: a review. *Circulation*, 1986; **74, (suppl. IV)**, 138–53.
9. Currin RT, Gores GJ, Thurman RG and Lemaster JJ: Protection by acidotic pH against anoxic cell killing in perfused rat liver: evidence for a pH paradox. *FASEB Journal*, 1991; **5,** 207–10.
10. Sander-Jensen K, Mehlsen J, Stadager C, Christensen NJ, Fahrenkrug J, Schwartz TW, Warberg J and Bie P: Increase in vagal activity during hypotensive lower-body negative pressure in humans. *American Journal of Physiology*, 1988; **255,** R149–56.
11. Sander-Jensen K, Secher NH, Astrup A, Christensen NJ, Giese J, Schwartz TW, Warberg J and Bie P: Hypotension induced by passive head-up tilt: endocrine and circulatory mechanisms. *American Journal of Physiology*, 1986; R742–8.
12. Sanders JS and Ferguson DW: Profound sympathoinhibition complicating hypovolemia in humans. *Annals of Internal Medicine*, 1989; **111,** 439–41.
13. Madsen P, Iversen H and Secher NH: Central venous oxygen saturation during hypovolaemic shock in man. *Scandinavian Journal of Clinical and Laboratory Investigations*, 1993; **53,** 67–72.
14. Matzen S and Secher NH: Cardioinhibitory–vasodepressor response to head-up tilt without hypoxaemia or myocardial ischaemia. *Clinical Physiology*, 1993; **13,** 281–8.
15. Anderson DP, Allen WJ, Barcroft H, Edholm OG and Manning GW: Circulatory changes during fainting and coma caused by oxygen lack. *Journal of Physiology (London)*, 1946; **104,** 426–34.
16. Caplan RA, Ward RJ, Posner K and Cheney FW: Unexpected cardiac arrest during spinal anesthesia: a closed claims analysis of predisposing factors. *Anesthesiology*, 1988; **68,** 5–11.
17. Morgan DA, Thoren P, Wilczynski EA, Victor RG and Mark AL: Serotonergic mechanisms mediate renal sympathoinhibition during severe hemorrhage in rats. *American Journal of Physiology*, 1988; **255,** H496–502.
18. Matzen S, Secher NH, Knigge U, Pawelczyk J, Perko G, Imersen H, Bach FW and Warberg J: Effect of serotonin receptor blockade on endocrine and cardiovascular responses to head-up tilt in humans. *Acta Physiologica Scandinavica*; in press (abstract).
19. Skoog P, Månsson J and Thoren P: Changes in renal sympathetic outflow during hypotensive haemorrhage in rats. *Acta Physiologica Scandinavica*, 1985; **125,** 655–60.
20. Matzen S, Secher NH, Knigge U, Bach FW and Warberg J: Effect of diazepam on endocrine and cardiovascular responses to head-up tilt in humans. *Acta Physiologica Scandinavica*, 1993; **148**, 143–51.
21. Matzen S, Secher NH, Knigge U, Bach FW and Warberg J: Pituitary–adrenal response to head-up tilt in humans: effect of H_1- and H_2-receptor blockade. *American Journal of Physiology*, 1992; **263,** R156–63.
22. Jacobsen J, Søfelt S, Fernandes A, Brocks V, Warberg J and Secher NH: Reduced left ventricular size at onset of bradycardia during epidural anaesthesia. *Acta Anaesthesiologica Scandinavica*, 1993; **36,** 831–6.
23. Gustafsson D, Andersson LO and Lundvall J: Decrease in survival time in β_2-adrenoreceptor blocked cats exposed to bleeding. *Acta Physiologica Scandinavica*, 1984; **122,** 181–6.
24. Holaday JW: Cardiovascular effects of endogenous opiate systems. *Annual Review of Pharmacology and Toxicology*, 1983; **23,** 541–94.
25. Evans RG, Ludbrook J and van Leeuwen AF: Role of central opiate receptor subtypes in the circulatory

responses of awake rabbits to graded caval occlusions. *Journal of Physiology (London)*, 1989; **419,** 15–31.
26. Evans RG, Ludbrook J and Potocnik SJ: Intercisternal naloxone and cardiac nerve blockade prevent vasodilatation during simulated haemorrhage in awake rabbits. *Journal of Physiology (London)*, 1989; **409,** 1–14.
27. Foldager N and Bonde-Petersen F: Human cardiovascular reactions to simulated hypovolaemia, modified by the opiate antagonist naloxone. *European Journal of Applied Physiology*, 1988; **57,** 507–13.
28. Feuerstein G and Siren A-L: Effect of naloxone and morphine on survival of conscious rats after hemorrhage. *Circulatory Shock*, 1986; **19,** 293–300.
29. Sjöstrand T: Circulatory control via vagal afferents. V. Impairment of the circulatory adjustment to hemorrhage by vagal deafferentation and prolonged hypotension. *Acta Physiologica Scandinavica*, 1973; **87,** 228–39.
30. Holaday JW, d'Amato RJ and Faden AL: Thyrotropin-releasing hormone improves cardiovascular function in experimental endotoxic and hemorrhagic shock. *Science Washington*, 1981; **213,** 216–18.
31. Velasco IT, Pontieri V, Rocha e Silva M and Lopes U: Hyperosmotic NaCl and severe hemorrhagic shock. *American Journal of Physiology*, 1980; **239,** H664–73.
32. Williamson JW, Mitchell JH, Olesen HL, Raven PB, Secher NH: Reflex increase in blood pressure induced by compression in man. *Journal of Physiology*; in press.
33. Haglund E and Haljamäe H: Failure of hypertonic saline to resuscitate intestinal ischemia shock in the rat. *Acta Anaesthesiologica Scandinavica*, 1992; **36,** 410–18.
34. Almquist A, Goldenberg IF, Milstein S, Chen M-Y, Chen X, Hansen R, Gornick CC and Benditt DG: Provocation of bradycardia and hypotension by isoproterenol and upright posture in patients with unexplained syncope. *New England Journal of Medicine*, 1989; **320,** 346–51.
35. Banner NR, Williams M, Patel N, Chalmers J, Lightman SL and Yacoub MH: Altered cardiovascular and neurohumoral responses to head-up tilt after heart–lung transplantation. *Circulation*, 1990; **82,** 863–71.
36. Hemmingsen C, Poulsen JA and Risbo A: Prophylactic ephedrine during spinal anaesthesia: double-blind study in patients in ASA group I–III. *British Journal of Anaesthesia*, 1989; **63,** 340–42.
37. Gaffney FA, Thal ER, Taylor WF, Bastian BC, Weigelt JA, Atkins JM and Blomqvist CG: Hemodynamic effects of medical anti-shock trousers (MAST garment). *Journal of Trauma*, 1981; **21,** 931–7.
38. Overman RR, Wang SC: The contributory role of the afferent nervous factor in experimental shock: sublethal hemorrhage and sciatic nerve stimulation. *American Journal of Physiology*, 1947; **148,** 289–95.
39. Little RA, Marchall HW and Kirkman E: Attenuation of the acute cardiovascular responses to haemorrhage by tissue injury in the conscious rat. *Journal of Experimental Physiology*, 1989; **74,** 825–33.
40. Secher NH, Perko G and Olesen HL: Effect of exercise on vasovagal (pre-)syncope. *Scandinavian Journal of Medicine and Science in Sports*, 1992; **2,** 160–61.
41. Ljungqvist O, Jansson E and Ware J: Effect of food deprivation on survival after hemorrhage in the rat. *Circulatory Shock*, 1987; **22,** 251–60.
42. Henriksen L and Paulson OB: The effects of sodium nitroprusside on cerebral blood flow and cerebral venous blood gases in man. *Acta Medica Scandinavica. Supplement*, 1983; **678,** 91–6.
43. Ahlquist RP: A study of adrenergic receptors. *American Journal of Physiology*, 1948; **153,** 596–600.
44. Sutherland EW, Robinson GA and Butcher RW: Some aspects of the biological role of adenosine 3′,5′-monophosphate (cyclic AMP). *Circulation*, 1968; **37,** 279–306.
45. Neer EJ and Clapham DE: Roles of G protein subunits in transmembrane signalling. *Nature*, 1988; **333,** 129–34.
46. Löllgren H and Drexler H: Use of inotropes in the critical care setting. *Critical Care Medicine*, 1990; **18,** 56–60.
47. Goldberg LI and Raifer SI: Dopamine receptors: applications in clinical cardiology. *Circulation*, 1985; **72,** 245–8.
48. Leffer AM, Cowgill R, Marchall FF, Hall LM and Brand ED: Characterization of mycardial depressant factor present in hemorrhagic shock. *American Journal of Physiology*, 1967; **213,** 492–8.
49. Gaffin SL, Grinberg Z, Abraham C, Birkham J and Shechter Y: Protection against hemorrhagic shock in the cat by human plasma containing endotoxin-specific antibodies. *Journal of Surgical Research*, 1981; **31,** 18–21.
50. Fleckenstein AE, Smith SL, Linseman KL, Beuving LJ and Hall ED: Comparison of the efficacy of mechanistically different antioxidants in the rat hemorrhagic shock model. *Circulatory Shock*, 1991; **35,** 223–30.
51. Hall ED, Yonkers PA and McCall JM: Attenuation of hemorrhagic shock by the non-glucocorticoid 21-aminosteroid U74006F. *European Journal of Pharmacology*, 1988; **147,** 299–303.

16

The treatment of hypovolaemic shock: volume therapy

Ole Michael Nielsen

Volume therapy was first addressed by WB O'Shaughnessy in a letter to the Lancet 1831.[1] He reported on the composition of blood in cholera victims and recommended an intravenous saline solution for replacement of the volume deficit. Almost 100 years later Penfield and Teplitsky[2] still recommended intermittent infusion of an isosmotic saline solution for volume therapy. They also considered that the infusion rate should be guided by the recording of CVP. Hereafter the composition of fluid to be administered was debated extensively. Thus, Coller *et al.*[3] emphasized salt restriction and the infusion of glucose solutions, while Shires *et al.*[4] suggested that fluid therapy should involve large amounts of sodium-containing solutions. This later approach remains the basis of modern volume replacement therapy.

In the early seventies reports indicated pulmonary complications with volume infusion based on sodium-containing solutions.[5–7] On the basis of Starling forces, the importance of maintaining plasma colloid osmotic pressure (COP) was emphazised. This led to the 'crystalloid–colloid' controversy. On the one side, proponents for the use of crystalloid solutions in resuscitation of haemorrhagic shock argued that changes in plasma COP are not well correlated with pulmonary function. The other side stressed the importance of COP for the distribution of extracellular fluid across the pulmonary capillary membrane.

Volume therapy

The most important therapeutic purpose for volume therapy in hypovolaemic patients is the restoration and maintenance of blood volume. However, the clinical signs of hypovolaemia are not reliable. They include increased, normal or decreased heart rate, and a reduced arterial pressure. Other parameters such as CVP, pulmonary capillary wedge pressure and haematocrit may be of value after acute haemorrhage, but are unreliable in critically ill patients when compared with blood volume.[8] Also, variables such as blood pressure, pulse, haematocrit, CVP, pulmonary capillary wedge pressure and urine output are useful after major surgery, but have limitations in their ability to reflect promptly alterations in circulating volume and the response to therapy.

The fluid challenge technique of Weil and Henning[9] is the standard for evaluating cardiovascular responses to fluid therapy while at the same time minimizing the risk for fluid overload resulting in pulmonary oedema. A bolus infusion of 500 ml isotonic saline is administered over 20 min. The infusion is discontinued if the haemodynamic parameters are normalized, or when a predetermined upper limit for the cardiac filling pressure as indicated by CVP and pulmonary capillary wedge pressure is reached. Alternatively, fluid infusion is controlled by comparison with preset cardiac filling pressures every tenth minute. Examples of such preset values are: (1) a change in CVP or pulmonary capillary wedge pressure of less than 3 mmHg – the infusion is continued; (2) a 3–5 mmHg increase in filling pressures – the infusion is interrupted and reevaluated after 10 min; and (3) filling pressure increases more than 5 mmHg – the infusion is discontinued.

Shoemaker *et al.*[10] recommended the recording of parameters related to patient outcome. These include cardiac index, oxygen delivery and oxygen consumption. Variables were derived from comparison of survivors and non survivors in a population of critically ill patients. A following clinical study demonstrated reduced morbidity and mortality when therapy normalized these variables.

Extracellular volume

The extracellular volume is both the immediate receiving 'organ' of the infused fluid via the plasma volume, and the volume through which the cells are nourished. Extracellular volume includes plasma volume and the interstitial volume separated by the capillary membrane. The exchange rate of fluid between these two compartments is rapid. Substances exchanged between the blood and cells pass through the interstitium. The composition of the interstitium is complex and cannot be considered merely to serve as a buffer capacity for the plasma volume.[11] It consists of a build up of fibrillar components (collagen, reticular and elastic fibres) embedded in an amorphous ground substance. This gel-like matrix contains several glucosaminoglycans such as hyaluronic acid, chondroitin sulphate and kerato-sulphate. The glucosaminoglycans have a low isoelectric point. Consequently, at physiologic pH there is a high negative colloidal charge within the interstitial ground substance.[12] The gel-phase may be subdivided into a colloid-rich phase from which proteins are excluded, and a water-rich phase available for transport of proteins.

When an isotonic sodium chloride solution is infused it is rapidly distributed in the extracellular volume. The plasma expanding effect is therefore approximately one-third to one-fourth of the infused volume, reflecting the relative size of plasma volume and intestitial volumes. However, not all of the infused sodium can be traced in the extracellular volume. The fate of the 'missing' sodium and its accompanying water is not well established. During haemorrhagic shock Shires *et al.*[13] found a marked decrease in extracellular water and a significant increase in the intracellular sodium concentration. Similar results were obtained in a septic shock model.[14,15] Another approach by Flear *et al.*[16] demonstrated that trauma is associated with cellular changes. Potassium and organic solutes are shifted from the cells with simultaneous influx of sodium and water. In partial ischaemic muscle cells dysfunction of the membrane N–K-ATPase, or altered ion permeability induced by free oxygen radicals or other substances, may cause sodium influx.[17,18] This 'sick cell syndrome' explains the fact that plasma sodium is low after resuscitation from haemorrhagic shock as well as after surgery in spite of positive sodium balance.

Plasma colloid osmotic pressure and extracellular fluid

Colloid osmotically active molecules retain water in the vascular compartment against the hydrostatic pressure gradient across the capillary membrane. Water is retained due to a decrease in its chemical potential normally referred to as the osmotic pressure. In the case of a system of dissolved proteins and membranes impermeable to these proteins, it is termed the colloid osmotic pressure. The relation between the hydrostatic pressures and opposing COP to the filtration of water through the capillary membrane was established as the 'Starling equation':[19]

$$Q = K \times S\ ((Pc - Pt) - z(COPc - COPt))$$

where Q is the amount of fluid filtered across the membrane, K the filtration coefficient for the membrane, S the surface area of the capillary bed, Pc and Pt the hydrostatic pressures in the capillary and the surrounding tissue respectively, COPc and COPt, the colloid osmotic pressures of the plasma and tissue respectively, and z the reflection coefficient of the capillary membrane.[20]

Changes in circulating plasma proteins and especially the level of albumin affect COP in plasma, and thus the distribution of fluid between plasma and the interstitium. Plasma albumin exerts approximately 75 per cent of the intravascular COP. During surgery several mechanisms lead to decreased plasma albumin, as is the case in other trauma such as burns, accidents and haemorrhage. A common denominator is the acute phase plasma protein response.[21] This consists of an increase in synthesis and concentration of several proteins with diverse functions. They include C-reactive protein, α_1-acid glucoprotein, α_1-antitrypsin, haptoglobin and fibrinogen. At the same time the concentrations of albumin and transferrin decrease, and remain low for several days.[22] This response *per se* decreases plasma COP, as do the protein immobilization developed during abdominal surgery,[23] the plasma loss after burns, dislocation of proteins to the traumatized area[24] and unreplaced blood loss.

Plasma is also lost when blood is replaced with an erythrocyte suspension.

These mechanisms relate to the disappearance of plasma proteins from the vascular space. However, the transport of proteins from the interstitial fluid to the circulation should also be considered. Ariel[25] found that following postoperative administration of 3 litres iso-osmotic saline, plasma proteins reenter the vascular volume, while this could not be achieved with glucose solutions. In sheep Kramer *et al.*[26] demonstrated that increased lymphatic flow carried albumin to the vascular compartment. Also, Mullins and Bell[27] demonstrated increased lymph flow and lymph albumin concentration after saline expansion; conversely, dehydration leads to a diminished volume available for protein molecules.[11] The acute phase protein response also helps in restoring the protein content of the circulation, although with a different protein composition.

Plasma colloid osmotic pressure and fluid distribution across the capillary membrane

In a study of 53 patients undergoing reconstructive surgery on the abdominal aorta, the preoperative compiled mean plasma COP was 27 mmHg and the standard deviation 2.4 mmHg.[28] Fig. 16.1 shows the calculated changes in interstitial fluid plotted against mean plasma COP on days 1 and 4 after surgery. Of the 32 patients with mean plasma COP lower than 22 mmHg (preoperative mean −2SD) interstitial fluid was elevated in 28 patients, and for those with levels less than 20 mmHg it was elevated in all patients. In contrast, in patients with a mean plasma COP of more than 22 mmHg interstitial fluid changes were evenly distributed.

The preoperative compiled mean plasma COP is in accordance with the most cited value of 26–28 mmHg. The unchanged interstitial fluid associated with values above 22 mmHg is consistent with results of Fadnes[29] and Reed[30] based on rats made hypoproteinaemic by induced nephrotic syndrome. Thus, the decline in mean plasma COP was paralleled by an identical decrease in interstitial COP until it was lowered to 20 mmHg, which inevitably led to formation of oedema. It should be noted, however, that the studied patients[28] were nutritionally healthy. In patients with preoperative protein depletion, chronic infections, cancer, nephrotic syndrome and chronic intestinal ischaemia, the safety margin may be smaller.

Based on the physiology of the extracellular fluid space and the changes in plasma protein compo-

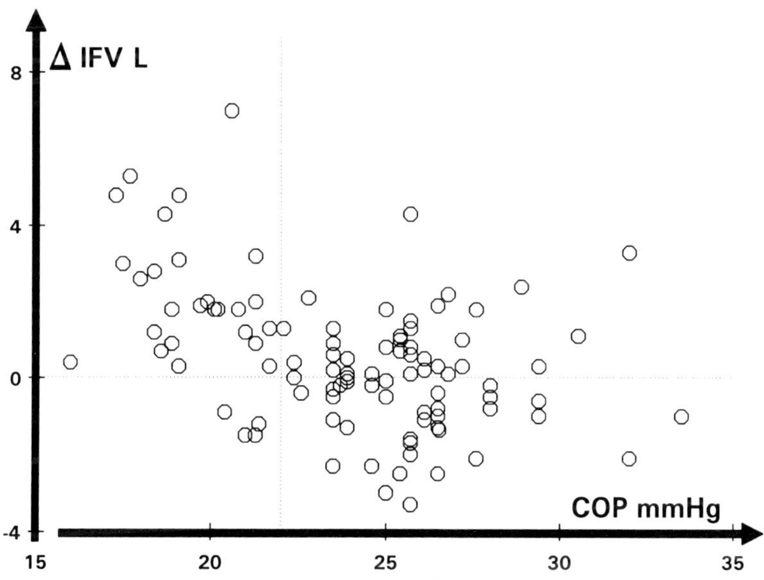

Fig. 16.1. Changes in interstitial fluid volume (Δ IFV) plotted against mean plasma colloid osmotic pressure (COP) on days 1 and 4 postoperative in 53 patients undergoing reconstructive surgery on the abdominal aorta.

sition following haemorrhagic shock, it is suggested that both isotonic sodium chloride solutions and colloid-rich solutions be used during the immediate resuscitation. Further, that the effects on haemodynamic variables be closely monitored. The type of colloid to be used is a matter of opinion, but human serum albumin is effective and can be used in large amounts. Artificial colloids such as dextran, gelatins and hydroxyethylstarch solutions are effective as plasma expanders but can only be administered in limited amounts. However, their price makes them attractive.

References

1. O'Shaughnessy WB: Experiments on the blood in cholera. *Lancet*, 1831; **32,** 490 (letter).
2. Penfield WG and Teplitsky D: Prolonged intravenous infusion and the clinical determination of venous pressure. *Archives of Surgery*, 1923; **7,** 111–15.
3. Coller FA, Campbell KN, Vaughan HH, Iob LV and Moyer CA: Post-operative salt intolerance. *Annals of Surgery*, 1944; **119,** 533–42.
4. Shires T, Williams J and Brown F: Acute change in extracellular fluids associated with major surgical procedures. *Annals of Surgery*, 1961; **154,** 803–10.
5. Berman IR and Spencer FC: The wet lung: diagnostic considerations. *Annals of Surgery*, 1972; **175,** 458 (editorial).
6. Gutierrez VS, Berman IR, Soloway HB and Hamit HF: Relationship of hypoproteinemia and prolonged mechanical ventilation to the development of pulmonary insufficiency in shock. *Annals of Surgery*, 1970; **171,** 385–93.
7. Fleming WH and Bowen JC: The use of diuretics in the treatment of early wet lung syndrome. *Annals of Surgery*, 1972; **175,** 505–9.
8. Shippy CR, Appel PL and Shoemaker WC: Reliability of clinical monitoring to assess blood volume in critically ill patients. *Critical Care Medicines*, 1984; **12,** 107–12.
9. Weil MH and Henning RJ: New concepts in the diagnosis and fluid treatment of circulatory shock. *Anaesthesia and Analgesia*, 1979; **58,** 124–32.
10. Shoemaker WC, Kram HB and Appel PL: Therapy of shock based on pathophysiology, monitoring, and outcome prediction. *Critical Care Medicines*, 1990; **18,** S19–25.
11. Auckland K and Nicolaysen G: Interstitial fluid volume: local regulatory mechanisms. *Physiological Reviews*, 1981; **61,** 556–643.
12. Haljamäe H: Anatomy of the interstitial tissue. *Lymphology*, 1978; **11,** 128–32.
13. Shires GT, Cunningham JN, Baker CRF, Illner H, Wagner IY and Maher J: Alterations in cellular membrane function during hemorrhagic shock in primates. *Annals of Surgery*, 1972; **176,** 288–95.
14. Trunkey DD, Illner H, Wagner IY and Shires GT: The effect of septic shock on skeletal muscle action potentials in the primate. *Surgery*, 1979; **85,** 938–43.
15. Illner HP and Shires GT: Membrane defect and energy status of rabbit muscle cells in sepsis and septic shock. *Archives of Surgery*, 1981; **116,** 1302–5.
16. Flear CTG, Bhattacharya SS and Singh CM: Solute and water exchanges between cells and extracellular fluids in health and disturbances after trauma. *Journal of Parental and Enteral Nutrition*, 1980; **4,** 98–120.
17. Perry MO, Shires GT and Albert SA: Cellular changes with graded limb ischemia and reperfusion. *Journal of Vascular Surgery*, 1981; **1,** 536–40.
18. Roberts JP, Perry MO, Hariri RJ and Shires GT: Incomplete recovery of muscle cell function following partial but not complete ischemia. *Circulatory Shock*, 1985; **5,** 253–8.
19. Pappenheimer JR and Soto-Rivera A: Effective osmotic pressure of the plasma proteins and other quantities associated with the capillary circulation in the hindlimbs of cats and dogs. *American Journal of Physiology*, 1948; **152,** 471–91.
20. Staverman AJ: The theory of measurement of osmotic pressure. *Recueil des Travaux Chimiques des Pays Bas*, 1951; **70,** 344–52.
21. Kushner I: The phenomenon of the acute phase response. *Annals of the New York Academy of Sciences*, 1982; **389,** 39–48.
22. Lebreton JP, Joisel F, Raoult JP, Lannuzel B, Rogez JP and Humbert G: Serum concentrations on human $alpha_2$ HS glucoprotein during the inflammatory process. Evidence that $alpha_2$ HS glucoprotein is a negative acute phase reactant. *Journal of Clinical Investigation*, 1979; **64,** 1118–29.
23. Jarnum S: Plasma protein exudation in the peritoneal cavity during laparotomy. *Gastroenterology*, 1961; **41,** 107–18.
24. Smith PC, Frank HA, Kasdon EJ, Dearborn EC and Skillman JJ: Albumin uptake by skin, skeletal muscle and lung in living and dying patients. *Annals of Surgery* 1978; **187,** 31–7.
25. Ariel IM: The internal balance of plasma protein in surgical patients. *Surgery, Gynecology and Obstetrics*, 1951; **92,** 405–13.
26. Kramer GC, Harms BA, Bodai BI, Demling RH and Renkin RH: Mechanisms for redistribution of plasma proteins following acute protein depletion. *American Journal of Physiology*, 1982; **243,** H803–9.
27. Mullins RJ and Bell DR: Changes in interstitial volume and masses of albumin and IgG in rabbit skin and skeletal muscle after saline volume loading. *Circulation Research*, 1982; **51,** 305–13.
28. Nielsen OM: Extracellular fluid volume and colloid

osmotic pressure in abdominal vascular surgery. A study of volume changes. *Danish Medical Bulletin*, 1991; **38,** 9–21.

29. Fadnes HO: Protein concentration and hydrostatic pressure in subcutaneous tissue of rats in hypoproteinemia. *Scandinavian Journal of Clinical and Laboratory Investigation*, **35,** 441–6.
30. Reed RK: Interstitial fluid volume, colloid osmotic pressure and hydrostatic pressure in rat skeletal muscle. Effect of hypoproteinemia. *Acta Physiologica Scandinavica*, 1981; **112,** 576–83.

Index

WITHDRAWN
University of Bristol
UNIVERSITY OF BRISTOL LIBRARY
MEDICAL